STATA SURVIVAL ANALYSIS AND EPIDEMIOLOGICAL TABLE REFERENCE MANUAL
RELEASE 10

A Stata Press Publication
StataCorp LP
College Station, Texas

Stata Press, 4905 Lakeway Drive, College Station, Texas 77845

The suggested citation for this software is

StataCorp. 2007. *Stata Statistical Software: Release 10*. College Station, TX: StataCorp LP.

Table of Contents

intro . . . . Introduction to survival analysis manual   1

survival analysis . . . . Introduction to survival analysis & epidemiological tables commands   4

ct . . . . Count-time data   11

ctset . . . . Declare data to be count-time data   12

cttost . . . . Convert count-time data to survival-time data   18

discrete . . . . Discrete-time survival analysis   21

epitab . . . . Tables for epidemiologists   23

estimation options . . . . Estimation options   79

ltable . . . . Life tables for survival data   80

snapspan . . . . Convert snapshot data to time-span data   93

st . . . . Survival-time data   96

st_is . . . . Survival analysis subroutines for programmers   98

stbase . . . . Form baseline dataset   103

stci . . . . Confidence intervals for means and percentiles of survival time   113

stcox . . . . Fit Cox proportional hazards model   122

stcox diagnostics . . . . stcox diagnostic plots   157

stcox postestimation . . . . Postestimation tools for stcox   166

stcurve . . . . Plot survivor, hazard, or cumulative hazard function   183

stdescribe . . . . Describe survival-time data   192

stfill . . . . Fill in by carrying forward values of covariates   196

stgen . . . . Generate variables reflecting entire histories   199

stir . . . . Report incidence-rate comparison   205

stpower . . . . Sample-size, power, and effect-size determination for survival analysis   208

stpower cox . . Sample size, power, and effect size for the Cox proportional hazards model   220

stpower exponential . . . . Sample size and power for the exponential test   236

stpower logrank . . . . Sample size, power, and effect size for the log-rank test   265

stptime . . . . Calculate person-time, incidence rates, and SMR   285

strate . . . . Tabulate failure rates and rate ratios   292

streg . . . . Fit parametric survival models   303

streg postestimation . . . . Postestimation tools for streg   334 sts . . . . Generate, graph, list, and test the survivor and cumulative hazard functions 343

sts generate . . . . Create variables containing survivor and related functions 359

sts graph . . . . Graph the survivor and cumulative hazard functions 362

sts list . . . . List the survivor or cumulative hazard function 380

sts test . . . . Test equality of survivor functions 385

stset . . . . Declare data to be survival-time data 400

stsplit . . . . Split and join time-span records 442

stsum . . . . Summarize survival-time data 460

sttocc . . . . Convert survival-time data to case–control data 465

sttoct . . . . Convert survival-time data to count-time data 470

stvary . . . . Report whether variables vary over time 472

glossary . . . . Glossary of terms 474

Cross-Referencing the Documentation

When reading this manual, you will find references to other Stata manuals. For example,

[U] **26 Overview of Stata estimation commands**

[R] **regress**

[D] **reshape**

The first is a reference to chapter 26, *Overview of Stata estimation commands* in the *Stata User's Guide*, the second is a reference to the `regress` entry in the *Base Reference Manual*, and the third is a reference to the `reshape` entry in the *Data Management Reference Manual*.

All the manuals in the Stata Documentation have a shorthand notation:

[GSM]	*Getting Started with Stata for Macintosh*
[GSU]	*Getting Started with Stata for Unix*
[GSW]	*Getting Started with Stata for Windows*
[U]	*Stata User's Guide*
[R]	*Stata Base Reference Manual*
[D]	*Stata Data Management Reference Manual*
[G]	*Stata Graphics Reference Manual*
[P]	*Stata Programming Reference Manual*
[XT]	*Stata Longitudinal/Panel-Data Reference Manual*
[MV]	*Stata Multivariate Statistics Reference Manual*
[SVY]	*Stata Survey Data Reference Manual*
[ST]	*Stata Survival Analysis and Epidemiological Tables Reference Manual*
[TS]	*Stata Time-Series Reference Manual*
[I]	*Stata Quick Reference and Index*
[M]	*Mata Reference Manual*

Detailed information about each of these manuals may be found online at

http://www.stata-press.com/manuals/

Title

> **intro** — Introduction to survival analysis manual

Description

This entry describes this manual and what has changed since Stata 9. See the next entry, [ST] **survival analysis**, for an introduction to Stata's survival analysis capabilities.

Remarks

This manual documents commands for survival analysis and epidemiological tables and is referred to as [ST] in cross-references. Following this entry, [ST] **survival analysis** provides an overview of the commands.

This manual is arranged alphabetically. If you are new to Stata's survival analysis and epidemiological tables commands, we recommend that you read the following sections first:

[ST] **survival analysis**	Introduction to survival analysis & epidemiological tables commands
[ST] **st**	Survival-time data
[ST] **stset**	Set variables for survival data

Stata is continually being updated, and Stata users are always writing new commands. To find out about the latest survival analysis features, type `search survival` after installing the latest official updates; see [R] **update**. To find out about the latest epidemiological features, type `search epi`.

What's new

This section is intended for previous Stata users. If you are new to Stata, you may as well skip it.

1. Existing estimation commands `stcox` and `streg` may now be used with the `svy:` prefix and so can fit models for complex survey data; see [ST] **stcox** and [ST] **streg**.

2. New command `stpower` provides sample-size and power calculations for survival studies that use Cox proportional hazards regressions, log-rank tests for two groups, or differences in exponentially distributed hazards or log hazards.

   a. `stpower cox` estimates required sample size (given power) or power (given sample size) or the minimal detectable coefficient (given power and sample size) for models with multiple covariates. The command provides options to account for possible correlation between the covariate of interest and other predictors and for withdrawal of subjects from the study. See [ST] **stpower cox**.

   b. `stpower logrank` estimates required sample size (given power) or power (given sample size) or the minimal detectable hazard ratio (given power and sample size) for studies comparing survivor functions of two groups by using the log-rank test. Both the Freedman (1982) and the Schoenfeld (1981) methods are provided. The command allows for unequal allocation of subjects between the groups and possible withdrawal of subjects. Estimates can be adjusted for uniform accrual. See [ST] **stpower logrank**.

c. `stpower exponential` estimates sample size (given power) or power (given sample size) of tests of the difference between hazards or log hazards of two groups under the assumption of exponential survivor functions (also known as the exponential test). Both the Lachin–Foulkes (1986) and Rubinstein–Gail–Santner (1981) methods are provided. Unequal group allocation, uniform or truncated exponential accrual, and different exponential losses due to follow-up in each group are allowed. See [ST] **stpower exponential**.

The `stpower` commands allow automated production of customizable tables and have options to assist with creating graphs of power curves. See [ST] **stpower**.

3. Concerning existing command `sts graph`,

   a. New option `risktable()` places a subjects-at-risk table underneath and aligned with the survivor or hazard plot.

   b. New option `ci` replaces old options `gwood`, `cna`, and `cihazard`. `sts graph` will choose the appropriate confidence interval on the basis of the function being graphed.

   c. Confidence intervals are now graphed using shaded areas and new options `plotopts()` and `ciopts()` allow you to control how plots and confidence intervals look.

   d. Overlaid confidence intervals are now allowed and are produced when new option `ci` is combined with existing option `by(varlist)`.

   e. New option `censopts()` controls the appearance of ticks and markers produced by existing option `censored()`.

   f. Boundary computations for smoothing hazards have been improved. New option `noboundary` specifies that no boundary correction be done.

   g. The lower bound of the range to plot the hazard function now extends to zero.

   h. Option `na` has been renamed `cumhaz`. `na` may still be used.

   See [ST] **sts graph**. Setting `version` to less than 10 restores previous behavior.

4. For `sts list`, option `na` has been renamed `cumhaz`. `na` may be used as a synonym for `cumhaz`. See [ST] **sts list**.

5. Improvements to `stcurve` analogous to those of `sts graph` have been made.

   a. Boundary computations for smoothing hazards have been improved. New option `noboundary` specifies that no boundary correction be done.

   b. The lower bound of the range to plot the hazard function now extends to zero.

   See [ST] **stcurve**.

6. All `st` estimation commands accept option `vce(vcetype)`. As mentioned in the [U] **1.3.3 What's new in statistics (general)**, `vce(robust)` and `vce(cluster varname)` are the right ways to specify the old `robust` and `cluster()` options, and option `vce()` now allows other VCE calculations as well.

7. Existing command `predict` after `stcox` has a new option, `scores`, that allows generating variables with the partial efficient score residuals; see [ST] **stcox postestimation**.

8. Existing command `ltable` has new options `byopts()`, `plotopts()`, `plot#opts()`, and `ci#opts()` that allow for more customization of the graph. New option `ci` adds confidence intervals to the graph. See [ST] **ltable**.

9. Existing command `stphplot` has a new option `plot#opts()` that allows for more customization of the graph. See [ST] **stcox diagnostics**.

10. Existing command `stcoxkm` has new options `byopts()`, `obsopts()`, `obs#opts()`, `predopts()`, and `pred#opts()` that allow for more customization of the graph. See [ST] **stcox diagnostics**.

11. Existing command `cc` has new option `tarone` that produces Tarone's (1985) adjustment of the Breslow–Day test for homogeneity of odds ratios. See [ST] **epitab**.

12. Existing command `stdes` has been renamed to `stdescribe`. `stdes` continues to work. See [ST] **stdescribe**.

13. The manual has an expanded glossary.

For a complete list of all the new features in Stata 10, see [U] **1.3 What's new**.

References

Freedman, L. S. 1982. Tables of the number of patients required in clinical trials using the logrank test. *Statistics in Medicine* 1: 121–129.

Lachin, J. M., and M. A. Foulkes. 1986. Evaluation of sample size and power for analysis of survival with allowance for nonuniform patient entry, losses to follow-up, noncompliance, and stratification. *Biometrics* 42: 507–519.

Rubinstein, L. V., M. H. Gail, and T. J. Santner. 1981. Planning the duration of a comparative clinical trial with loss to follow-up and a period of continued observation. *Journal of Chronic Diseases* 34: 469–479.

Schoenfeld, D. 1981. The asymptotic properties of nonparametric tests for comparing survival distributions. *Biometrika* 68: 316–319.

Tarone, R. E. 1985. On heterogeneity tests based on efficient scores. *Biometrika* 72: 91–95.

Also See

[U] **1.3 What's new**

[R] **intro** — Introduction to base reference manual

Title

survival analysis — Introduction to survival analysis & epidemiological tables commands

Description

Stata's survival analysis routines are used to compute sample size, power, and effect size and to declare, convert, manipulate, summarize, and analyze survival data. Survival data is time-to-event data, and survival analysis is full of jargon: truncation, censoring, hazard rates, etc. See the glossary in this manual. For a good Stata-specific introduction to survival analysis, see Cleves, Gould, and Gutierrez (2004).

Stata also has several commands for analyzing contingency tables resulting from various forms of observational studies, such as cohort or matched case–control studies.

This manual documents the following commands, which are described in detail in their respective manual entries.

Declaring and converting count data

ctset	[ST] **ctset**	Declare data to be count-time data
cttost	[ST] **cttost**	Convert count-time data to survival-time data

Converting snapshot data

snapspan	[ST] **snapspan**	Convert snapshot data to time-span data

Declaring and summarizing survival-time data

stset	[ST] **stset**	Declare data to be survival-time data
stdescribe	[ST] **stdescribe**	Describe survival-time data
stsum	[ST] **stsum**	Summarize survival-time data

Manipulating survival-time data

stvary	[ST] **stvary**	Report whether variables vary over time
stfill	[ST] **stfill**	Fill in by carrying forward values of covariates
stgen	[ST] **stgen**	Generate variables reflecting entire histories
stsplit	[ST] **stsplit**	Split time-span records
stjoin	[ST] **stsplit**	Join time-span records
stbase	[ST] **stbase**	Form baseline dataset

Obtaining summary statistics, confidence intervals, tables, etc.

sts	[ST] **sts**	Generate, graph, list, and test the survivor and cumulative hazard functions
stir	[ST] **stir**	Report incidence-rate comparison
stci	[ST] **stci**	Confidence intervals for means and percentiles of survival time
strate	[ST] **strate**	Tabulate failure rate
stptime	[ST] **stptime**	Calculate person-time, incidence rates, and SMR
stmh	[ST] **strate**	Calculate rate ratios with the Mantel–Haenszel method
stmc	[ST] **strate**	Calculate rate ratios with the Mantel–Cox method
ltable	[ST] **ltable**	Display and graph life tables

Fitting regression models

stcox	[ST] **stcox**	Fit Cox proportional hazards model
estat concordance	[ST] **stcox postestimation**	Calculate Harrell's C
estat phtest	[ST] **stcox postestimation**	Test Cox proportional-hazards assumption
stphplot	[ST] **stcox diagnostics**	Graphically assess the Cox proportional-hazards assumption
stcoxkm	[ST] **stcox diagnostics**	Graphically assess the Cox proportional-hazards assumption
streg	[ST] **streg**	Fit parametric survival models
stcurve	[ST] **stcurve**	Plot survivor, hazard, or cumulative hazard function

Sample-size and power determination for survival analysis

stpower cox	[ST] **stpower cox**	Sample size, power, and effect size for the Cox proportional hazards model
stpower exponential	[ST] **stpower exponential**	Sample size and power for the exponential test
stpower logrank	[ST] **stpower logrank**	Sample size, power, and effect size for the log-rank test

Converting survival-time data

sttocc	[ST] **sttocc**	Convert survival-time data to case–control data
sttoct	[ST] **sttoct**	Convert survival-time data to count-time data

Programmer's utilities

st_*	[ST] **st_is**	Survival analysis subroutines for programmers

Epidemiological tables

ir	[ST] **epitab**	Incidence rates for cohort studies
iri	[ST] **epitab**	Immediate form of ir
cs	[ST] **epitab**	Risk differences, risk ratios, and odds ratios for cohort studies
csi	[ST] **epitab**	Immediate form of cs
cc	[ST] **epitab**	Odds ratios for case–control data
cci	[ST] **epitab**	Immediate form of cc
tabodds	[ST] **epitab**	Tests of log odds for case–control data
mhodds	[ST] **epitab**	Odds ratios controlled for confounding
mcc	[ST] **epitab**	Analysis of matched case–control data
mcci	[ST] **epitab**	Immediate form of mcc

(Continued on next page)

Remarks

Remarks are presented under the following headings:

> *Introduction*
> *Declaring and converting count data*
> *Converting snapshot data*
> *Declaring and summarizing survival-time data*
> *Manipulating survival-time data*
> *Obtaining summary statistics, confidence intervals, tables, etc.*
> *Fitting regression models*
> *Sample size and power determination for survival analysis*
> *Converting survival-time data*
> *Programmer's utilities*
> *Epidemiological tables*

Introduction

All but one entry in this manual deals with the analysis of survival data, which is used to measure the time to an event of interest such as death or failure. Survival data can be organized in two ways. The first way is as *count data*, which refers to observations on populations, whether people or generators, with observations recording the number of units at a given time that failed or were lost because of censoring. The second way is as *survival-time*, or *time-span* data. In survival-time data, the observations represent periods and contain three variables that record the start time of the period, the end time, and an indicator of whether failure or right-censoring occurred at the end of the period. The representation of the response of these three variables makes survival data unique in terms of implementing the statistical methods in the software.

Survival data may also be organized as *snapshot data* (a small variation of the survival-time format), in which observations depict an instance in time rather than an interval. When you have snapshot data, you simply use the `snapspan` command to convert it to survival-time data before proceeding.

Stata commands that begin with `ct` are used to convert count data to survival-time data. Survival-time data is analyzed using Stata commands that begin with `st`, known in our terminology as st commands. You can express all the information contained in count data in an equivalent survival-time dataset, but the converse is not true. Thus Stata commands are made to work with survival-time data since it is the more general representation.

The one remaining entry is [ST] **epitab**, which describes epidemiological tables. [ST] **epitab** covers many commands dealing with analyzing contingency tables arising from various observational studies, such as case–control or cohort studies. [ST] **epitab** is included in this manual because the concepts presented there are related to concepts of survival analysis, and both topics use the same terminology and are of equal interest to many researchers.

Declaring and converting count data

Count data must first be converted to survival-time data before Stata's st commands can be used. Count data can be thought of as aggregated survival-time data. Rather than having observations that are specific to a subject and a period, you have data that, at each recorded time, record the number lost because of failure and, optionally, the number lost because of right-censoring.

`ctset` is used to tell Stata the names of the variables in your count data that record the time, the number failed, and the number censored. You `ctset` your data before typing `cttost` to convert it to survival-time data. Because you `ctset` your data, you can type `cttost` without any arguments to perform the conversion. Stata remembers how the data are `ctset`.

Converting snapshot data

Snapshot data are data in which each observation records the status of a given subject at a certain point in time. Usually you have multiple observations on each subject that chart the subject's progress through the study.

Before using Stata's survival analysis commands with snapshot data, you must first convert the data to survival-time data; that is, the observations in the data should represent intervals. When you convert snapshot data, the existing time variable in your data is used to record the end of a time span, and a new variable is created to record the beginning. Time spans are created using the recorded snapshot times as breakpoints at which new intervals are to be created. Before converting snapshot data to time-span data, you must understand the distinction between *enduring variables* and *instantaneous variables*. Enduring variables record characteristics of the subject that endure throughout the time span, such as sex or smoking status. Instantaneous variables describe events that occur at the end of a time span, such as failure or censoring. When you convert snapshots to intervals, enduring variables obtain their values from the previous recorded snapshot or are set to missing for the first interval. Instantaneous variables obtain their values from the current recorded snapshot since the existing time variable now records the end of the span.

Stata's snapspan makes this whole process easy. You specify an ID variable identifying your subjects, the snapshot time variable, the name of the new variable to hold the beginning times of the spans, and any variables that you want to treat as instantaneous variables. Stata does the rest for you.

Declaring and summarizing survival-time data

Stata does not automatically recognize survival-time data, so you must declare your survival-time data to Stata by using stset. Every st command relies on the information that is provided when you stset your data. Survival-time data come in different forms. For example, your time variables may be dates, time measured from a fixed date, or time measured from some other point unique to each subject, such as enrollment in the study. You can also consider the following questions. What is the onset of risk for the subjects in your data? Is it time zero? Is it enrollment in the study or some other event, such as a heart transplant? Do you have censoring, and if so, which variable records it? What values does this variable record for censoring/failure? Do you have delayed entry? That is, were some subjects at risk of failure before you actually observed them? Do you have simple data and wish to treat everyone as entering and at risk at time zero?

Whatever the form of your data, you must first stset it before analyzing it, and so if you are new to Stata's st commands, we highly recommend that you take the time to learn about stset. It is really easy once you get the hang of it, and [ST] **stset** has many examples to help. For more discussion of stset, see chapter 6 of Cleves, Gould, and Gutierrez (2004).

Once you stset the data, you can use stdescribe to describe the aspects of your survival data. For example, you'll see the number of subjects you were successful in declaring, the total number of records associated with these subjects, the total time at risk for these subjects, time gaps for any of these subjects, any delayed entry, etc. You can use stsum to summarize your survival data, for example, to obtain the total time at risk and the quartiles of time-to-failure in analysis time units.

Manipulating survival-time data

Once your data have been stset, you may want to clean them up a bit before beginning your analysis. Suppose that you had an enduring variable and snapspan recorded it as missing for the interval leading up to the first recorded snapshot time. You can use stfill to fill in missing values of covariates, either by carrying forward the values from previous periods or by making the covariate equal to its earliest recorded (nonmissing) value for all time spans. You can use stvary to check for time-varying covariates or to confirm that certain variables, such as sex, are not time varying. You can use stgen to generate new covariates based on functions of the time spans for each given subject. For example, you can create a new variable called eversmoked that equals one for all a subject's observations, if the variable smoke in your data is equal to one for *any* of the subject's time spans. Think of stgen as just a convenient way to do things that could be done using by *subject_id*: with survival-time data.

stsplit is useful for creating data that have multiple records per subject from data that have one record per subject. Suppose that you have already stset your data and wish to introduce a time-varying covariate. You would first need to stsplit your data so that separate time spans could be created for each subject, allowing the new covariate to assume different values over time within a subject. stjoin is the opposite of stsplit. Suppose that you have data with multiple records per subject but then realize that the data could be collapsed into single-subject records with no loss of information. Using stjoin would speed up any subsequent analysis using the st commands without changing the results.

stbase can be used to set every variable in your multiple-record st data to the value at baseline, defined as the earliest time at which each subject was observed. It can also be used to convert st data to cross-sectional data.

Obtaining summary statistics, confidence intervals, tables, etc.

Stata provides several commands for nonparametric analysis of survival data that can produce a wide array of summary statistics, inference, tables, and graphs. sts is a truly powerful command, used to obtain nonparametric estimates, inference, tests, and graphs of the survivor function, cumulative hazard function, and the hazard function. You can compare estimates across groups, such as smoking versus nonsmoking, and you can adjust these estimates for the effects of other covariates in your data. sts can present these estimates as tables and graphs. sts can also be used to test the equality of survivor functions across groups.

stir is used to estimate incidence rates and to compare incidence rates across groups. stci is the survival-time data analog of ci and is used to obtain confidence intervals for means and percentiles of time to failure. strate is used to tabulate failure rates. stptime is used to calculate person-time and standardized mortality/morbidity ratios (SMRs). stmh calculates rate ratios by using the Mantel–Haenszel method, and stmc calculates rate ratios by using the Mantel–Cox method.

ltable displays and graphs life tables for individual-level or aggregate data.

Fitting regression models

Stata has commands for fitting both semiparametric and parametric regression models to survival data. stcox fits the Cox proportional hazards model and can be used to retrieve estimates of the baseline survival function, the baseline cumulative hazard function, and the baseline hazard contributions. stcox can also calculate a myriad of Cox regression diagnostic quantities, such as martingale residuals, efficient score residuals, and Schoenfeld residuals. stcox has four options for handling tied failures. stcox can be used to fit stratified Cox models, where the baseline hazard is allowed to differ over the strata, and it can be used to model multivariate survival data by using a *shared-frailty* model, which can be thought of as a Cox model with random effects. After stcox, you can use estat phtest to test the proportional-hazards assumption or estat concordance to calculate Harrell's C. With stphplot and stcoxkm, you can graphically assess the proportional-hazards assumption.

Stata offers six parametric regression models for survival data: exponential, Weibull, log-normal, log-logistic, Gompertz, and gamma. All six models are fitted using `streg`, and you can specify the model you want with the `distribution()` option. All these models, except for the exponential, have ancillary parameters that are estimated (along with the linear predictor) from the data. By default, these ancillary parameters are treated as constant, but you may optionally model the ancillary parameters as functions of a linear predictor. Stratified models may also be fitted using `streg`. You can also fit frailty models with `streg` and specify whether you want the frailties to be treated as spell-specific or shared across groups of observations.

`stcurve` is for use after `stcox` and `streg` and will plot the estimated survivor, hazard, and cumulative hazard function for the fitted model. Covariates, by default, are held fixed at their mean values, but you can specify other values if you wish. `stcurve` is useful for comparing these functions across different levels of covariates.

Sample size and power determination for survival analysis

Stata has commands for computing sample size, power, and effect size for survival analysis using the log-rank test, the Cox proportional hazards model, and the exponential test comparing exponential hazard rates.

`stpower logrank` estimates required sample size, power, and effect size for survival analysis comparing survivor functions in two groups using the log-rank test. It provides options to account for unequal allocation of subjects between the two groups, possible withdrawal of subjects from the study (loss to follow-up), and uniform accrual of subjects into the study.

`stpower cox` estimates required sample size, power, and effect size for survival analysis using Cox proportional hazards (PH) models with possibly multiple covariates. It provides options to account for possible correlation between the covariate of interest and other predictors and for withdrawal of subjects from the study.

`stpower exponential` estimates required sample size and power for survival analysis comparing two exponential survivor functions using the exponential test (in particular, the Wald test of the difference between hazards or, optionally, of the difference between log hazards). It accommodates unequal allocation between the two groups, flexible accrual of subjects into the study (uniform and truncated exponential), and group-specific losses to follow-up.

The `stpower` commands allow automated production of customizable tables and have options to assist with the creation of graphs of power curves and more.

Converting survival-time data

Stata has commands for converting survival-time data to case–control and count data. These commands are rarely used, since most of the analyses are performed using data in the survival-time format. `sttocc` is useful for converting survival data to case–control data suitable for estimation with `clogit`. `sttoct` is the opposite of `cttost` and will convert survival-time data to count data.

Programmer's utilities

Stata also provides routines for programmers interested in writing their own st commands. These are basically utilities for setting, accessing, and verifying the information saved by `stset`. For example, `st_is` verifies that the data have in fact been `stset` and gives the appropriate error if not. `st_show` is used to preface the output of a program with key information on the st variables used in the analysis. Programmers interested in writing st code should see [ST] **st_is**.

Epidemiological tables

See the *Description* section of [ST] **epitab** for an overview of Stata's commands for calculating statistics and performing lists that are useful for epidemiologists.

Reference

Cleves, M. A., W. W. Gould, and R. G. Gutierrez. 2004. *An Introduction to Survival Analysis Using Stata*. Rev. ed. College Station, TX: Stata Press.

Also See

[ST] **stset** — Declare data to be survival-time data

[ST] **intro** — Introduction to survival analysis manual

Title

> **ct** — Count-time data

Description

The term *ct* refers to count-time data and the commands—all of which begin with the letters "ct"—for analyzing them. If you have data on populations, whether people or generators, with observations recording the number of units under test at time t (subjects alive) and the number of subjects that failed or were lost because of censoring, you have what we call count-time data.

If, on the other hand, you have data on individual subjects with observations recording that this subject came under observation at time t_0 and that, later, at t_1 a failure or censoring was observed, you have what we call survival-time data. If you have survival-time data, see [ST] **st**.

Do not confuse count-time data with counting-process data, which can be analyzed using the st commands; see [ST] **st**.

There are two ct commands:

ctset	[ST] **ctset**	Declare data to be count-time data
cttost	[ST] **cttost**	Convert count-time data to survival-time data

The key is the `cttost` command. Once you have converted your count-time data to survival-time data, you can use the st commands to analyze the data. The entire process is as follows:

1. `ctset` your data so that Stata knows that they are count-time data; see [ST] **ctset**.

2. Type `cttost` to convert your data to survival-time data; see [ST] **cttost**.

3. Use the st commands; see [ST] **st**.

Also See

[ST] **ctset** — Declare data to be count-time data

[ST] **cttost** — Convert count-time data to survival-time data

[ST] **st** — Survival-time data

[ST] **survival analysis** — Introduction to survival analysis & epidemiological tables commands

Title

> **ctset** — Declare data to be count-time data

Syntax

Declare data in memory to be count-time data and run checks on data

    ctset *timevar nfailvar* [*ncensvar* [*nentvar*]] [, by(*varlist*) <u>nosh</u>ow]

Specify whether to display identities of key ct variables

    ctset, { <u>sh</u>ow | <u>nosh</u>ow }

Clear ct setting

    ctset, clear

Display identity of key ct variables and rerun checks on data

    { ctset | ct }

where *timevar* refers to the time of failure, censoring, or entry. It should contain times ≥ 0.

nfailvar records the number failing at time *timevar*.

ncensvar records the number censored at time *timevar*.

nentvar records the number entering at time *timevar*.

Stata sequences events at the same time as

at *timevar*	*nfailvar* failures occurred,
then at *timevar* + 0	*ncensvar* censorings occurred,
finally at *timevar* + 0 + 0	*nentvar* subjects entered the data.

Description

ct refers to count-time data and is described here and in [ST] **ct**. Do not confuse count-time data with counting-process data, which can be analyzed using the st commands; see [ST] **st**.

In the first syntax, ctset declares the data in memory to be ct data, informing Stata of the key variables. When you ctset your data, ctset also checks that what you have declared makes sense.

In the second syntax, ctset changes the value of show/noshow. In show mode—the default—the other ct commands display the identities of the key ct variables before their normal output. If you type ctset, noshow, they will not do this. If you type ctset, noshow and then wish to restore the default behavior, type ctset, show.

In the third syntax, ctset, clear causes Stata to no longer consider the data to be ct data. The dataset itself remains unchanged. It is not necessary to type ctset, clear before doing another ctset. ctset, clear is used mostly by programmers.

In the fourth syntax, ctset—which can be abbreviated ct here—displays the identities of the key ct variables and reruns the checks on your data. Thus, ct can remind you of what you have ctset (especially if you have ctset, noshow) and reverify your data if you make changes to the data.

Options

by(*varlist*) indicates that counts are provided by group. For instance, consider data containing records such as

t	fail	cens	sex	agecat
5	10	2	0	1
5	6	1	1	1
5	12	0	0	2

These data indicate that, in the category sex = 0 and agecat = 1, 10 failed and 2 were censored at time 5; for sex = 1, 1 was censored and 6 failed; and so on.

The above data would be declared

    . ctset t fail cens, by(sex agecat)

The order of the records is not important, nor is it important that there be a record at every time for every group or that there be only one record for a time and group. However, the data must contain the full table of events.

noshow and show specify whether the identities of the key ct variables are to be displayed at the start of every ct command. Some users find the report reassuring; others find it repetitive. In any case, you can set and unset show, and you can always type ct to see the summary.

clear makes Stata no longer consider the data to be ct data.

Remarks

Remarks are presented under the following headings:

> *Examples*
> *Data errors flagged by ctset*

Examples

About all you can do with ct data in Stata is convert it to survival-time (st) data so that you can use the survival analysis commands. To analyze count-time data with Stata,

    . ctset ...
    . cttost
    . (*now use any of the st commands*)

(*Continued on next page*)

▷ Example 1: Simple ct data

We have data on generators that are run until they fail:

```
. use http://www.stata-press.com/data/r10/ctset1
. list, sep(0)
```

	failtime	fail
1.	22	1
2.	30	1
3.	40	2
4.	52	1
5.	54	4
6.	55	2
7.	85	7
8.	97	1
9.	100	3
10.	122	2
11.	140	1

For instance, at time 54, four generators failed. To `ctset` these data, we could type

```
. ctset failtime fail
       dataset name:  http://www.stata-press.com/data/r10/ctset1.dta
               time:  failtime
           no. fail:  fail
           no. lost:  --              (meaning 0 lost)
          no. enter:  --              (meaning all enter at time 0)
```

It is not important that there be only 1 observation per failure time. For instance, according to our data, at time 85 there were seven failures. We could remove that observation and substitute two in its place—one stating that at time 85 there were five failures and another that at time 85 there were two more failures. `ctset` would interpret that data just as it did the previous data.

In more realistic examples, the generators might differ from one another. For instance, the following data show the number failing with old-style (bearings = 0) and new-style (bearings = 1) bearings:

```
. use http://www.stata-press.com/data/r10/ctset2
. list, sepby(bearings)
```

	bearings	failtime	fail
1.	0	22	1
2.	0	40	2
3.	0	54	1
4.	0	84	2
5.	0	97	2
6.	0	100	1
7.	1	30	1
8.	1	52	1
9.	1	55	1
10.	1	100	3
11.	1	122	2
12.	1	140	1

That the data are sorted on bearings is not important. The `ctset` command for these data is

```
. ctset failtime fail, by(bearings)
    dataset name:  http://www.stata-press.com/data/r10/ctset2.dta
           time:  failtime
        no. fail:  fail
        no. lost:  --                    (meaning 0 lost)
       no. enter:  --                    (meaning all enter at time 0)
             by:  bearings
```
                                                                        ◁

▷ Example 2: ct data with censoring

In real data, not all units fail in the time allotted. Say that the generator experiment was stopped after 150 days. The data might be

```
. use http://www.stata-press.com/data/r10/ctset3
. list
```

	bearings	failtime	fail	censored
1.	0	22	1	0
2.	0	40	2	0
3.	0	54	1	0
4.	0	84	2	0
5.	1	97	2	0
6.	0	100	1	0
7.	0	150	0	2
8.	1	30	1	0
9.	1	52	1	0
10.	1	55	1	0
11.	1	122	2	0
12.	1	140	1	0
13.	1	150	0	3

The ctset command for these data is

```
. ctset failtime fail censored, by(bearings)
    dataset name:  http://www.stata-press.com/data/r10/ctset3.dta
           time:  failtime
        no. fail:  fail
        no. lost:  censored
       no. enter:  --                    (meaning all enter at time 0)
             by:  bearings
```

In some other data, observations might also be censored along the way; that is, the value of censored would not be 0 before time 150. For instance, a record might read

bearings	failtime	fail	censored
0	84	2	1

This would mean that at time 84, two failed and one was lost because of censoring. The failure and censoring occurred at the same time, and when we analyze these data, Stata will assume that the censored observation could have failed, that is, that the censoring occurred after the two failures.
                                                                        ◁

▷ Example 3: ct data with delayed entry

Data on survival time of patients with a particular kind of cancer are collected. Time is measured as time since diagnosis. After data collection started, the sample was enriched with some patients from hospital records who had been previously diagnosed. Some of the data are

```
time    die    cens    ent     other variables
   0      0       0     50
   1      0       0      5      . . .
   .
   .
  30      0       0      3      . . .
  31      0       1      2      . . .
  32      1       0      1      . . .
   .
   .
 100      1       1      0      . . .
   .
   .
```

Fifty patients entered at time 0 (time of diagnosis); five patients entered 1 day after diagnosis; and three, two, and one entered 30, 31, and 32 days after diagnosis, respectively. On the 32nd day, one of the previously entering patients died.

If the other variables are named sex and agecat, the ctset command for these data is

```
. ctset time die cens ent, by(sex agecat)
          time:   time
      no. fail:   die
      no. lost:   cens
     no. enter:   ent
            by:   sex agecat
```

◁

The count-time format is an inferior way to record data like these—data in which every subject does not enter at time 0—because some information is already lost. When did the patient who died on the 32nd day enter? There is no way of telling.

For traditional survival analysis calculations, it does not matter. More modern methods of estimating standard errors, however, seek to identify each patient, and these data do not support using such methods.

This issue concerns the robust estimates of variance and the vce(robust) options on some of the st analysis commands. After converting the data, you must not use the vce(robust) option, even if an st command allows it, because the identities of the subjects—tying together when a subject starts and ceases to be at risk—are assigned randomly by cttost when you convert your ct to st data. When did the patient who died on the 32nd day enter? For conventional calculations, it does not matter, and cttost chooses a time randomly from the available entry times.

Data errors flagged by ctset

ctset requires only two things of your data: that the counts all be positive or zero and, if you specify an entry variable, that the entering and exiting (failure + censored) balance.

If all subjects enter at time 0, we recommend that you do not specify a number-that-enter variable. ctset can determine for itself the number who enter at time 0 by summing the failures and censorings.

Also See

[ST] **ct** — Count-time data

[ST] **cttost** — Convert count-time data to survival-time data

Title

cttost — Convert count-time data to survival-time data

Syntax

cttost [, *options*]

options	description
t0(*t0var*)	name of entry-time variable
wvar(*wvar*)	name of frequency-weighted variable
clear	overwrite current data in memory
† nopreserve	do not save the original data; programmer's command

† nopreserve is not shown in the dialog box.

You must ctset your data before using cttost; see [ST] **ctset**.

Description

cttost converts count-time data to their survival-time format so that they can be analyzed with Stata. Do not confuse count-time data with counting-process data, which can also be analyzed with the st commands; see [ST] **ctset** for a definition and examples of count data.

Options

t0(*t0var*) specifies the name of the new variable to create that records entry time. (For most ct data, no entry-time variable is necessary because everyone enters at time 0.)

Even if an entry-time variable is necessary, you need not specify this option. cttost will, by default, choose t0, time0, or etime according to which name does not already exist in the data.

wvar(*wvar*) specifies the name of the new variable to be created that records the frequency weights for the new pseudoobservations. Count-time data are actually converted to frequency-weighted st data, and a variable is needed to record the weights. This sounds more complicated than it is. Understand that cttost needs a new variable name, which will become a permanent part of the st data.

If you do not specify wvar(), cttost will, by default, choose w, pop, weight, or wgt according to which name does not already exist in the data.

clear specifies that it is okay to proceed with the conversion, even though the current dataset has not been saved on disk.

The following option is available with cttost but is not shown in the dialog box:

nopreserve speeds the conversion by not saving the original data that can be restored should things go wrong or should you press *Break*. nopreserve is intended for use by programmers who use cttost as a subroutine. Programmers can specify this option if they have already preserved the original data. nopreserve does not affect the conversion.

Remarks

Converting ct to st data is easy. We have some count-time data,

```
. use http://www.stata-press.com/data/r10/cttost
. ct
    dataset name:  http://www.stata-press.com/data/r10/cttost.dta
           time:  time
       no. fail:  ndead
       no. lost:  ncens
      no. enter:  --                      (meaning all enter at time 0)
             by:  agecat treat
. list in 1/5
```

	agecat	treat	time	ndead	ncens
1.	2	1	464	4	0
2.	3	0	268	3	1
3.	2	0	638	2	0
4.	1	0	803	1	4
5.	1	0	431	2	0

and to convert it we type cttost:

```
. cttost
       failure event:  ndead != 0 & ndead < .
 obs. time interval:  (0, time]
 exit on or before:  failure
              weight:  [fweight=w]
```

```
      33  total obs.
       0  exclusions

      33  physical obs. remaining, equal to
      82  weighted obs., representing
      39  failures in single record/single failure data
   48726  total analysis time at risk, at risk from t =          0
                              earliest observed entry t =         0
                               last observed exit t =         1227
```

Now that it is converted, we can use any of the st commands:

```
. sts test treat, logrank
         failure _d:  ndead
   analysis time _t:  time
              weight:  [fweight=w]
```

Log-rank test for equality of survivor functions

treat	Events observed	Events expected
0	22	17.05
1	17	21.95
Total	39	39.00

```
          chi2(1) =       2.73
          Pr>chi2 =     0.0986
```

Also See

[ST] **ct** — Count-time data

[ST] **ctset** — Declare data to be count-time data

Title

---

discrete — Discrete-time survival analysis

As of the date that this manual was printed, Stata does not have a suite of built-in commands for discrete-time survival models matching the `st` suite for continuous-time models, but a good case could be made that it should. Instead, these models can be fitted easily using other existing estimation commands and data manipulation tools.

Discrete-time survival analysis concerns analysis of time-to-event data whenever survival times are either (a) intrinsically discrete (e.g., numbers of machine cycles) or (b) grouped into discrete intervals of time ("interval censoring"). If intervals are of equal length, the same methods can be applied to both (a) and (b); survival times will be positive integers.

You can fit discrete-time survival models with the maximum likelihood method. Data may contain completed or right-censored spells, and late entry (left truncation) can also be handled, as well as unobserved heterogeneity (also termed "frailty"). Estimation makes use of the property that the sample likelihood can be rewritten in a form identical to the likelihood for a binary dependent variable multiple regression model and applied to a specially organized dataset (Allison 1984, Jenkins 1995). For models without frailty, you can use, for example, `logistic` (or `logit`) to fit the discrete-time logistic hazard model or `cloglog` to fit the discrete-time proportional hazards model (Prentice and Gloeckler 1978). Models incorporating normal frailty may be fitted using `xtlogit` and `xtcloglog`. A model with gamma frailty (Meyer 1990) may be fitted using `pgmhaz` (Jenkins 1997).

Estimation consists of three steps:

1. *Data organization*: The dataset must be organized so that there is 1 observation for each period when a subject is at risk of experiencing the transition event. For example, if the original dataset contains one row for each subject, i, with information about their spell length, T_i, the new dataset requires T_i rows for each subject, one row for each period at risk. This may be accomplished using `expand` or `stsplit`. (This step is episode splitting at each and every interval.) The result is data of the same form as a discrete panel (`xt`) dataset with repeated observations on each panel (subject).

2. *Variable creation*: You must create at least three types of variables. First, you will need an interval identification variable, which is a sequence of positive integers $t = 1, \ldots, T_i$. For example,

   ```
   . sort subject_id
   . by subject_id: generate t = _n
   ```

   Second, you need a period-specific censoring indicator, d_i. If $d_i = 1$ if subject i's spell is complete and $d_i = 0$ if the spell is right-censored, the new indicator $d_{it}^* = 1$ if $d_i = 1$ and $t = T_i$ and $d_{it}^* = 0$ otherwise.

   Third, you must define variables (as functions of t) to summarize the pattern of duration dependence. These variables are entered as covariates in the regression. For example, for a duration dependence pattern analogous to that in the continuous-time Weibull model, you could define a new variable $x_1 = \log t$. For a quadratic specification, you define variables $x_1 = t$ and $x_2 = t^2$. We can achieve a piecewise constant specification by defining a set of dummy variables, with each group of periods sharing the same hazard rate, or a semiparametric model (analogous to the Cox regression model for continuous survival-time data) using separate dummy variables for each and every duration interval. No duration variable need be defined if you want to fit a model with a constant hazard rate.

   In addition to these three essentials, you may define other time-varying covariates.

21

3. *Estimation*: You fit a binary dependent variable multiple regression model, with d_{it}^* as the dependent variable and covariates, including the duration variables and any other covariates.

For estimation using spell data with late entry, the stages are the same as those outlined above, with one modification and one warning. To fit models without frailty, you must drop all intervals prior to each subject's entry to the study. For example, if entry is in period e_i, you drop it if $t < e_i$. If you want to fit frailty models on the basis of discrete-time data with late entry, then be aware that the estimation procedure outlined does not lead to correct estimates. (The sample likelihood in the reorganized data does not account for conditioning for late entry here. You will need to write your own likelihood function by using `ml`; see [R] **maximize**.)

To derive predicted hazard rates, use the `predict` command. For example, after `logistic` or `cloglog`, use `predict, pr`. After `xtlogit` or `xtcloglog`, use `predict, pu0` (which predicts the hazard assuming the individual effect is equal to the mean value). Estimates of the survivor function, S_{it}, can then be derived from the predicted hazard rates, p_{it}, since $S_{it} = (1 - p_{i1})(1 - p_{i2})(\cdots)(1 - p_{it})$.

Acknowledgment

We thank Stephen Jenkins, University of Essex, UK, for drafting this initial entry.

References

Allison, P. D. 1984. *Event History Analysis: Regression for Longitudinal Event Data*. Newbury Park, CA: Sage.

Jenkins, S. P. 1995. Easy estimation methods for discrete-time duration models. *Oxford Bulletin of Economics and Statistics* 57: 129–138.

——. 1997. sbe17: Discrete time proportional hazards regression. *Stata Technical Bulletin* 39: 22–32. Reprinted in *Stata Technical Bulletin Reprints*, vol. 7, pp. 109–121.

Meyer, B. D. 1990. Unemployment insurance and unemployment spells. *Econometrica* 58: 757–782.

Prentice, R. L., and L. Gloeckler. 1978. Regression analysis of grouped survival data with application to breast cancer data. *Biometrics* 34: 57–67.

Also See

[D] **expand** — Duplicate observations

[ST] **stcox** — Fit Cox proportional hazards model

[ST] **streg** — Fit parametric survival models

[R] **cloglog** — Complementary log-log regression

[R] **logistic** — Logistic regression, reporting odds ratios

[XT] **xtcloglog** — Random-effects and population-averaged cloglog models

[XT] **xtlogit** — Fixed-effects, random-effects, and population-averaged logit models

Title

---

epitab — Tables for epidemiologists

Syntax

Cohort studies

ir var_{case} var_{exposed} var_{time} $\begin{bmatrix} if \end{bmatrix}$ $\begin{bmatrix} in \end{bmatrix}$ $\begin{bmatrix} weight \end{bmatrix}$ $\begin{bmatrix} , & ir\_options \end{bmatrix}$

iri $\#_a$ $\#_b$ $\#_{N_1}$ $\#_{N_2}$ $\begin{bmatrix} , & \text{tb} & \underline{\text{level}}(\#) \end{bmatrix}$

cs var_{case} var_{exposed} $\begin{bmatrix} if \end{bmatrix}$ $\begin{bmatrix} in \end{bmatrix}$ $\begin{bmatrix} weight \end{bmatrix}$ $\begin{bmatrix} , & cs\_options \end{bmatrix}$

csi $\#_a$ $\#_b$ $\#_c$ $\#_d$ $\begin{bmatrix} , & csi\_options \end{bmatrix}$

Case–control studies

cc var_{case} var_{exposed} $\begin{bmatrix} if \end{bmatrix}$ $\begin{bmatrix} in \end{bmatrix}$ $\begin{bmatrix} weight \end{bmatrix}$ $\begin{bmatrix} , & cc\_options \end{bmatrix}$

cci $\#_a$ $\#_b$ $\#_c$ $\#_d$ $\begin{bmatrix} , & cci\_options \end{bmatrix}$

tabodds var_{case} $\begin{bmatrix} expvar \end{bmatrix}$ $\begin{bmatrix} if \end{bmatrix}$ $\begin{bmatrix} in \end{bmatrix}$ $\begin{bmatrix} weight \end{bmatrix}$ $\begin{bmatrix} , & tabodds\_options \end{bmatrix}$

mhodds var_{case} $expvar$ $\begin{bmatrix} vars_{\text{adjust}} \end{bmatrix}$ $\begin{bmatrix} if \end{bmatrix}$ $\begin{bmatrix} in \end{bmatrix}$ $\begin{bmatrix} weight \end{bmatrix}$ $\begin{bmatrix} , & mhodds\_options \end{bmatrix}$

Matched case–control studies

mcc $var_{\text{exposed\_case}}$ $var_{\text{exposed\_control}}$ $\begin{bmatrix} if \end{bmatrix}$ $\begin{bmatrix} in \end{bmatrix}$ $\begin{bmatrix} weight \end{bmatrix}$ $\begin{bmatrix} , & \text{tb} & \underline{\text{level}}(\#) \end{bmatrix}$

mcci $\#_a$ $\#_b$ $\#_c$ $\#_d$ $\begin{bmatrix} , & \text{tb} & \underline{\text{level}}(\#) \end{bmatrix}$

ir_options	description
Options	
by(*varname*)	stratify on *varname*
e̲standard	combine external weights with within-stratum statistics
i̲standard	combine internal weights with within-stratum statistics
s̲tandard(*varname*)	combine user-specified weights with within-stratum statistics
p̲ool	display pooled estimate
noc̲rude	do not display crude estimate
noh̲om	do not display homogeneity test
ird	calculate standard incidence-rate difference
tb	calculate test-based confidence intervals
l̲evel(#)	set confidence level; default is level(95)

cs_options	description
Options	
by(*varlist*)	stratify on *varlist*
estandard	combine external weights with within-stratum statistics
istandard	combine internal weights with within-stratum statistics
standard(*varname*)	combine user-specified weights with within-stratum statistics
pool	display pooled estimate
nocrude	do not display crude estimate
nohom	do not display homogeneity test
rd	calculate standardized risk difference
binomial(*varname*)	number of subjects variable
or	report odds ratio
woolf	use Woolf approximation for calculating SE of the odds ratio
tb	calculate test-based confidence intervals
exact	calculate Fisher's exact p
level(#)	set confidence level; default is level(95)

csi_options	description
or	report odds ratio
woolf	use Woolf approximation for calculating SE of the odds ratio
tb	calculate test-based confidence intervals
exact	calculate Fisher's exact p
level(#)	set confidence level; default is level(95)

cc_options	description
Options	
by(*varname*)	stratify on *varname*
estandard	combine external weights with within-stratum statistics
istandard	combine internal weights with within-stratum statistics
standard(*varname*)	combine user-specified weights with within-stratum statistics
pool	display pooled estimate
nocrude	do not display crude estimate
nohom	do not display homogeneity test
bd	perform Breslow–Day homogeneity test
tarone	perform Tarone's homogeneity test
binomial(*varname*)	number of subjects variable
cornfield	use Cornfield approximation for calculating SE of the odds ratio
woolf	use Woolf approximation for calculating SE of the odds ratio
tb	calculate test-based confidence intervals
exact	calculate Fisher's exact p
level(#)	set confidence level; default is level(95)

cci_options	description
<u>c</u>ornfield	use Cornfield approximation for calculating SE of the odds ratio
<u>w</u>oolf	use Woolf approximation for calculating SE of the odds ratio
tb	calculate test-based confidence intervals
<u>e</u>xact	calculate Fisher's exact p
<u>l</u>evel(#)	set confidence level; default is level(95)

tabodds_options	description
Main	
<u>b</u>inomial(*varname*)	number of subjects variable
<u>l</u>evel(#)	set confidence level; default is level(95)
or	report odds ratio
<u>adj</u>ust(*varlist*)	report odds ratios adjusted for the variables in *varlist*
base(#)	reference group of control variable for odds ratio
<u>c</u>ornfield	use Cornfield approximation for calculating SE of the odds ratio
<u>w</u>oolf	use Woolf approximation for calculating SE of the odds ratio
tb	calculate test-based confidence intervals
<u>g</u>raph	graph odds against categories
<u>ci</u>plot	same as graph option, except include confidence intervals
CI plot	
<u>ci</u>opts(*rcap_options*)	affect rendition of the confidence bands
Plot	
marker_options	change look of markers (color, size, etc.)
marker_label_options	add marker labels; change look or position
cline_options	affect rendition of the plotted points
Add plots	
<u>addp</u>lot(*plot*)	add other plots to the generated graph
Y axis, X axis, Titles, Legend, Overall	
twoway_options	any options other than by() documented in [G] ***twoway_options***

mhodds_options	description
Options	
by(*varlist*)	stratify on *varlist*
<u>b</u>inomial(*varname*)	number of subjects variable
<u>c</u>ompare(v_1,v_2)	override categories of the control variable
<u>l</u>evel(#)	set confidence level; default is level(95)

fweights are allowed; see [U] **11.1.6 weight**.

Description

ir is used with incidence-rate (incidence density or person-time) data. It calculates point estimates and confidence intervals for the incidence-rate ratio and difference, along with attributable or prevented fractions for the exposed and total population. iri is the immediate form of ir; see [U] **19 Immediate commands**. Also see [R] **poisson** and [ST] **stcox** for related commands.

cs is used with cohort study data with equal follow-up time per subject and sometimes with cross-sectional data. Risk is then the proportion of subjects who become cases. It calculates point estimates and confidence intervals for the risk difference, risk ratio, and (optionally) the odds ratio, along with attributable or prevented fractions for the exposed and total population. csi is the immediate form of cs; see [U] **19 Immediate commands**. Also see [R] **logistic** and [R] **glogit** for related commands.

cc is used with case–control and cross-sectional data. It calculates point estimates and confidence intervals for the odds ratio, along with attributable or prevented fractions for the exposed and total population. cci is the immediate form of cc; see [U] **19 Immediate commands**. Also see [R] **logistic** and [R] **glogit** for related commands.

tabodds is used with case–control and cross-sectional data. It tabulates the odds of failure against a categorical explanatory variable *expvar*. If *expvar* is specified, tabodds performs an approximate χ^2 test of homogeneity of odds and a test for linear trend of the log odds against the numerical code used for the categories of *expvar*. Both tests are based on the score statistic and its variance; see *Methods and Formulas*. When *expvar* is absent, the overall odds are reported. The variable var_{case} is coded 0/1 for individual and simple frequency records and equals the number of cases for binomial frequency records.

Optionally, tabodds tabulates adjusted or unadjusted odds ratios, using either the lowest levels of *expvar* or a user-defined level as the reference group. If adjust(*varlist*) is specified, it produces odds ratios adjusted for the variables in *varlist* along with a (score) test for trend.

mhodds is used with case–control and cross-sectional data. It estimates the ratio of the odds of failure for two categories of *expvar*, controlled for specified confounding variables, $vars_{adjust}$, and tests whether this odds ratio is equal to one. When *expvar* has more than two categories but none are specified with the compare() option, mhodds assumes that *expvar* is a quantitative variable and calculates a 1-degree-of-freedom test for trend. It also calculates an approximate estimate of the rate ratio for a one-unit increase in *expvar*. This is a one-step Newton–Raphson approximation to the maximum likelihood estimate calculated as the ratio of the score statistic, U, to its variance, V (Clayton and Hills 1993, 103).

mcc is used with matched case–control data. It calculates McNemar's chi-squared; point estimates and confidence intervals for the difference, ratio, and relative difference of the proportion with the factor; and the odds ratio. mcci is the immediate form of mcc; see [U] **19 Immediate commands**. Also see [R] **clogit** and [R] **symmetry** for related commands.

Options

Options are listed in the order that they appear in the syntax tables above. The commands for which the option is valid are indicated in parentheses immediately after the option name.

Options (ir, cs, cc, and mhodds) / Main (tabodds)

by(*varname*) (ir, cs, cc, and mhodds) specifies that the tables be stratified on *varname*. Within-stratum statistics are shown and then combined with Mantel–Haenszel weights. If estandard, istandard, or standard() is also specified (see below), the weights specified are used in place of Mantel–Haenszel weights. cs and mhodds will accept a *varlist*.

estandard, istandard, and standard(*varname*) (ir, cs, and cc) request that within-stratum statistics be combined with external, internal, or user-specified weights to produce a standardized estimate. These options are mutually exclusive and can be used only when by() is also specified. (When by() is specified without one of these options, Mantel–Haenszel weights are used.)

estandard external weights are the person-time for the unexposed (ir), the total number of unexposed (cs), or the number of unexposed controls (cc).

istandard internal weights are the person-time for the exposed (ir), the total number of exposed (cs), or the number of exposed controls (cc). istandard can be used to produce, among other things, standardized mortality ratios (SMRs).

standard(*varname*) allows user-specified weights. *varname* must contain a constant within stratum and be nonnegative. The scale of *varname* is irrelevant.

pool (ir, cs, and cc) specifies that, in a stratified analysis, the directly pooled estimate also be displayed. The pooled estimate is a weighted average of the stratum-specific estimates using inverse-variance weights, which are the inverse of the variance of the stratum-specific estimate. pool is relevant only if by() is also specified.

nocrude (ir, cs, and cc) specifies that in a stratified analysis the crude estimate—an estimate obtained without regard to strata—not be displayed. nocrude is relevant only if by() is also specified.

nohom (ir, cs, and cc) specifies that a χ^2 test of homogeneity not be included in the output of a stratified analysis. This tests whether the exposure effect is the same across strata and can be performed for any pooled estimate—directly pooled or Mantel–Haenszel. nohom is relevant only if by() is also specified.

ird (ir) may be used only with estandard, istandard, or standard(). It requests that ir calculate the standardized incidence-rate difference rather than the default incidence-rate ratio.

rd (cs) may be used only with estandard, istandard, or standard(). It requests that cs calculate the standardized risk difference rather than the default risk ratio.

bd (cc) specifies that Breslow and Day's χ^2 test of homogeneity be included in the output of a stratified analysis. This tests whether the exposure effect is the same across strata. bd is relevant only if by() is also specified.

tarone (cc) specifies that Tarone's χ^2 test of homogeneity, which is a correction to the Breslow–Day test, be included in the output of a stratified analysis. This tests whether the exposure effect is the same across strata. tarone is relevant only if by() is also specified.

binomial(*varname*) (cs, cc, tabodds, and mhodds) supplies the number of subjects (cases plus controls) for binomial frequency records. For individual and simple frequency records, this option is not used.

or (cs, csi, and tabodds), for cs and csi, reports the calculation of the odds ratio in addition to the risk ratio if by() is not specified. With by(), or specifies that a Mantel–Haenszel estimate of the combined odds ratio be made rather than the Mantel–Haenszel estimate of the risk ratio. In either case, this is the same calculation that would be made by cc and cci. Typically, cc, cci, or tabodds is preferred for calculating odds ratios. For tabodds, or specifies that odds ratios be produced; see base() for details about selecting a reference category. By default, tabodds will calculate odds.

adjust(*varlist*) (tabodds) specifies that odds ratios adjusted for the variables in *varlist* be calculated.

base(*#*) (tabodds) specifies that the *#*th category of *expvar* be used as the reference group for calculating odds ratios. If base() is not specified, the first category, corresponding to the minimum value of *expvar*, is used as the reference group.

cornfield (cc, cci, and tabodds) requests that the Cornfield (1956) approximation be used to calculate the standard error of the odds ratio. Otherwise, standard errors are obtained as the square root of the variance of the score statistic or exactly for cc and cci.

woolf (cs, csi, cc, cci, and tabodds) requests that the Woolf (1955) approximation, also known as the Taylor expansion, be used for calculating the standard error of the odds ratio. Otherwise, with the exception of tabodds and mhodds, the Cornfield (1956) approximation is used. The Cornfield approximation takes substantially longer (a few seconds) to calculate than the Woolf approximation. For tabodds and mhodds, standard errors of the odds ratios are obtained as the square root of the variance of the score statistic. This standard error is used in calculating a confidence interval for the odds ratio. (For matched case–control data, exact confidence intervals are always calculated.)

tb (ir, iri, cs, csi, cc, cci, tabodds, mcc, and mcci) requests that test-based confidence intervals (Miettinen 1976) be calculated wherever appropriate in place of confidence intervals based on other approximations or exact confidence intervals. We recommend that test-based confidence intervals be used only for pedagogical purposes and never for research work.

exact (cs, csi, cc, and cci) requests that Fisher's exact p be calculated rather than the χ^2 and its significance level. We recommend specifying exact whenever samples are small. A conservative rule of thumb for 2×2 tables is to specify exact when the least-frequent cell contains fewer than 1,000 cases. When the least-frequent cell contains 1,000 cases or more, there will be no appreciable difference between the exact significance level and the significance level based on the χ^2, but the exact significance level will take considerably longer to calculate. exact does not affect whether exact confidence intervals are calculated. Commands always calculate exact confidence intervals where they can, unless tb or woolf is specified.

compare(v_1, v_2) (mhodds) indicates the categories of *expvar* to be compared; v_1 defines the numerator and v_2, the denominator. When compare() is not specified and there are only two categories, the second is compared to the first; when there are more than two categories, an approximate estimate of the odds ratio for a unit increase in *expvar*, controlled for specified confounding variables, is given.

level(*#*) (ir, iri, cs, cc, cci, tabodds, mhodds, mcc, and mcci) specifies the confidence level, as a percentage, for confidence intervals. The default is level(95) or as set by set level; see [R] **level**.

The following options are for use only with tabodds.

──┤ Main ├───

graph (tabodds) produces a graph of the odds against the numerical code used for the categories of *expvar*. All graph options except connect() are allowed. This option is not allowed with the or option or the adjust() option.

ciplot (tabodds) produces the same plot as the graph option, except that it also includes the confidence intervals. This option may not be used with either the or option or the adjust() option.

──┤ CI plot ├───

ciopts(*rcap_options*) (tabodds) is allowed only with the ciplot option. It affects the rendition of the confidence bands; see [G] *rcap_options*.

⌐ Plot └

marker_options (tabodds) affect the rendition of markers drawn at the plotted points, including their shape, size, color, and outline; see [G] *marker_options*.

marker_label_options (tabodds) specify if and how the markers are to be labeled; see [G] *marker_label_options*.

cline_options (tabodds) affect whether lines connect the plotted points and the rendition of those lines; see [G] *cline_options*.

⌐ Add plots └

addplot(*plot*) (tabodds) provides a way to add other plots to the generated graph; see [G] *addplot_option*.

⌐ Y axis, X axis, Titles, Legend, Overall └

twoway_options (tabodds) are any of the options documented in [G] *twoway_options*, excluding by(). These include options for titling the graph (see [G] *title_options*) and options for saving the graph to disk (see [G] *saving_option*).

Remarks

Remarks are presented under the following headings:

> *Incidence-rate data*
> *Stratified incidence-rate data*
> *Standardized estimates with stratified incidence-rate data*
> *Cumulative incidence data*
> *Stratified cumulative incidence data*
> *Standardized estimates with stratified cumulative incidence data*
> *Case–control data*
> *Stratified case–control data*
> *Case–control data with multiple levels of exposure*
> *Case–control data with confounders and possibly multiple levels of exposure*
> *Standardized estimates with stratified case–control data*
> *Matched case–control data*

To calculate appropriate statistics and suppress inappropriate statistics, the ir, cs, cc, tabodds, mhodds, and mcc commands, along with their immediate counterparts, are organized in the way epidemiologists conceptualize data. ir processes incidence-rate data from prospective studies; cs, cohort study data with equal follow-up time (cumulative incidence); cc, tabodds, and mhodds, case–control or cross-sectional (prevalence) data; and mcc, matched case–control data. With the exception of mcc, these commands work with both simple and stratified tables.

Epidemiological data are often summarized in a contingency table from which various statistics are calculated. The rows of the table reflect cases and noncases or cases and person-time, and the columns reflect exposure to a *risk factor*. To an epidemiologist, *cases* and *noncases* refer to the outcomes of the process being studied. For instance, a case might be a person with cancer and a noncase a person without cancer.

A *factor* is something that might affect the chances of being ultimately designated a case or a noncase. Thus, a case might be a cancer patient and the factor, smoking behavior. A person is said to be *exposed* or *unexposed* to the factor. Exposure can be classified as a dichotomy, smokes or does not smoke, or as multiple levels, such as number of cigarettes smoked per week.

For an introduction to epidemiological methods, see Walker (1991). For an intermediate treatment, see Clayton and Hills (1993) and Lilienfeld and Stolley (1994). For other advanced discussions, see van Belle et al. (2004); Kleinbaum, Kupper, and Morgenstern (1982); and Rothman and Greenland (1998). For an anthology of writings on epidemiology since World War II, see Greenland (1987b). See Jewell (2004) for a text aimed at graduate students in the medical professions, which uses Stata for much of the analysis. See Dohoo, Martin, and Stryhn (2003) for a graduate-level text on the principles and methods of veterinary epidemiologic research, and Stata datasets and do-files are available.

❏ Technical Note

Many of the examples in this section provide output after we specified the `level(90)` option, obtaining 90% confidence intervals. This was done so that the results in our examples will be the same as those given in various texts, especially Rothman and Greenland (1998). This should not be taken as an endorsement that a 90% confidence interval is somehow appropriate in professional work.

❏

Incidence-rate data

In incidence-rate data from a prospective study, you observe the transformation of noncases into cases. Starting with a group of noncase subjects, you monitor them to determine whether they become cases (e.g., struck by lightning or, more likely, stricken with cancer). You monitor two populations: those exposed and those unexposed to the factor. A summary of the data is

	Exposed	Unexposed	Total
Cases	a	b	$a + b$
Person-time	N_1	N_0	$N_1 + N_0$

▷ Example 1: iri

It will be easiest to understand these commands if we start with the immediate forms. Remember, in the immediate form, we specify the data on the command line rather than specifying names of variables containing the data; see [U] **19 Immediate commands**. We have data (Boice and Monson 1977, reported in Rothman and Greenland 1998, 238) on breast cancer cases and person-years of observation for women with tuberculosis repeatedly exposed to multiple X-ray fluoroscopies, and those not so exposed:

	X-ray fluoroscopy	
	Exposed	Unexposed
Breast cancer cases	41	15
Person-years	28,010	19,017

Using the immediate form of `ir`, we specify the values in the table following the command:

```
. iri 41 15 28010 19017
```

	Exposed	Unexposed	Total
Cases	41	15	56
Person-time	28010	19017	47027

	Exposed	Unexposed	Total
Incidence Rate	.0014638	.0007888	.0011908

	Point estimate	[95% Conf. Interval]	
Inc. rate diff.	.000675	.0000749	.0012751
Inc. rate ratio	1.855759	1.005684	3.6093 (exact)
Attr. frac. ex.	.4611368	.0056519	.722938 (exact)
Attr. frac. pop	.337618		

(midp) Pr(k>=41) =	0.0177	(exact)
(midp) 2*Pr(k>=41) =	0.0355	(exact)

iri shows the table, reports the incidence rates for the exposed and unexposed populations, and then shows the point estimates of the difference and ratio of the two incidence rates along with their confidence intervals. The incidence rate is simply the frequency with which noncases are transformed into cases.

Next iri reports the attributable fraction among the exposed population, an estimate of the proportion of exposed cases attributable to exposure. We estimate that 46.1% of the 41 breast cancer cases among the exposed were due to exposure. (Had the incidence-rate ratio been less than 1, iri would have reported the prevented fraction in the exposed population, an estimate of the net proportion of all potential cases in the exposed population that was prevented by exposure; see the following technical note.)

After that, the table shows the attributable fraction in the total population, which is the net proportion of all cases attributable to exposure. This number, of course, depends on the proportion of cases that are exposed in the base population, which here is taken to be 41/56 and may not be relevant in all situations. We estimate that 33.8% of the 56 cases were due to exposure. We estimate that 18.9 cases were caused by exposure; that is, $.338 \times 56 = .461 \times 41 = 18.9$.

At the bottom of the table, iri reports both one- and two-sided exact significance tests. For the one-sided test, the probability that the number of exposed cases is 41 or greater is .0177. This is a "midp" calculation; see *Methods and Formulas* below. The two-sided test is $2 \times .0177 = .0354$.

◁

❏ Technical Note

When the incidence rate is less than 1, iri (and ir, cs, csi, cc, and cci) substitutes the prevented fraction for the attributable fraction. Let us reverse the roles of exposure in the above data, treating as exposed a person who did not receive the X-ray fluoroscopy. You can think of this as a new treatment for preventing breast cancer—the suggested treatment being not to use fluoroscopy.

(*Continued on next page*)

```
. iri 15 41 19017 28010
```

	Exposed	Unexposed	Total
Cases	15	41	56
Person-time	19017	28010	47027

Incidence Rate	.0007888	.0014638	.0011908

	Point estimate	[95% Conf. Interval]	
Inc. rate diff.	-.000675	-.0012751	-.0000749
Inc. rate ratio	.5388632	.277062	.9943481 (exact)
Prev. frac. ex.	.4611368	.0056519	.722938 (exact)
Prev. frac. pop	.1864767		

```
            (midp)   Pr(k<=15) =                       0.0177 (exact)
            (midp) 2*Pr(k<=15) =                       0.0355 (exact)
```

The prevented fraction among the exposed is the net proportion of all potential cases in the exposed population that were prevented by exposure. We estimate that 46.1% of potential cases among the women receiving the new "treatment" were prevented by the treatment. (Previously, we estimated that the same percentage of actual cases among women receiving the X-rays was caused by the X-rays.)

The prevented fraction for the population, which is the net proportion of all potential cases in the total population that was prevented by exposure, as with the attributable fraction, depends on the proportion of cases that are exposed in the base population—here taken as 15/56—so it may not be relevant in all situations. We estimate that 18.6% of the potential cases were prevented by exposure.

See Greenland and Robins (1988) for a discussion of how to interpret attributable and prevented fractions.

❑

▷ Example 2: ir

ir works like iri, except that it obtains the entries in the tables by summing data. You specify three variables: the first represents the number of cases represented by this observation, the second indicates whether the observation is for subjects exposed to the factor, and the third records the total time the subjects in this observation were observed. An observation may reflect one subject or a group of subjects.

For instance, here is a 2-observation dataset for the table in the previous example:

```
. use http://www.stata-press.com/data/r10/irxmpl
. list
```

	cases	exposed	time
1.	41	0	28010
2.	15	1	19017

If we typed ir cases exposed time, we would obtain the same output that we obtained above. Another way the data might be recorded is

```
. use http://www.stata-press.com/data/r10/irxmpl2
. list
```

	cases	exposed	time
1.	20	0	14000
2.	21	0	14010
3.	15	1	19017

Here the first 2 observations will be automatically summed by `ir` since both are exposed. Finally, the data might be individual-level data:

```
. list in 1/5
```

	cases	exposed	time
1.	1	1	10
2.	0	1	8
3.	0	0	9
4.	1	0	2
5.	0	1	1

The first observation represents a woman who got cancer, was exposed, and was observed for 10 years. The second is a woman who did not get cancer, was exposed, and was observed for 8 years, and so on.

◁

❑ Technical Note

`ir` (and all the other commands) assume that a subject was exposed if the exposed variable is nonzero and not missing, assume the subject was not exposed if the variable is zero, and ignore the observation if the variable is missing. For `ir`, the case variable and the time variable are restricted to nonnegative integers and are summed within the exposed and unexposed groups to obtain the entries in the table.

❑

Stratified incidence-rate data

▷ Example 3: ir with stratified data

`ir` can work with stratified tables as well as single tables. For instance, Rothman (1986, 185) discusses data from Rothman and Monson (1973) on the mortality by sex and age for patients with trigeminal neuralgia:

	Age through 64		Age 65+	
	Males	Females	Males	Females
Deaths	14	10	76	121
Person-years	1516	1701	949	2245

Entering the data into Stata, we have the dataset:

```
. use http://www.stata-press.com/data/r10/rm
(Rothman and Monson 1973 data)
. list
```

	age	male	deaths	pyears
1.	<65	1	14	1516
2.	<65	0	10	1701
3.	65+	1	76	949
4.	65+	0	121	2245

The stratified analysis of the incidence-rate ratio is

```
. ir deaths male pyears, by(age) level(90)
```

Age category	IRR	[90% Conf. Interval]		M-H Weight	
<65	1.570844	.7380544	3.431878	4.712465	(exact)
65+	1.485862	1.153559	1.907441	35.95147	(exact)
Crude	1.099794	.8688097	1.388891		(exact)
M-H combined	1.49571	1.191914	1.876938		

```
Test of homogeneity (M-H)    chi2(1) =     0.02  Pr>chi2 = 0.8992
```

Here we also specified level(90) to obtain 90% confidence intervals. The row labeled M-H combined reflects the combined Mantel–Haenszel estimates.

As with the previous example, it is not important that each entry in the table correspond to 1 observation in the data—ir sums the time (pyears) and case (deaths) variables within the exposure (male) category.

From the output, we learn that the Mantel–Haenszel estimate differs from the simple crude estimate—that incidence rates appear to vary by age category—and from the test of homogeneity. We find that the exposure effect (the effect of trigeminal neuralgia) is the same across age categories; i.e., we cannot reject the hypothesis that the effects do not differ. Thus we are justified in using the Mantel–Haenszel estimate.

◁

❑ Technical Note

Stratification is one way to deal with confounding; that is, perhaps sex affects the incidence of trigeminal neuralgia and so does age, so the table was stratified by age in an attempt to uncover the sex effect. (We are concerned that age may confound the true association between sex and the incidence of trigeminal neuralgia because the less-than-65/65+ age distributions are so different for males and females. If age affects incidence, the difference in the age distributions would induce different incidences for males and females and thus confound the true effect of sex.)

We do not, however, have to use tables to uncover effects; the estimation alternative when we have aggregate data is Poisson regression, and we can use the same data on which we ran ir with poisson. With individual-level data, Poisson regression is an alternative, but so is Cox regression; see below.

(Although age in the previous example appears to be a string, it is actually a numeric variable taking on values 0 and 1. We attached a value label to produce the labels <65 and 65+ to make ir's output look better; see [U] **12.6.3 Value labels**. Stata's estimation commands will ignore this labeling.)

```
. poisson deaths male age, exposure(pyears) level(90) irr

Iteration 0:   log likelihood = -10.836732
Iteration 1:   log likelihood = -10.734087
Iteration 2:   log likelihood = -10.733944
Iteration 3:   log likelihood = -10.733944
```

Poisson regression				Number of obs	=	4
				LR chi2(2)	=	164.01
				Prob > chi2	=	0.0000
Log likelihood = -10.733944				Pseudo R2	=	0.8843

deaths	IRR	Std. Err.	z	P>|z|	[90% Conf. Interval]	
male	1.495096	.2060997	2.92	0.004	1.191779	1.875611
age	8.888775	1.934943	10.04	0.000	6.213541	12.71583
pyears	(exposure)					

Compare these results with the Mantel–Haenszel estimates produced by `ir`:

Source	IR Ratio	90% Conf. Int.	
Mantel–Haenszel (ir)	1.50	1.19	1.88
poisson	1.50	1.19	1.88

Results are identical to two decimal places. Moreover, in addition to obtaining the incidence-rate ratio for the `male` exposure variable, we also obtain an estimate and confidence interval for the incidence rate of being 65 and over relative to being less than age 65. Here the number is not of much interest since the outcome variable is total mortality and we already knew that older people have a higher mortality rate. In other contexts, however, the number may be of greater interest.

See [R] **poisson** for an explanation of the `poisson` command.

❏

❏ Technical Note

Both the model fitted above and the preceding table asserted that exposure effects are the same across age categories and, if they are not, then both of the previous results are equally inappropriate. The table presented a test of homogeneity, reassuring us that the exposure effects do indeed appear to be constant. The Poisson-regression alternative can be used to reproduce that test by including interactions between the groups and exposure:

```
. generate maleXage = male*age
. poisson deaths male age maleXage, exp(pyears) level(90) irr

Iteration 0:   log likelihood = -10.898799
Iteration 1:   log likelihood = -10.726225
Iteration 2:   log likelihood = -10.725904
Iteration 3:   log likelihood = -10.725904
```

Poisson regression				Number of obs	=	4
				LR chi2(3)	=	164.03
				Prob > chi2	=	0.0000
Log likelihood = -10.725904				Pseudo R2	=	0.8843

deaths	IRR	Std. Err.	z	P>|z|	[90% Conf. Interval]	
male	1.660688	1.396496	0.60	0.546	.4164666	6.622099
age	9.167973	3.01659	6.73	0.000	5.33613	15.75144
maleXage	.9459	.41539	-0.13	0.899	.4593455	1.947829
pyears	(exposure)					

The significance level of the `maleXage` effect is 0.899, the same as previously reported by `ir`.

Here forming the male-times-age interaction was easy because there were only two age groups. Had there been more groups, the test would have been slightly more difficult—see the next technical note.

❑

❑ Technical Note

A word of caution is in order when applying `poisson` (or any estimation technique) to more than two age categories. Say that in our data, we had three age categories, which we will call categories 0, 1, and 2, and that they are stored in the variable `agecat`. We might think of the categories as corresponding to age less than 35, 35–64, and 65 and above.

With such data, we might type `ir deaths male pyears, by(agecat)`, but we would *not* type `poisson deaths male agecat, exposure(pyears)` to obtain the equivalent Poisson-regression estimated results. Such a model might be reasonable, but it is not equivalent because we would be constraining the age effect in category 2 to be (multiplicatively) twice the effect in category 1.

To `poisson` (and all Stata's estimation commands other than `anova`), `agecat` is simply one variable, and only one estimated coefficient is associated with it. Thus the model is

$$\text{Poisson index} = P = \beta_0 + \beta_1 \texttt{male} + \beta_2 \texttt{agecat}$$

The expected number of deaths is then e^P, and the incidence-rate ratio associated with a variable is e^β; see [R] **poisson**. Thus the value of the Poisson index when `male==0` and `agecat==1` is $\beta_0 + \beta_2$, and the possibilities are

	male==0	male==1
agecat==0	β_0	$\beta_0 + \beta_1$
agecat==1	$\beta_0 + \beta_2$	$\beta_0 + \beta_2 + \beta_1$
agecat==2	$\beta_0 + 2\beta_2$	$\beta_0 + 2\beta_2 + \beta_1$

The age effect for `agecat==2` is constrained to be twice the age effect for `agecat==1`—the only difference between lines 3 and 2 of the table is that β_2 is replaced with $2\beta_2$. Under certain circumstances, such a constraint might be reasonable, but it does not correspond to the assumptions made in generating the Mantel–Haenszel combined results.

To obtain results equivalent to the Mantel–Haenszel result, we must estimate a separate effect for each age group, meaning that we must replace $2\beta_2$, the constrained effect, with β_3, a new coefficient that is free to take on any value. We can achieve this by creating two new variables and using them in place of `agecat`. `agecat1` will take on the value 1 when `agecat` is 1 and 0 otherwise; `agecat2` will take on the value 1 when `agecat` is 2 and 0 otherwise:

```
. generate agecat1 = (agecat==1)
. generate agecat2 = (agecat==2)
. poisson deaths male agecat1 agecat2 [freq=pop], exposure(pyears) irr
```

In Stata, we do not have to generate these variables for ourselves. We could use Stata's expand-interaction command `xi`:

```
. xi: poisson deaths male i.agecat [freq=pop], exposure(pyears) irr
```

See [R] **xi** and [U] **25 Dealing with categorical variables**. Although that discussion is in terms of linear regression, it applies equally to Poisson regression.

To reproduce the homogeneity test with multiple age categories, we could type

```
. xi: poisson deaths i.agecat*male [freq=pop], exp(pyears) irr
. testparm _Ia*Xm*
```

Poisson regression combined with xi generalizes to multiway tables. Suppose that there are three exposure categories. Assume exposure variable burn takes on the values 1, 2, and 3 for first-, second-, and third-degree burns. The table itself is estimated by typing

```
. xi: poisson deaths i.burn i.agecat [freq=pop], exp(pyears) irr
```

and the test of homogeneity by typing

```
. xi: poisson deaths i.burn*i.agecat [freq=pop], exp(pyears) irr
. testparm _Ib*Xa*
```

❑

❑ Technical Note

When you have individual-level data, Cox regression and Poisson regression are alternatives to stratified tables. For instance, if we had the individual-level data for deaths by sex and age for the patients with trigeminal neuralgia, the first few observations might be

```
. list in 1/3
```

	patient	male	age	died	studyt~e
1.	1	0	64	0	2
2.	2	1	58	1	3.5
3.	3	1	44	0	3

Patient 1 is a female, age 64, who did not die and was monitored for 2 years. Patient 2 is a male, age 58, who died after being monitored for 3.5 years. With these data, we could obtain the same incidence-rate table we obtained previously by typing

```
. generate agecat = age>=65
. ir died male studytime, by(agecat)
```

but there would be a problem. We would be assuming that patient 1 contributes 2 person-years to the age 64 group, which is not true. Patient 1 contributes 1 person-year to the age 64 group and one more person-year to the age 65 group. We would not have this problem if age did not vary over time, so for the moment, pretend that age is really something else—say, race—that does not vary over time. Then the Cox regression alternative could be obtained by typing

```
. stset studytime, failure(died)
. stcox male agecat
```

Now let's deal with the fact that age does vary over time. The following commands will transform our data:

```
. expand studytime+cond(int(studytime)==studytime,0,1)
. by patient, sort: generate time=cond(_n!=_N,1,studytime-(_N-1))
. by patient: generate cumtime=sum(time)
. by patient: replace died=0 if _n!=_N
. by patient: replace age=age+_n-1
```

See [D] **expand** and [U] **13 Functions and expressions**. For an explanation of cond() and sum(), see [U] **13.3 Functions**. After we issue these commands, our data are

```
. list in 1/10, sepby(patient)
```

	patient	male	age	died	studyt~e	time	cumtime
1.	1	0	64	0	2	1	1
2.	1	0	65	0	2	1	2
3.	2	1	58	0	3.5	1	1
4.	2	1	59	0	3.5	1	2
5.	2	1	60	0	3.5	1	3
6.	2	1	61	0	3.5	1	4
7.	2	1	62	1	3.5	-.5	3.5
8.	3	1	44	0	3	1	1
9.	3	1	45	0	3	1	2
10.	3	1	46	0	3	1	3

That is, there are now two observations for patient 1, one at age 64 and another at age 65. In neither case did the patient die. For patient 2, there are now 4 observations, three corresponding to ages 58–60, during which the patient did not die, and one more (contributing half a year) corresponding to age 61, at which time the patient died. The variable time records the contribution of the observation to exposure; cumtime records the total time from entry into the study (diagnosis of trigeminal neuralgia) to the end of the observation.

We can obtain our original table from these data by typing

```
. generate agecat = age>=65
. ir died male studytime, by(agecat)
```

The corresponding Cox regression model could be estimated by typing

```
. stset cumtime, failure(died) id(patient)
. stcox male agecat
```

We use the stset command to specify that this is a dataset with repeated observations on patients; see [ST] **stset**. Once the dataset is stset, stcox knows to estimate a time-varying regression. As an aside, it might be better to replace agecat with age since, with Cox regression, we can estimate continuous effects, so there is no reason to categorize the data.

So what would happen if we did all this? We do not have the original data, so results must be speculative. We can make up various datasets that correspond to the aggregate data in the table. One possibility, for instance, is that the 6,411 person-years reported in the aggregate table correspond to 6,411 patients, each observed for 1 year. In that case:

```
. use http://www.stata-press.com/data/r10/rm2, clear
(Rothman and Monson 1973 data)

. stcox male agecat, level(90)

        failure _d:  dead
  analysis time _t:  cumtime

Iteration 0:   log likelihood = -1937.2353
Iteration 1:   log likelihood = -1858.8456
Iteration 2:   log likelihood = -1855.3196
Iteration 3:   log likelihood = -1855.2292
Iteration 4:   log likelihood = -1855.2291
Refining estimates:
Iteration 0:   log likelihood = -1855.2291

Cox regression -- Breslow method for ties

No. of subjects =        6411              Number of obs   =       6411
No. of failures =         221
Time at risk    =        6411
                                          LR chi2(2)      =     164.01
Log likelihood  =   -1855.2291            Prob > chi2     =     0.0000
```

_t	Haz. Ratio	Std. Err.	z	P>|z|	[90% Conf. Interval]	
male	1.495096	.2060997	2.92	0.004	1.191779	1.875611
agecat	8.888775	1.934943	10.04	0.000	6.213541	12.71583

Thus comparing these results with those previously obtained:

Source	IR Ratio	90% Conf. Int.	
Mantel–Haenszel (ir)	1.50	1.19	1.88
poisson	1.50	1.19	1.88
stcox	1.50	1.19	1.88

Remember that we obtained the Cox regression estimates assuming that each patient was observed for only 1 year (that is, outside this technical note, we concocted a dataset that would yield the same results as the aggregate data if we ran the ir command on them, and we concocted those data assuming that each patient was observed for 1 year). If we had the real underlying data, so we knew exactly how long each patient was observed, the stcox estimates would be preferable to those of ir or poisson.   ❏

Standardized estimates with stratified incidence-rate data

The by() option specifies that the data are stratified and, by default, will produce a Mantel–Haenszel combined estimate of the incidence-rate ratio. With the estandard, istandard, or standard(*varname*) options, you can specify your own weights and obtain standardized estimates of the incidence-rate ratio or difference.

▷ Example 4: ir with stratified data, using standardized estimates

Rothman and Greenland (1998, 259) report results from Doll and Hill (1966) on age-specific coronary disease deaths among British male doctors from cigarette smoking:

Age	Smokers		Nonsmokers	
	Deaths	Person-years	Deaths	Person-years
35–44	32	52,407	2	18,790
45–54	104	43,248	12	10,673
55–64	206	28,612	28	5,710
65–74	186	12,663	28	2,585
75–84	102	5,317	31	1,462

We have entered these data into Stata:

```
. use http://www.stata-press.com/data/r10/dollhill2
. list
```

	age	smokes	deaths	pyears
1.	35-44	1	32	52407
2.	35-44	0	2	18790
3.	45-54	1	104	43248
4.	45-54	0	12	10673
5.	55-64	1	206	28612
6.	55-64	0	28	5710
7.	65-74	1	186	12663
8.	65-74	0	28	2585
9.	75-84	1	102	5317
10.	75-84	0	31	1462

We can obtain the Mantel–Haenszel combined estimate along with the crude estimate for ignoring stratification of the incidence rate ratio and 90% confidence intervals by typing

```
. ir deaths smokes pyears, by(age) level(90)
```

age	IRR	[90% Conf. Interval]		M-H Weight	
35-44	5.736638	1.704271	33.61646	1.472169	(exact)
45-54	2.138812	1.274552	3.813282	9.624747	(exact)
55-64	1.46824	1.044915	2.110422	23.34176	(exact)
65-74	1.35606	.9626026	1.953505	23.25315	(exact)
75-84	.9047304	.6375194	1.305412	24.31435	(exact)
Crude	1.719823	1.437544	2.0688		(exact)
M-H combined	1.424682	1.194375	1.699399		

Test of homogeneity (M-H)   chi2(4) =   10.41 Pr>chi2 = 0.0340

Note the presence of heterogeneity revealed by the test; the effect of smoking is not the same across age categories. Moreover, the listed stratum-specific estimates show an effect that appears to be declining with age. (Even if the test of homogeneity is not significant, you should always examine estimates carefully when stratum-specific effects occur on both sides of 1 for ratios and 0 for differences.)

Rothman and Greenland (1998, 264) obtain the standardized incidence-rate ratio and 90% confidence intervals weighting each age category by the population of the exposed group, thus producing the standardized mortality ratio (SMR). This calculation can be reproduced by specifying by(age) to indicate that the table is stratified and istandard to specify we want the internally standardized rate. We may also specify that we would like to see the pooled estimate (weighted average where the weights are based on the variance of the strata calculations):

```
. ir deaths smokes pyears, by(age) level(90) istandard pool
```

age	IRR	[90% Conf. Interval]		Weight	
35-44	5.736638	1.704271	33.61646	52407	(exact)
45-54	2.138812	1.274552	3.813282	43248	(exact)
55-64	1.46824	1.044915	2.110422	28612	(exact)
65-74	1.35606	.9626026	1.953505	12663	(exact)
75-84	.9047304	.6375194	1.305412	5317	(exact)
Crude	1.719823	1.437544	2.0688		(exact)
Pooled (direct)	1.355343	1.134356	1.619382		
I. Standardized	1.417609	1.186541	1.693676		

```
Test of homogeneity (direct) chi2(4) =     10.20  Pr>chi2 = 0.0372
```

We obtained the simple pooled results because we specified the pool option. Note the significance of the homogeneity test; it provides the motivation for standardizing the rate ratios.

If we wanted the externally standardized ratio (weights proportional to the population of the unexposed group), we would substitute estandard for istandard in the above command.

Not shown by Rothman and Greenland but as easily obtained are the internally and externally weighted standardized incidence-rate differences. We will obtain the internally weighted difference:

```
. ir deaths smokes pyears, by(age) level(90) istandard ird
```

age	IRD	[90% Conf. Interval]		Weight
35-44	.0005042	.0002877	.0007206	52407
45-54	.0012804	.0006205	.0019403	43248
55-64	.0022961	.0005628	.0040294	28612
65-74	.0038567	.0000521	.0076614	12663
75-84	-.0020201	-.0090201	.00498	5317
Crude	.0018537	.001342	.0023654	
I. Standardized	.0013047	.000712	.0018974	

◁

▷ Example 5: ir with user-specified weights

In addition to calculating results by using internal or external weights, ir (and cs and cc) can calculate results for arbitrary weights. If we wanted to obtain the incidence-rate ratio weighting each age category equally, we would type

```
. generate conswgt=1
. ir deaths smokes pyears, by(age) level(90) standard(conswgt)
```

age	IRR	[90% Conf. Interval]		Weight	
35-44	5.736638	1.704271	33.61646	1	(exact)
45-54	2.138812	1.274552	3.813282	1	(exact)
55-64	1.46824	1.044915	2.110422	1	(exact)
65-74	1.35606	.9626026	1.953505	1	(exact)
75-84	.9047304	.6375194	1.305412	1	(exact)
Crude	1.719823	1.437544	2.0688		(exact)
Standardized	1.155026	.9373745	1.423214		

◁

❑ Technical Note

estandard and istandard are convenience features; they do nothing different from what you could accomplish by creating the appropriate weights and using the standard() option. For instance, we could duplicate the previously shown results of istandard (example before last) by typing

. sort age smokes

. by age: generate wgt=pyears[_N]

. list in 1/4

	age	smokes	deaths	pyears	conswgt	wgt
1.	35-44	0	2	18790	1	52407
2.	35-44	1	32	52407	1	52407
3.	45-54	0	12	10673	1	43248
4.	45-54	1	104	43248	1	43248

. ir deaths smokes pyears, by(age) level(90) standard(wgt) ird
 (output omitted)

sort age smokes made the exposed group (smokes = 1) the last observation within each age category. by age: gen wgt=pyears[_N] created wgt equal to the last observation in each age category.

❑

Cumulative incidence data

In cumulative incidence (follow-up or longitudinal) data, rather than using the time a subject was at risk to normalize ratios, you use the number of subjects. A group of noncases is monitored for some time, during which some become cases. Each subject is also known to be exposed or unexposed. A summary of the data is

	Exposed	Unexposed	Total
Cases	a	b	$a + b$
Noncases	c	d	$c + d$
Total	$a + c$	$b + d$	$a + b + c + d$

Data of this type are generally summarized using the risk ratio. A ratio of 2 means that an exposed subject is twice as likely to become a case than is an unexposed subject, a ratio of one-half means half as likely, and so on. The "null" value—the number corresponding to no effect—is a ratio of 1. If cross-sectional data are analyzed in this format, a prevalence ratio can be obtained.

▷ Example 6: csi

We have data on diarrhea during a 10-day follow-up period among 30 breast-fed infants colonized with *Vibrio cholerae* 01 according to antilipopolysaccharide antibody titers in the mother's breast milk (Glass et al. 1983, reported in Rothman and Greenland 1998, 243):

	Antibody level	
	High	Low
Diarrhea	7	12
No diarrhea	9	2

The `csi` command works much like the `iri` command. We recommend specifying the `exact` option, however, whenever the least-frequent cell contains fewer than 1,000 observations. We have few observations here:

```
. csi 7 12 9 2, exact
```

	Exposed	Unexposed	Total
Cases	7	12	19
Noncases	9	2	11
Total	16	14	30
Risk	.4375	.8571429	.6333333

	Point estimate	[95% Conf. Interval]	
Risk difference	-.4196429	-.7240828	-.1152029
Risk ratio	.5104167	.2814332	.9257086
Prev. frac. ex.	.4895833	.0742914	.7185668
Prev. frac. pop	.2611111		

```
                1-sided Fisher's exact P = 0.0212
                2-sided Fisher's exact P = 0.0259
```

We find that high antibody levels reduce the risk of diarrhea (the risk falls from .86 to .44). The difference is just significant at the 2.59% two-sided level. (Had we not specified the `exact` option, a χ^2 value and its significance level would have been reported in place of Fisher's exact p. The calculated χ^2 two-sided significance level would have been .0173, but this calculation is inferior for small samples.)

◁

❑ Technical Note

By default, `cs` and `csi` do not report the odds ratio, but they will if you specify the `or` option. If you want odds ratios, however, use the `cc` or `cci` commands—the commands appropriate for case–control data—because `cs` and `csi` calculate the attributable (prevented) fraction with the risk ratio, even if you specify `or`:

```
. csi 7 12 9 2, or exact
```

	Exposed	Unexposed	Total
Cases	7	12	19
Noncases	9	2	11
Total	16	14	30
Risk	.4375	.8571429	.6333333

	Point estimate	[95% Conf. Interval]		
Risk difference	-.4196429	-.7240828	-.1152029	
Risk ratio	.5104167	.2814332	.9257086	
Prev. frac. ex.	.4895833	.0742914	.7185668	
Prev. frac. pop	.2611111			
Odds ratio	.1296296	.0246233	.7180882	(Cornfield)

```
                1-sided Fisher's exact P = 0.0212
                2-sided Fisher's exact P = 0.0259
```

Sometimes, the lower or upper confidence bound for the odds ratio will be missing, meaning that the Cornfield approximation did not converge. This can occur when the number of observations is quite small. Two other approximations, however, are available—the Woolf confidence intervals (obtained by specifying woolf) and the test-based intervals (obtained by specifying tb).

❏

❏ Technical Note

As with iri and ir, csi and cs report either the attributable or the prevented fraction for the exposed and total populations; see the discussion under *Incidence-rate data* above. In the previous example, we estimated that 49% of potential cases in the exposed population were prevented by exposure. We also estimated that exposure accounted for a 26% reduction in cases over the entire population, but that is based on the exposure distribution of the (small) population (16/30) and probably is of little interest.

Fleiss, Levin, and Paik (2003, 128) reports infant mortality by birthweight for 72,730 live white births in 1974 in New York City:

```
. csi 618 422 4597 67093
```

	Exposed	Unexposed	Total
Cases	618	422	1040
Noncases	4597	67093	71690
Total	5215	67515	72730
Risk	.1185043	.0062505	.0142995

	Point estimate	[95% Conf. Interval]	
Risk difference	.1122539	.1034617	.121046
Risk ratio	18.95929	16.80661	21.38769
Attr. frac. ex.	.9472554	.9404996	.9532441
Attr. frac. pop	.5628883		

```
                 chi2(1) =   4327.92  Pr>chi2 = 0.0000
```

In these data, exposed means a premature baby (birthweight $\leq$2,500 g), and a case is a baby who is dead at the end of 1 year. We find that being premature accounts for 94.7% of deaths among the premature population. We also estimate, paraphrasing from Fleiss, Levin, and Paik (2003, 128), that 56.3% of all white infant deaths in New York City in 1974 could have been prevented if prematurity had been eliminated. (Moreover, Fleiss, Levin, and Paik put a standard error on the attributable fraction for the population. The formula is given in *Methods and Formulas* but is appropriate only for the population on which the estimates are based.)

❏

▷ Example 7: cs

cs works like csi, except that it obtains its information from the data. The data equivalent to typing csi 7 12 9 2 are

```
. use http://www.stata-press.com/data/r10/csxmpl, clear
. list
```

	case	exp	pop
1.	1	1	7
2.	1	0	12
3.	0	1	9
4.	0	0	2

We could then type `cs case exp [freq=pop]`. If we had individual-level data, so that each observation reflected a patient and we had 30 observations, we would type `cs case exp`.

◁

Stratified cumulative incidence data

▷ Example 8: cs with stratified data

Rothman and Greenland (1998, 255) reprints the following age-specific information for deaths from all causes for tolbutamide and placebo treatment groups (University Group Diabetes Program 1970):

	Age through 54		Age 55 and above	
	Tolbutamide	Placebo	Tolbutamide	Placebo
Dead	8	5	22	16
Surviving	98	115	76	79

The data corresponding to these results are

```
. use http://www.stata-press.com/data/r10/ugdp
. list
```

	age	case	exposed	pop
1.	<55	0	0	115
2.	<55	0	1	98
3.	<55	1	0	5
4.	<55	1	1	8
5.	55+	0	0	69
6.	55+	0	1	76
7.	55+	1	0	16
8.	55+	1	1	22

The order of the observations is unimportant. If we were now to type `cs case exposed [freq=pop]`, we would obtain a summary for all the data, ignoring the stratification by age. To incorporate the stratification, we type

(Continued on next page)

```
. cs case exposed [freq=pop], by(age)
  Age category |        RR     [95% Conf. Interval]    M-H Weight
  ------------+--------------------------------------+-----------
          <55 |  1.811321    .6112044    5.367898      2.345133
          55+ |  1.192602    .6712664     2.11883      8.568306
  ------------+--------------------------------------+-----------
        Crude |  1.435574    .8510221    2.421645
  M-H combined |  1.325555     .797907    2.202132
  ------------+--------------------------------------+-----------

  Test of homogeneity (M-H)      chi2(1) =     0.447  Pr>chi2 = 0.5037
```

Mantel–Haenszel weights are appropriate when the risks may differ according to the strata but the risk ratio is believed to be the same (homogeneous across strata). Under these assumptions, Mantel–Haenszel weights are designed to use the information efficiently. They are not intended to measure a composite risk ratio when the within-stratum risk ratios differ. Then we want a standardized ratio (see below).

The risk ratios above appear to differ markedly, but the confidence intervals are also broad because of the small sample sizes. The test of homogeneity shows that the differences can be attributed to chance; the use of the Mantel–Haenszel combined is probably justified.

◁

❑ Technical Note

Using stratified cumulative incidence tables, as with stratified incidence-rate tables, is only one way to control for the effect of a confounding factor. The estimation alternative is logistic regression, although this requires using the odds ratio rather than the risk ratio as the measure of risk. For the above data, the odds ratio is

```
. cs case exposed [freq=pop], by(age) or
  Age category |        OR     [95% Conf. Interval]    M-H Weight
  ------------+--------------------------------------+--------------------
          <55 |  1.877551    .6238165    5.637046      2.168142 (Cornfield)
          55+ |  1.248355    .6112772    2.547411      6.644809 (Cornfield)
  ------------+--------------------------------------+--------------------
        Crude |  1.510673    .8381198    2.722012
  M-H combined |  1.403149    .7625152    2.582015
  ------------+--------------------------------------+--------------------

  Test of homogeneity (M-H)      chi2(1) =     0.347  Pr>chi2 = 0.5556
             Test that combined OR = 1:
                          Mantel-Haenszel chi2(1) =      1.19
                                     Pr>chi2 =    0.2750
```

Here the event is sufficiently unlikely to proceed; the risk ratio is 1.33, and the odds ratio is 1.40. We also present the crude estimate obtained for analyzing the data without stratifying.

Recasting the problem in the language of modeling, the outcome variable is case and is explained by age and exposed. (As in the incidence-rate example, age may appear to be a string variable in our data—we listed the data in the previous example—but it is actually a numeric variable taking on values 0 and 1 with value labels disguising that fact; see [U] **12.6.3 Value labels**.)

```
. logistic case exposed age [freq=pop]
Logistic regression                              Number of obs   =        409
                                                 LR chi2(2)      =      22.47
                                                 Prob > chi2     =     0.0000
Log likelihood =  -142.6212                      Pseudo R2       =     0.0730
```

case	Odds Ratio	Std. Err.	z	P>|z|	[95% Conf. Interval]	
exposed	1.404674	.4374454	1.09	0.275	.7629451	2.586175
age	4.216299	1.431519	4.24	0.000	2.167361	8.202223

Compare these results with the Mantel–Haenszel estimates obtained with cs:

Source	Odds Ratio	95% Conf. Int.	
Mantel–Haenszel (cs)	1.40	0.76	2.58
logistic	1.40	0.76	2.59

They are virtually identical.

Logistic regression has advantages over the stratified-table approach. First, we obtained an estimate of the age effect: being 55 years or over significantly increases the odds of death. In addition to the point estimate, 4.22, we have a confidence interval for the effect: 2.17 to 8.20.

Given the measured age effect, we would expect that it does not apply only to persons on either side of the 55-year cutoff. It would be more reasonable to assume that a 54-year-old patient has a higher probability of death, due merely to age, than a 53-year-old patient; a 53-year-old, a higher probability than a 52-year-old; and so on. If we had the underlying data, where each patient's age is presumably known, we could include the actual age in the model and so better control for the age effect. This would improve our estimate of the effect of being exposed to tolbutamide.

See [R] **logistic** for an explanation of the logistic command. Also see the technical note in *Incidence-rate data* concerning categorical variables, which applies to logistic regression as well as Poisson regression.

❑

Standardized estimates with stratified cumulative incidence data

As with ir, cs can produce standardized estimates, and the method is basically the same, although the options for which estimates are to be combined or standardized make it confusing. We showed above that cs can produce Mantel–Haenszel weighted estimates of the risk ratio (the default) or the odds ratio (obtained by specifying or). cs can also produce standardized estimates of the risk ratio (the default) or the risk difference (obtained by specifying rd).

▷ Example 9: cs with stratified data, using standardized estimates

To produce an estimate of the internally standardized risk ratio by using our age-specific data on deaths from all causes for tolbutamide and placebo treatment groups (example above), we type

```
. cs case exposed [freq=pop], by(age) istandard
```

Age category	RR	[95% Conf. Interval]		Weight
<55	1.811321	.6112044	5.367898	106
55+	1.192602	.6712664	2.11883	98
Crude	1.435574	.8510221	2.421645	
I. Standardized	1.312122	.7889772	2.182147	

We could obtain externally standardized estimates by substituting `estandard` for `istandard`.

To produce an estimate of the risk ratio weighting each age category equally, we could type

```
. generate wgt=1
. cs case exposed [freq=pop], by(age) standard(wgt)
```

Age category	RR	[95% Conf. Interval]		Weight
<55	1.811321	.6112044	5.367898	1
55+	1.192602	.6712664	2.11883	1
Crude	1.435574	.8510221	2.421645	
Standardized	1.304737	.7844994	2.169967	

If we instead wanted the rate difference, we would type

```
. cs case exposed [freq=pop], by(age) standard(wgt) rd
```

Age category	RD	[95% Conf. Interval]		Weight
<55	.033805	-.0278954	.0955055	1
55+	.0362545	-.0809204	.1534294	1
Crude	.0446198	-.0192936	.1085332	
Standardized	.0350298	-.0311837	.1012432	

If we wanted to weight the less-than-55 age group five times as heavily as the 55-and-over group, we would create `wgt` to contain 5 for the first age group and 1 for the second (or 10 for the first group and 2 for the second—the scale of the weights does not matter).

◁

Case–control data

In case–control data, you select a sample on the basis of the outcome under study; i.e., cases and noncases are sampled at different rates. If you were examining the link between coffee consumption and heart attacks, for instance, you could select a sample of subjects with and without the heart problem and then examine their coffee-drinking behavior. A subject who has suffered a heart attack is called a *case* just as with cohort study data. A subject who has never suffered a heart attack, however, is called a *control* rather than merely a noncase, emphasizing that the sampling was performed with respect to the outcome.

In case–control data, all hope of identifying the risk (i.e., incidence) of the outcome (heart attacks) associated with the factor (coffee drinking) vanishes, at least without information on the underlying sampling fractions, but you can examine the proportion of coffee drinkers among the two populations and reason that, if there is a difference, that coffee drinking may be associated with the risk of heart attacks. Remarkably, even without the underlying sampling fractions, you can also measure the ratio of the odds of heart attacks if a subject drinks coffee to the odds if a subject does not—the so-called odds ratio.

What is lost is the ability to compare absolute rates, which is not always the same as comparing relative rates; see Fleiss, Levin, and Paik (2003, 123).

▷ Example 10: cci

cci calculates the odds ratio and the attributable risk associated with a 2 × 2 table. Rothman et al. (1979) (reprinted in Rothman 1986, 161, and Rothman and Greenland 1998, 245) presents case–control data on the history of chlordiazopoxide use in early pregnancy for mothers of children born with and without congenital heart defects:

	Chlordiazopoxide use	
	Yes	No
Case mothers	4	386
Control mothers	4	1250

We will use the level(90) option to obtain 90% confidence intervals as reported by Rothman and Greenland:

```
. cci 4 386 4 1250, level(90)
                                                         Proportion
                   |  Exposed   Unexposed  |    Total    Exposed
-------------------+-----------------------+-----------------------
            Cases  |      4         386    |     390      0.0103
         Controls  |      4        1250    |    1254      0.0032
-------------------+-----------------------+-----------------------
            Total  |      8        1636    |    1644      0.0049

                   |  Point estimate       |   [90% Conf. Interval]
-------------------+-----------------------+-----------------------
       Odds ratio  |     3.238342          |    .7698467   13.59664 (exact)
   Attr. frac. ex. |       .6912           |   -.2989599    .9264524 (exact)
   Attr. frac. pop |     .0070892          |
                                     chi2(1) =    3.07  Pr>chi2 = 0.0799
```

We obtain a point estimate of the odds ratio as 3.24 and a χ^2 value, which is a test that the odds ratio is 1, significant at the 10% level.

◁

❏ Technical Note

Although we tend to think of statistical tests and confidence intervals as different ways of presenting the same information, that is not exactly true. The statistical test is derived under the assumption of the null hypothesis that the odds ratio is 1. A "test-based" confidence interval is a direct transformation of the statistical test, and there can be no disagreement between them. If you specify the tb option, csi and the other epitab commands will produce test-based confidence intervals. When you do not specify this option, however, the epitab commands calculate either exact or approximate confidence intervals. Exact confidence intervals are unbeatable—if there is a disagreement between the exact interval and the test statistic, you can believe the interval. (Within exact results, midp intervals more closely approximate asymptotic test statistics.) All the classical test statistics are derived under various simplifying assumptions that are not present in exact calculations. (The epitab commands always place the word "exact" next to exact calculation results.)

The Cornfield confidence intervals, on the other hand, are an example of an approximation. The Cornfield approximation, along with the other approximations, attempts to produce confidence intervals around a point central to the confidence interval, producing intervals that should more accurately reflect the exact confidence interval when the parameter deviates from the null hypothesis. This makes the confidence interval focus on estimation rather than statistical testing.

In this case, here is the result of calculating the confidence interval for the odds ratio by using various methods:

Method	90% Conf. Int.		Source
exact	0.77	13.60	Rothman 1986, 174 or cci
Woolf	1.01	10.40	Rothman 1986, 175 or cci, woolf
test-based	1.07	9.77	Rothman 1986, 175 or cci, tb
Cornfield	1.07	9.83	Rothman 1986, 175 or cci, cornfield

There are only eight exposed patients here, and the differences shown above are larger than typically observed. That they are also on both sides of the knife edge of 1 is (pedagogically speaking) fortuitous. The exact answer, which is just that, includes 1 in the interval, so we cannot reject (at the 10% level) the hypothesis that the odds ratio is 1. That is the "right" answer (but see the next technical note). The Woolf, test-based, and Cornfield intervals exclude 1 and reassuringly conform to the χ^2 value. In any case, all results are so close to 1 that we should still think about chance as an explanation. ❏

❏ Technical Note

If you specify the exact option, cc and cci will report the exact significance of the table. We could have—and should have—done that above because of the small number of cases. We did not do this for expositional purposes, but we will do so now:

```
. cci 4 386 4 1250, level(90) exact
```

	Exposed	Unexposed		Total	Proportion Exposed
Cases	4	386		390	0.0103
Controls	4	1250		1254	0.0032
Total	8	1636		1644	0.0049

	Point estimate	[90% Conf. Interval]		
Odds ratio	3.238342	.7698467	13.59664	(exact)
Attr. frac. ex.	.6912	-.2989599	.9264524	(exact)
Attr. frac. pop	.0070892			

```
                    1-sided Fisher's exact P = 0.0964
                    2-sided Fisher's exact P = 0.0964
```

In this table the one- and two-sided significance values are equal. This is not a mistake, but it does not happen often. Exact significance values are calculated by summing the probabilities for tables that have the same marginals (row and column sums) but that are less likely (given an odds ratio of 1) than the observed table. When considering each possible table, we might ask if the table is in the same or opposite tail as the observed table. If it is in the same tail, we would count the table under consideration in the one-sided test and, either way, we would count it in the two-sided test. Here all the tables more extreme than this table are in the same tail, so the one- and two-sided tests are the same.

The exact p is .096 < .100; that is, the table is significant at the 10% level. In the previous example, we said that "exact confidence intervals are unbeatable—if there is a disagreement between the exact interval and the test statistic, you can believe the interval". We also reported (Rothman 1986, 174) that the exact confidence interval for the odds ratio is 0.77 to 13.6, which includes 1. How can both statements be true and yet both statistics be exact?

Confidence intervals and test statistics measure different things. The .0964 is the fraction of all tables that are less likely than the observed table conditional on the odds ratio being 1. The lower bound of the confidence interval 0.77 corresponds to the statement that the probability of observing tables with four or more exposed cases, conditional on the odds ratio being .77, is 0.05. The upper bound of the confidence interval 13.6 corresponds to the statement that the probability of observing tables with four or fewer exposed cases, conditional on the odds ratio being 13.6, is 0.05. No two of these are the same, and there is no reason why they should somehow agree.

You expect them to agree because you are used to thinking in large-sample approximations. For infinite-sized samples, the answers above will agree, and for large but finite samples, the answers will tend to agree. If we had many exposed individuals (as we do not), we would not have had this problem.

❏

❏ Technical Note

The reported value of the attributable or prevented fraction among the exposed is calculated on using the odds ratio as a proxy for the risk ratio. This can be justified only if the outcome is exceedingly unlikely in the population. The extrapolation to the attributable or prevented fraction for the population assumes that the control group is a random sample of the corresponding group in the underlying population.

❏

▷ Example 11: cc equivalent to cci

Equivalent to typing `cci 4 386 4 1250` would be typing `cc case exposed [freq=pop]` with the data:

```
. use http://www.stata-press.com/data/r10/ccxmpl

. list
```

	case	exposed	pop
1.	1	1	4
2.	1	0	386
3.	0	1	4
4.	0	0	1250

◁

Stratified case–control data

▷ Example 12: cc with stratified data

cc can work with stratified tables. Rothman and Greenland (1998, 273) reprint and discuss data from a case–control study on infants with congenital heart disease and Down's syndrome and healthy controls, according to maternal spermicide use before conception and maternal age at delivery (Rothman 1982):

| | Maternal age to 34 | | Maternal age 35+ | |
	Spermicide used	not used	Spermicide used	not used
Down's syndrome	3	9	1	3
Controls	104	1059	5	86

The data corresponding to these tables are

```
. use http://www.stata-press.com/data/r10/downs
. list
```

	case	exposed	pop	age
1.	1	1	3	<35
2.	1	0	9	<35
3.	0	1	104	<35
4.	0	0	1059	<35
5.	1	1	1	35+
6.	1	0	3	35+
7.	0	1	5	35+
8.	0	0	86	35+

The stratified results for the odds ratio are

```
. cc case exposed [freq=pop], by(age) woolf
```

Maternal age	OR	[95% Conf. Interval]		M-H Weight	
<35	3.394231	.9048403	12.73242	.7965957	(Woolf)
35+	5.733333	.5016418	65.52706	.1578947	(Woolf)
Crude	3.501529	1.110362	11.04208		(Woolf)
M-H combined	3.781172	1.18734	12.04142		

```
Test of homogeneity (M-H)      chi2(1) =     0.14  Pr>chi2 = 0.7105
                    Test that combined OR = 1:
                          Mantel-Haenszel chi2(1) =      5.81
                                         Pr>chi2 =    0.0159
```

For no particular reason, we also specified the woolf option to obtain Woolf approximations to the within-stratum confidence intervals rather than Cornfield approximations. Had we wanted test-based confidence intervals and the crude estimate, we would have used

```
. cc case exposed [freq=pop], by(age) tb tarone
```

Maternal age	OR	[95% Conf. Interval]		M-H Weight	
<35	3.394231	.976611	11.79672	.7965957	(tb)
35+	5.733333	.6402941	51.33752	.1578947	(tb)
Crude	3.501529	1.189946	10.30358		(tb)
M-H combined	3.781172	1.282056	11.15183		(tb)

```
Test of homogeneity (M-H)        chi2(1) =     0.14  Pr>chi2 = 0.7105
Test of homogeneity (Tarone)     chi2(1) =     0.14  Pr>chi2 = 0.7092
                    Test that combined OR = 1:
                          Mantel-Haenszel chi2(1) =      5.81
                                         Pr>chi2 =    0.0159
```

We recommend that test-based confidence intervals be used only for pedagogical reasons and never for research work.

Whatever method you choose for calculating confidence intervals, Stata will report a test of homogeneity, which here is $\chi^2(1) = .14$ and "insignificant". That is, the odds of Down's syndrome might vary with maternal age, but we cannot reject the hypothesis that the odds ratios of those exposed to spermicide and those not exposed are the same in the two maternal age strata. This is thus a test to reject the appropriateness of the single, Mantel–Haenszel combined odds ratio—a rejection not justified by these data.

◁

❑ Technical Note

In the last example, we requested that Tarone's test of homogeneity be reported by specifying the `tarone` option. For this dataset, both the Mantel–Haenszel and the Tarone tests produced virtually identical results, but this is not always the case. When data are sparse, you may have strata with a zero count in one or more cells. The Mantel–Haenszel test will not include these strata in the homogeneity test because the odds ratios for these strata cannot be estimated. On the other hand, the Tarone homogeneity test includes all strata in its calculation. Although Tarone's test of homogeneity is more appropriate when data are sparse, if the number of strata is large and there are few observations per strata, the distribution of the test statistic may not approximate the nominal chi-squared, even if the null hypothesis is true.

❑

❑ Technical Note

As with cohort study data, an alternative to stratified tables for uncovering effects is logistic regression. From the logistic point of view, case–control data are no different from cohort study data—you must merely ignore the estimated intercept, which is not reported by `logistic` in any case. (`logit`, on the other hand, makes the same estimates as `logistic` but displays the coefficients rather than transforming them to odds ratios, so it does display the estimated intercept. The intercept is meaningless in case–control data because it reflects the baseline prevalence of the outcome, which you controlled by sampling.)

The data we used with `cc` can be used directly by `logistic`. (The `age` variable, which appears to be a string, is really numeric with an associated value label; see [U] **12.6.3 Value labels**. age takes on the value 0 for the age-less-than-35 group and 1 for the 35+ group.)

```
. logistic case exposed age [freq=pop]
Logistic regression                              Number of obs   =       1270
                                                 LR chi2(2)      =       8.74
                                                 Prob > chi2     =     0.0127
Log likelihood = -81.517532                      Pseudo R2       =     0.0509
```

case	Odds Ratio	Std. Err.	z	P>|z|	[95% Conf. Interval]	
exposed	3.787779	2.241922	2.25	0.024	1.187334	12.0836
age	4.582857	2.717351	2.57	0.010	1.433594	14.65029

We compare the results with those presented by `cc` in the previous example:

Source	Odds ratio	95% CI	
Mantel–Haenszel (cc)	3.78	1.19	12.04
logistic	3.79	1.19	12.08

As with the cohort study data, results are virtually identical, and all the same comments we made previously apply once again.

To demonstrate, let us now ask a question that would be difficult to answer on the basis of a stratified table analysis. We now know that spermicide use appears to increase the risk of having a baby with Down's syndrome, and we also know that the mother's age also increases the risk. Is the effect of spermicide use statistically different for mothers in the two age groups?

```
. generate ageXex = age*exposed
. logistic case exposed age ageXex [freq=pop]
Logistic regression                             Number of obs   =       1270
                                                LR chi2(3)      =       8.87
                                                Prob > chi2     =     0.0311
Log likelihood = -81.451332                     Pseudo R2       =     0.0516
```

case	Odds Ratio	Std. Err.	z	P>|z|	[95% Conf. Interval]	
exposed	3.394231	2.289544	1.81	0.070	.9048403	12.73242
age	4.104651	2.774868	2.09	0.037	1.091034	15.44237
ageXex	1.689141	2.388785	0.37	0.711	.1056563	27.0045

The answer is no. The odds ratio and confidence interval reported for `exposed` now measure the spermicide effect for an `age==0` (age < 35) mother. The odds ratio and confidence interval reported for `ageXex` are the (multiplicative) difference in the odds ratio for an `age==1` (age 35+) mother relative to a young mother. The point estimate is that the effect is larger for older mothers, suggesting grounds for future research, but the difference is not significant.

See [R] **logistic** for an explanation of the `logistic` command. Also see the technical note under *Incidence-rate data* above concerning Poisson regression, which applies equally to logistic regression.

❏

Case–control data with multiple levels of exposure

In a case–control study, subjects with the disease of interest (cases) are compared to disease-free individuals (controls) to assess the relationship between exposure to one or more risk factors and disease incidence. Often exposure is measured qualitatively at several discrete levels or measured on a continuous scale and then grouped into three or more levels. The data can be summarized as

	Exposure level				
	1	2	...	k	Total
Cases	a_1	a_2	...	a_k	M_1
Controls	c_1	c_2	...	c_k	M_0
Total	N_1	N_2	...	N_k	T

An advantage afforded by having multiple levels of exposure is the ability to examine dose–response relationships. If the association between a risk factor and a disease or outcome is real, we expect the strength of that association to increase with the level and duration of exposure. Demonstrating the existence of a dose–response relationship provides strong support for a direct or even causal relationship between the risk factor and the outcome. On the other hand, the lack of a dose–response is usually seen as an argument against causality.

We can use the `tabodds` command to tabulate and examine the odds of failure or odds ratios against a categorical exposure variable. The test for trend calculated by `tabodds` can serve as a test for dose–response if the exposure variable is at least ordinal. If the exposure variable has no natural ordering, the trend test is meaningless and should be ignored. See the technical note at the end of this section for more information regarding the test for trend.

Before looking at an example, consider three possible data arrangements for case–control and prevalence studies. The most common data arrangement is individual records, where each subject in the study has his or her own record. Closely related are frequency records where identical individual records are included only once, but with a variable giving the frequency with which the record occurs. The *weight* option is used for these data to specify the frequency variable. Data can also be arranged as binomial frequency records where each record contains a variable D, the number of cases; another variable N, the number of total subjects (cases plus controls); and other variables. An advantage of binomial frequency records is that large datasets can be entered succinctly into a Stata database.

▷ Example 13: tabodds

Consider the following data from the Ille-et-Villaine study of esophageal cancer discussed in Breslow and Day (1980, chap. 4):

| | Alcohol consumption (g/day) | | | | |
	0–39	40–79	80–119	120+	Total
Cases	2	9	9	5	25
Controls	47	31	9	5	92
Total	49	40	18	10	117

corresponding to subjects age 55–64 who use from 0 to 9 g of tobacco per day. There are 24 such tables, each representing one of four levels of tobacco use and one of six age categories. The data can be used to create a binomial frequency record dataset by simply entering each table's data by typing

```
. input alcohol D N agegrp tobacco
           alcohol        D         N       agegrp        tobacco
   1.            1         2        49            4              1
   2.            2         9        40            4              1
   3.            3         9        18            4              1
   4.            4         5        10            4              1
   5. end

.
```

where D is the number of esophageal cancer cases and N is the number of total subjects (cases plus controls) for each combination of six age groups (agegrp), four levels of alcohol consumption in g/day (alcohol), and four levels of tobacco use in g/day (tobacco).

Both the tabodds and mhodds commands can correctly handle all three data arrangements. Binomial frequency records require that the number of total subjects (cases plus controls) represented by each record N be specified with the binomial() option.

We could also enter the data as frequency-weighted data:

```
. input alcohol case freq agegrp tobacco
           alcohol       case      freq       agegrp        tobacco
   1.            1         1         2            4              1
   2.            1         0        47            4              1
   3.            2         1         9            4              1
   4.            2         0        31            4              1
   5.            3         1         9            4              1
   6.            3         0         9            4              1
   7.            4         1         5            4              1
   8.            4         0         5            4              1
   9. end

.
```

If you are planning on using any of the other estimation commands, such as `poisson` or `logistic`, we recommend that you enter your data either as individual records or as frequency-weighted records and not as binomial frequency records because the estimation commands currently do not recognize the `binomial` option.

We have entered all the esophageal cancer data into Stata as a frequency-weighted record dataset as previously described. In our data, `case` indicates the esophageal cancer cases and controls, and `freq` is the number of subjects represented by each record (the weight).

We added value labels to the variables `agegrp`, `alcohol`, and `tobacco` in our dataset to ease interpretation in outputs, but these variables are numeric.

We are interested in the association between alcohol consumption and esophageal cancer. We first use `tabodds` to tabulate the odds of esophageal cancer against alcohol consumption:

```
. use http://www.stata-press.com/data/r10/bdesop, clear
. tabodds case alcohol [fweight=freq]
```

alcohol	cases	controls	odds	[95% Conf. Interval]	
0-39	29	386	0.07513	0.05151	0.10957
40-79	75	280	0.26786	0.20760	0.34560
80-119	51	87	0.58621	0.41489	0.82826
120+	45	22	2.04545	1.22843	3.40587

```
Test of homogeneity (equal odds):  chi2(3)  =    158.79
                                   Pr>chi2  =     0.0000
Score test for trend of odds:      chi2(1)  =    152.97
                                   Pr>chi2  =     0.0000
```

The test of homogeneity clearly indicates that the odds of esophageal cancer differ by level of alcohol consumption, and the test for trend indicates a significant increase in odds with increasing alcohol use. This suggests a strong dose–response relation. The `graph` option can be used to study the shape of the relationship of the odds with alcohol consumption. Most of the heterogeneity in these data can be "explained" by the linear increase in risk of esophageal cancer with increased dosage (alcohol consumption).

We also could have requested that the odds ratios at each level of alcohol consumption be calculated by specifying the `or` option. For example, `tabodds case alcohol [fweight=freq], or` would produce odds ratios using the minimum value of alcohol—i.e., alcohol = 1 (0–39)—as the reference group, and the command `tabodds case alcohol [fweight=freq], or base(2)` would use alcohol = 2 (40–79) as the reference group.

Although our results appear to provide strong evidence supporting an association between alcohol consumption and esophageal cancer, we need to be concerned with the possible existence of confounders, specifically age and tobacco use, in our data. We can again use `tabodds` to tabulate and examine the odds of esophageal cancer against age and against tobacco use, independently:

```
. tabodds case agegrp [fweight=freq]
```

agegrp	cases	controls	odds	[95% Conf.	Interval]
25-34	1	115	0.00870	0.00121	0.06226
35-44	9	190	0.04737	0.02427	0.09244
45-54	46	167	0.27545	0.19875	0.38175
55-64	76	166	0.45783	0.34899	0.60061
65-74	55	106	0.51887	0.37463	0.71864
75+	13	31	0.41935	0.21944	0.80138

```
Test of homogeneity (equal odds): chi2(5)  =     96.94
                                   Pr>chi2  =    0.0000

Score test for trend of odds:      chi2(1)  =     83.37
                                   Pr>chi2  =    0.0000
```

```
. tabodds case tobacco [fweight=freq]
```

tobacco	cases	controls	odds	[95% Conf.	Interval]
0-9	78	447	0.17450	0.13719	0.22194
10-19	58	178	0.32584	0.24228	0.43823
20-29	33	99	0.33333	0.22479	0.49428
30+	31	51	0.60784	0.38899	0.94983

```
Test of homogeneity (equal odds): chi2(3)  =     29.33
                                   Pr>chi2  =    0.0000

Score test for trend of odds:      chi2(1)  =     26.93
                                   Pr>chi2  =    0.0000
```

We can see that there is evidence to support our concern that both age and tobacco use are potentially important confounders. Clearly, before we can make any statements regarding the association between esophageal cancer and alcohol use, we must examine and, if necessary, adjust for the effect of any confounder. We will return to this example in the following section.

◁

❑ Technical Note

The score test for trend performs a test for linear trend of the log odds against the numerical code used for the exposure variable. The test depends not only on the relationship between dose level and the outcome but also on the numeric values assigned to each level or, to be more accurate, to the distance between the numeric values assigned. For example, the trend test on a dataset with four exposure levels coded 1, 2, 3, and 4 gives the same results as coding the levels 10, 20, 30, and 40 because the distance between the levels in each case is constant. In the first case, the distance is one unit, and in the second case, it is 10 units. However, if we code the exposure levels as 1, 10, 100, and 1,000, we would obtain different results because the distance between exposure levels is not constant. Thus, be careful when assigning values to exposure levels. You must determine whether equally spaced numbers make sense for your data or if other more meaningful values should be used.

Remember that we are testing whether a log-linear relationship exists between the odds and the outcome variable. For your particular problem, this relationship may not be correct or even make sense, so you must be careful in interpreting the output of this trend test.

❑

Case–control data with confounders and possibly multiple levels of exposure

In the esophageal cancer data example introduced earlier, we determined that the apparent association between alcohol consumption and esophageal cancer could be confounded by age and tobacco use. You can adjust for the effect of possible confounding factors by stratifying on these factors. This is the method used by both `tabodds` and `mhodds` to adjust for other variables in the dataset. We will compare and contrast these two commands in the following example.

▷ Example 14: tabodds, adjusting for confounding factors

We begin by using `tabodds` to tabulate unadjusted odd ratios. We do this to compare the adjusted and unadjusted odds ratios.

```
. tabodds case alcohol [fweight=freq], or
```

alcohol	Odds Ratio	chi2	P>chi2	[95% Conf. Interval]	
0-39	1.000000	.	.	.	.
40-79	3.565271	32.70	0.0000	2.237981	5.679744
80-119	7.802616	75.03	0.0000	4.497054	13.537932
120+	27.225705	160.41	0.0000	12.507808	59.262107

```
Test of homogeneity (equal odds): chi2(3)  =    158.79
                                   Pr>chi2  =    0.0000
Score test for trend of odds:      chi2(1)  =    152.97
                                   Pr>chi2  =    0.0000
```

The `alcohol = 1` group (0–39) was used by `tabodds` as the reference category for calculating the odds ratios. We could have selected a different group by specifying the `base()` option; however, because the lowest dosage level is most often the adequate reference group, as it is in these data, the `base()` option is seldom used.

We use `tabodds` with the `adjust()` option to tabulate Mantel–Haenszel age-adjusted odds ratios:

```
. tabodds case alcohol [fweight=freq], adjust(age)
Mantel-Haenszel odds ratios adjusted for age
```

alcohol	Odds Ratio	chi2	P>chi2	[95% Conf. Interval]	
0-39	1.000000	.	.	.	.
40-79	4.268155	37.36	0.0000	2.570025	7.088314
80-119	8.018305	59.30	0.0000	4.266893	15.067922
120+	28.570426	139.70	0.0000	12.146409	67.202514

```
Score test for trend of odds: chi2(1)  =   135.09
                              Pr>chi2  =   0.0000
```

We observe that the age-adjusted odds ratios are just slightly higher than the unadjusted ones, so it appears that age is not as strong a confounder as it first appeared. Even after adjusting for age, the dose–response relationship, as measured by the trend test, remains strong.

We now perform the same analysis but this time adjust for tobacco use instead of age.

```
. tabodds case alcohol [fweight=freq], adjust(tobacco)
Mantel-Haenszel odds ratios adjusted for tobacco
```

alcohol	Odds Ratio	chi2	P>chi2	[95% Conf. Interval]	
0-39	1.000000	.	.	.	.
40-79	3.261178	28.53	0.0000	2.059764	5.163349
80-119	6.771638	62.54	0.0000	3.908113	11.733306
120+	19.919526	123.93	0.0000	9.443830	42.015528

```
Score test for trend of odds: chi2(1)  =  135.04
                              Pr>chi2  =   0.0000
```

Again we observe a significant dose–response relationship and not much difference between the adjusted and unadjusted odds ratios. We could also adjust for the joint effect of both age and tobacco use by specifying adjust(tobacco age), but we will not bother here. ◁

A different approach to analyzing these data is to use the mhodds command. This command estimates the ratio of the odds of failure for two categories of an exposure variable, controlling for any specified confounding variables, and it tests whether this odds ratio is equal to one. For multiple exposures, if two exposure levels are not specified with compare(), mhodds assumes that exposure is quantitative and calculates a 1-degree-of-freedom test for trend. This test for trend is the same one that tabodds reports.

▷ Example 15: mhodds, controlling for confounding factors

We first use mhodds to estimate the effect of alcohol controlled for age:

```
. mhodds case alcohol agegrp [fweight=freq]
Score test for trend of odds with alcohol
controlling for agegrp
(The Odds Ratio estimate is an approximation to the odds ratio
for a one unit increase in alcohol)
```

Odds Ratio	chi2(1)	P>chi2	[95% Conf. Interval]	
2.845895	135.09	0.0000	2.385749	3.394792

Because alcohol has more than two levels, mhodds estimates and reports an approximate age-adjusted odds ratio for a one-unit increase in alcohol consumption. The χ^2 value reported is identical to that reported by tabodds for the score test for trend on the previous page.

We now use mhodds to estimate the effect of alcohol controlled for age, and while we are at it, we do this by levels of tobacco consumption:

(Continued on next page)

```
. mhodds case alcohol agegrp [fweight=freq], by(tobacco)
```

```
Score test for trend of odds with alcohol
controlling for agegrp
by tobacco
```

```
note: only 19 of the 24 strata formed in this analysis contribute
      information about the effect of the explanatory variable
```

```
(The Odds Ratio estimate is an approximation to the odds ratio
for a one unit increase in alcohol)
```

tobacco	Odds Ratio	chi2(1)	P>chi2	[95% Conf. Interval]	
0-9	3.579667	75.95	0.0000	2.68710	4.76871
10-19	2.303580	25.77	0.0000	1.66913	3.17920
20-29	2.364135	13.27	0.0003	1.48810	3.75589
30+	2.217946	8.84	0.0029	1.31184	3.74992

Mantel-Haenszel estimate controlling for agegrp and tobacco

Odds Ratio	chi2(1)	P>chi2	[95% Conf. Interval]	
2.751236	118.37	0.0000	2.292705	3.301471

```
Test of homogeneity of ORs (approx): chi2(3)   =     5.46
                                      Pr>chi2   =   0.1409
```

Again because `alcohol` has more than two levels, `mhodds` estimates and reports an approximate Mantel–Haenszel age and tobacco-use adjusted odds ratio for a one-unit increase in alcohol consumption. The χ^2 test for trend reported with the Mantel–Haenszel estimate is again the same one that `tabodds` produces if `adjust(agegrp tobacco)` is specified.

The results from this analysis also show an effect of alcohol, controlled for age, of about $\times 2.7$, which is consistent across different levels of tobacco consumption. Similarly,

```
. mhodds case tobacco agegrp [fweight=freq], by(alcohol)
```

```
Score test for trend of odds with tobacco
controlling for agegrp
by alcohol
```

```
note: only 18 of the 24 strata formed in this analysis contribute
      information about the effect of the explanatory variable
```

```
(The Odds Ratio estimate is an approximation to the odds ratio
for a one unit increase in tobacco)
```

alcohol	Odds Ratio	chi2(1)	P>chi2	[95% Conf. Interval]	
0-39	2.420650	15.61	0.0001	1.56121	3.75320
40-79	1.427713	5.75	0.0165	1.06717	1.91007
80-119	1.472218	3.38	0.0659	0.97483	2.22339
120+	1.214815	0.59	0.4432	0.73876	1.99763

Mantel-Haenszel estimate controlling for agegrp and alcohol

Odds Ratio	chi2(1)	P>chi2	[95% Conf. Interval]	
1.553437	20.07	0.0000	1.281160	1.883580

```
Test of homogeneity of ORs (approx): chi2(3)   =     5.26
                                      Pr>chi2   =   0.1540
```

shows an effect of tobacco, controlled for age, of about $\times 1.5$, which is consistent across different levels of alcohol consumption.

Comparisons between particular levels of alcohol and tobacco consumption can be made by generating a new variable with levels corresponding to all combinations of alcohol and tobacco, as in

```
. egen alctob = group(alcohol tobacco)
. mhodds case alctob [fweight=freq], compare(16,1)
Maximum likelihood estimate of the odds ratio
Comparing alctob==16 vs. alctob==1
```

Odds Ratio	chi2(1)	P>chi2	[95% Conf. Interval]
93.333333	103.21	0.0000	14.766136 589.938431

which yields an odds ratio of 93 between subjects with the highest levels of alcohol and tobacco and those with the lowest levels. Similar results can be obtained simultaneously for all levels of alctob using alctob = 1 as the comparison group by specifying tabodds D alctob, bin(N) or.

◁

Standardized estimates with stratified case–control data

▷ Example 16: cc with stratified data, using standardized estimates

You obtain standardized estimates (here for the odds ratio) using cc just as you obtain standardized estimates using ir or cs. Along with the by() option, you specify one of estandard, istandard, or standard(*varname*).

Rothman and Greenland (1998, 272) report the standardized mortality rate (SMR) along with a 90% confidence interval for the case–control study on infants with congenital heart disease and Down's syndrome. We can reproduce their estimates along with the pooled estimates by typing

```
. use http://www.stata-press.com/data/r10/downs, clear
. cc case exposed [freq=pop], by(age) istandard level(90) pool
```

Maternal age	OR	[90% Conf. Interval]		Weight	
<35	3.394231	.7761116	11.5405	104	(exact)
35+	5.733333	.1856098	61.20937	5	(exact)
Crude	3.501529	1.024302	10.04068		(exact)
Pooled (direct)	3.824166	1.442194	10.14028		
I. Standardized	3.779749	1.423445	10.03657		

Test of homogeneity (direct)   chi2(1) =   0.14 Pr>chi2 = 0.7109

Using the distribution of the nonexposed subjects in the source population as the standard, we can obtain an estimate of the standardized risk ratio (SRR):

```
. cc case exposed [freq=pop], by(age) estandard level(90)
```

Maternal age	OR	[90% Conf. Interval]		Weight	
<35	3.394231	.7761116	11.5405	1059	(exact)
35+	5.733333	.1856098	61.20937	86	(exact)
Crude	3.501529	1.024302	10.04068		(exact)
E. Standardized	3.979006	1.430689	11.06634		

Finally, if we wanted to weight the two age groups equally, we could type

```
. generate wgt=1
  cc case exposed [freq=pop], by(age) level(90) standard(wgt)
  Maternal age |        OR        [90% Conf. Interval]        Weight

           <35 |  3.394231     .7761116      11.5405              1 (exact)
           35+ |  5.733333     .1856098     61.20937              1 (exact)

         Crude |  3.501529     1.024302     10.04068                (exact)
  Standardized |  5.275104     .8787523     31.66617
```

◁

Matched case–control data

Matched case–control studies are performed to gain sample-size efficiency and to control for important confounding factors. In a matched case–control design, each case is matched with a control on the basis of demographic characteristics, clinical characteristics, etc. Thus their difference with respect to the outcome must be due to something other than the matching variables. If the only difference between them was exposure to the factor, we could attribute any difference in outcome to the factor.

A summary of the data is

Cases	Controls Exposed	Unexposed	Total
Exposed	a	b	$a + b$
Unexposed	c	d	$c + d$
Total	$a + c$	$b + d$	$n = a + b + c + d$

Each entry in the table represents the number of case–control pairs. For instance, in a of the pairs, both members were exposed; in b of the pairs, the case was exposed but the control was not; and so on. In total, n pairs were observed.

▷ Example 17: mcci

Rothman (1986, 257) discusses data from Jick et al. (1973) on a matched case–control study of myocardial infarction and drinking six or more cups of coffee per day (persons drinking from one to five cups per day were excluded):

Cases	Controls 6+ cups	0 cups
6+ cups	8	8
0 cups	3	8

mcci analyzes matched case–control data:

```
. mcci 8 8 3 8
                │   Controls
Cases           │ Exposed   Unexposed        Total
────────────────┼──────────────────────┼─────────────
       Exposed  │    8          8        │     16
     Unexposed  │    3          8        │     11
────────────────┼──────────────────────┼─────────────
         Total  │   11         16        │     27

McNemar's chi2(1) =      2.27    Prob > chi2 = 0.1317
Exact McNemar significance probability      = 0.2266

Proportion with factor
      Cases         .5925926
      Controls      .4074074     [95% Conf. Interval]
                   ──────────
      difference    .1851852    -.0822542    .4526246
      ratio        1.454545      .891101    2.374257
      rel. diff.    .3125       -.0243688    .6493688

      odds ratio   2.666667      .6400364   15.6064    (exact)
```

The relationship is not significant at better than the 13.17% level, but if we justify a one-sided test, the table is significant at the $13.17/2 = 6.59\%$ level. The point estimate is that drinkers of 6+ cups of coffee per day are 2.67 times more likely to suffer myocardial infarction. The interpretation of the relative difference is that, for every 100 controls who fail to have heart attacks, 31.25 might be expected to get heart attacks if they became heavy coffee drinkers.

◁

mcc works like the other nonimmediate commands but does not handle stratified data. If you have stratified matched case–control data, you can use conditional logistic regression to estimate odds ratios; see [R] **clogit**.

Matched case–control studies can also be analyzed using mhodds by controlling on the variable used to identify the matched sets. For example, if the variable set is used to identify the matched set for each subject,

```
. mhodds fail xvar set
```

will do the job. Any attempt to control for further variables will restrict the analysis to the comparison of cases and matched controls that share the same values of these variables. In general, this would lead to the omission of many records from the analysis. Similar considerations usually apply when investigating effect modification using the by() option. An important exception to this rule is that a variable used in matching cases to controls may appear in the by() option without loss of data.

▷ Example 18: mhodds with matched case–control data

Let us use mhodds to analyze matched case–control studies using the study of endometrial cancer and exposure to estrogen described in Breslow and Day (1980, chap. 5). In this study, there are four controls matched to each case. Cases and controls are matched on age, marital status, and time living in the community. The data collected include information on the daily dose of conjugated estrogen therapy. Breslow and Day created four levels of the dose variable and began by analyzing the 1:1 study formed by using the first control in each set. We examine the effect of exposure to estrogen:

```
. use http://www.stata-press.com/data/r10/bdendo11, clear

. describe

Contains data from http://www.stata-press.com/data/r10/bdendo11.dta
  obs:           126
  vars:           13                              3 Mar 2007 23:29
  size:         2,898 (99.9% of memory free)

              storage   display    value
variable name   type    format     label      variable label

set             int     %8.0g                  Set number
fail            byte    %8.0g                  Case=1/Control=0
gall            byte    %8.0g                  Gallbladder dis
hyp             byte    %8.0g                  Hypertension
ob              byte    %8.0g                  Obesity
est             byte    %8.0g                  Estrogen
dos             byte    %8.0g                  Ordinal dose
dur             byte    %8.0g                  Ordinal duration
non             byte    %8.0g                  Non-estrogen drug
duration        int     %8.0g                  months
age             int     %8.0g                  years
cest            byte    %8.0g                  Conjugated est dose
agegrp          float   %9.0g                  age group of set

Sorted by:  set

. mhodds fail est set

Mantel-Haenszel estimate of the odds ratio
Comparing est==1 vs. est==0, controlling for set

note: only 32 of the 63 strata formed in this analysis contribute
      information about the effect of the explanatory variable
```

Odds Ratio	chi2(1)	P>chi2	[95% Conf. Interval]	
9.666667	21.12	0.0000	2.944702	31.733072

For the 1:1 matched study, the Mantel–Haenszel methods are equivalent to conditional likelihood methods. The maximum conditional likelihood estimate of the odds ratio is given by the ratio of the off-diagonal frequencies in the two-way (case–control) table below. The data must be in the 1-observation-per-group format; that is, the matched case and control must appear in 1 observation (the sample format as required by the mcc command; see also [R] **clogit**).

```
. keep fail est set

. reshape wide est, i(set) j(fail)
(note: j = 0 1)

Data                                long    ->    wide

Number of obs.                       126    ->      63
Number of variables                    3    ->       3
j variable (2 values)               fail    ->    (dropped)
xij variables:
                                     est    ->    est0 est1

. rename est1 case

. rename est0 control

. label variable case case

. label variable control control
```

```
. tabulate case control
                  control
       case         0          1  |     Total
          0         4          3  |        7
          1        29         27  |       56
      Total        33         30  |       63
```

This is $29/3 = 9.67$, which agrees with the value obtained from mhodds and from mcci. In the more general $1:m$ matched study, however, the Mantel–Haenszel methods are no longer equal to the maximum conditional likelihood, although they are usually close.

To illustrate the use of the by() option in matched case–control studies, we look at the effect of exposure to estrogen, stratified by age3, which codes the sets into three age groups (55–64, 65–74, and 75+) as follows:

```
. use http://www.stata-press.com/data/r10/bdendo11, clear
. generate age3 = agegrp
. recode age3 1/2=1 3/4=2 5/6=3
(age3: 124 changes made)
. mhodds fail est set, by(age3)
Mantel-Haenszel estimate of the odds ratio
Comparing est==1 vs. est==0, controlling for set
by age3
note: only 32 of the 63 strata formed in this analysis contribute
      information about the effect of the explanatory variable
```

age3	Odds Ratio	chi2(1)	P>chi2	[95% Conf. Interval]	
1	6.000000	3.57	0.0588	0.72235	49.83724
2	15.000000	12.25	0.0005	1.98141	113.55557
3	8.000000	5.44	0.0196	1.00059	63.96252

Mantel-Haenszel estimate controlling for set and age3

Odds Ratio	chi2(1)	P>chi2	[95% Conf. Interval]	
9.666667	21.12	0.0000	2.944702	31.733072

```
Test of homogeneity of ORs (approx): chi2(2)  =     0.41
                                      Pr>chi2  =   0.8128
```

There is no further loss of information when we stratify by age3 because age was one of the matching variables.

The full set of matched controls can be used in the same way. For example, the effect of exposure to estrogen is obtained (using the full dataset) by

(Continued on next page)

```
. use http://www.stata-press.com/data/r10/bdendo, clear

. mhodds fail est set

Mantel-Haenszel estimate of the odds ratio
Comparing est==1 vs. est==0, controlling for set

note: only 58 of the 63 strata formed in this analysis contribute
      information about the effect of the explanatory variable
```

Odds Ratio	chi2(1)	P>chi2	[95% Conf. Interval]
8.461538	31.16	0.0000	3.437773 20.826746

The effect of exposure to estrogen, stratified by age3, is obtained by

```
. generate age3 = agegrp

. recode age3 1/2=1 3/4=2 5/6=3
(age3: 310 changes made)

. mhodds fail est set, by(age3)

Mantel-Haenszel estimate of the odds ratio
Comparing est==1 vs. est==0, controlling for set
by age3

note: only 58 of the 63 strata formed in this analysis contribute
      information about the effect of the explanatory variable
```

age3	Odds Ratio	chi2(1)	P>chi2	[95% Conf. Interval]
1	3.800000	3.38	0.0660	0.82165 17.57438
2	10.666667	18.69	0.0000	2.78773 40.81376
3	13.500000	9.77	0.0018	1.59832 114.02620

```
Mantel-Haenszel estimate controlling for set and age3
```

Odds Ratio	chi2(1)	P>chi2	[95% Conf. Interval]
8.461538	31.16	0.0000	3.437773 20.826746

```
Test of homogeneity of ORs (approx): chi2(2)  =    1.41
                                      Pr>chi2  =  0.4943
```

◁

Saved Results

ir and iri save the following in r():

Scalars

r(p)	one-sided p-value	r(afe)	attributable (prev.) fraction among exposed
r(ird)	incidence-rate difference	r(lb_afe)	lower bound of CI for afe
r(lb_ird)	lower bound of CI for ird	r(ub_afe)	upper bound of CI for afe
r(ub_ird)	upper bound of CI for ird	r(afp)	attributable fraction for the population
r(irr)	incidence-rate ratio	r(chi2_mh)	Mantel–Haenszel heterogeneity χ^2 (ir only)
r(lb_irr)	lower bound of CI for irr	r(chi2_p)	pooled heterogeneity χ^2 (pool only)
r(ub_irr)	upper bound of CI for irr	r(df)	degrees of freedom (ir only)

cs and csi save the following in r():

Scalars

r(p)	two-sided p-value	r(ub_or)	upper bound of CI for or
r(rd)	risk difference	r(afe)	attributable (prev.) fraction among exposed
r(lb_rd)	lower bound of CI for rd	r(lb_afe)	lower bound of CI for afe
r(ub_rd)	upper bound of CI for rd	r(ub_afe)	upper bound of CI for afe
r(rr)	risk ratio	r(afp)	attributable fraction for the population
r(lb_rr)	lower bound of CI for rr	r(chi2_mh)	Mantel–Haenszel heterogeneity χ^2 (cs only)
r(ub_rr)	upper bound of CI for rr	r(chi2_p)	pooled heterogeneity χ^2 (pool only)
r(or)	odds ratio	r(df)	degrees of freedom
r(lb_or)	lower bound of CI for or	r(chi2)	χ^2

cc and cci save the following in r():

Scalars

r(p)	two-sided p-value	r(ub_afe)	upper bound of CI for afe
r(p1_exact)	χ^2 or one-sided exact significance	r(afp)	attributable fraction for the population
r(p_exact)	two-sided significance (χ^2 or exact)	r(chi2_p)	pooled heterogeneity χ^2
		r(chi2_bd)	Breslow–Day χ^2
r(or)	odds ratio	r(df_bd)	degrees of freedom for Breslow–Day χ^2
r(lb_or)	lower bound of CI for or	r(chi2_t)	Tarone χ^2
r(ub_or)	upper bound of CI for or	r(df_t)	degrees of freedom for Tarone χ^2
r(afe)	attributable (prev.) fraction among exposed	r(df)	degrees of freedom
r(lb_afe)	lower bound of CI for afe	r(chi2)	χ^2

tabodds saves the following in r():

Scalars

r(odds)	odds	r(p_hom)	p-value for test of homogeneity
r(lb_odds)	lower bound for odds	r(df_hom)	degrees of freedom for χ^2 test of homogeneity
r(ub_odds)	upper bound for odds	r(chi2_tr)	χ^2 for score test for trend
r(chi2_hom)	χ^2 test of homogeneity	r(p_trend)	p-value for score test for trend

mhodds saves the following in r():

Scalars

r(p)	two-sided p-value	r(chi2_hom)	χ^2 test of homogeneity
r(or)	odds ratio	r(df_hom)	degrees of freedom for χ^2 test of homogeneity
r(lb_or)	lower bound of CI for or	r(chi2)	χ^2
r(ub_or)	upper bound of CI for or		

mcc and mcci save the following in r():

Scalars

r(p_exact)	two-sided significance (χ^2 or exact)	r(R_f)	ratio of proportion with factor
		r(lb_R_f)	lower bound of CI for R_f
r(or)	odds ratio	r(ub_R_f)	upper bound of CI for R_f
r(lb_or)	lower bound of CI for or	r(RD_f)	relative difference in proportion with factor
r(ub_or)	upper bound of CI for or		
r(D_f)	difference in proportion with factor	r(lb_RD_f)	lower bound of CI for RD_f
r(lb_D_f)	lower bound of CI for D_f	r(ub_RD_f)	upper bound of CI for RD_f
r(ub_D_f)	upper bound of CI for D_f	r(chi2)	χ^2

Methods and Formulas

All the epitab commands are implemented as ado-files.

The notation for incidence-rate data is

	Exposed	Unexposed	Total
Cases	a	b	M_1
Person-time	N_1	N_0	T

The notation for $2 \times k$ tables is

	\multicolumn{4}{c}{Exposure level}
	1	2	...	k	Total
Cases	a_1	a_2	...	a_k	M_1
Controls	c_1	c_2	...	c_k	M_0
Total	N_1	N_2	...	N_k	T

If tables are stratified, all quantities are indexed by i, the stratum number.

We will refer to Fleiss, Levin, and Paik (2003); Kleinbaum, Kupper, and Morgenstern (1982); and Rothman (1986) so often that we will adopt the notation F-23 to mean Fleiss, Levin, and Paik (2003) page 23, KKM-52 to mean Kleinbaum, Kupper, and Morgenstern (1982) page 52, and R-164 to mean Rothman (1986) page 164.

We have always avoided making the continuity corrections to χ^2 statistics, following the advice of KKM-292: "... the use of a continuity correction has been the subject of considerable debate in the statistical literature .... On the basis of our evaluation of this debate and other evidence, we do *not* recommend the use of the continuity correction." Breslow and Day (1980, 133), on the other hand, argue for inclusion of the correction, but not strongly. Their summary is that for small datasets, one should use exact statistics. In practice, we believe that the adjustment makes little difference for reasonably sized datasets.

Unstratified incidence-rate data

The incidence-rate difference is defined as $I_d = a/N_1 - b/N_0$ (R-164). The standard error of the incidence rate is $s_{I_d} \approx \sqrt{a/N_1^2 + b/N_0^2}$ (R-170), from which confidence intervals are calculated. For test-based confidence intervals, define

$$\chi = \frac{a - N_1 M_1/T}{\sqrt{M_1 N_1 N_0/T^2}}$$

(R-155). Test-based confidence intervals are $I_d(1 \pm z/\chi)$ (R-171), where z is obtained from the normal distribution.

The incidence-rate ratio is defined as $I_r = (a/N_1)/(b/N_0)$ (R-164). Let p_l and p_h be the exact confidence interval of the binomial probability for observing a successes of M_1 trials (obtained from cii, see [R] ci). The exact confidence interval for the incidence ratio is then $(p_l N_0)/\{(1 - p_l)N_1\}$ to $(p_u N_0)/\{(1 - p_u)N_1\}$ (R-166). Test-based confidence intervals are $I_r^{1 \pm z/\chi}$ (R-172).

The attributable fraction among the exposed is defined as AFE $= (I_r - 1)/I_r$ for $I_r \geq 1$ (KKM-164, R-38); the confidence interval is obtained by similarly transforming the interval values of I_r. The attributable fraction for the population is AF $=$ AFE $\cdot a/M_1$ (KKM-161); no confidence interval is reported. For $I_r < 1$, the prevented fraction among exposed is defined as PFE $= 1 - I_r$ (KKM-166, R-39); the confidence interval is obtained by similarly transforming the interval values of I_r. The prevented fraction for the population is PF $=$ PFE $\cdot N_1/T$ (KKM-165); no confidence interval is reported.

The "midp" one-sided exact significance (R-155) is calculated as the binomial probability (with $n = M_1$ and $p = N_1/T$) $\Pr(k = a)/2 + \Pr(k > a)$ if $I_r >= 1$ and $\Pr(k = a)/2 + \Pr(k < a)$, otherwise. The two-sided significance is twice the one-sided significance (R-155). If preferred, you can obtain nonmidp exact probabilities (and, to some ways of thinking, a more reasonable definition of two-sided significance) using `bitest`; see [R] **bitest**.

Unstratified cumulative incidence data

The risk difference is defined as $R_d = a/N_1 - b/N_0$ (R-164). Its standard error is

$$s_{R_d} \approx \left\{ \frac{a(N_1 - a)}{N_1^3} + \frac{b(N_0 - b)}{N_0^3} \right\}^{1/2}$$

(R-172), from which confidence intervals are calculated. For test-based confidence intervals, define

$$\chi = \frac{a - N_1 M_1/T}{\sqrt{(M_1 M_0 N_1 N_0)/\{T^2(T - 1)\}}}$$

(R-163). Test-based confidence intervals are $R_d(1 \pm z/\chi)$ (R-172).

The risk ratio is defined as $R_r = (a/N_1)/(b/N_0)$ (R-165). The standard error of $\ln R_r$ is

$$s_{\ln R_r} \approx \left(\frac{c}{aN_1} + \frac{d}{bN_0} \right)^{1/2}$$

(R-173), from which confidence intervals are calculated. Test-based confidence intervals are $R_r^{1 \pm z/\chi}$ (R-173).

For $R_r \geq 1$, the attributable fraction among the exposed is calculated as AFE $= (R_r - 1)/R_r$ (KKM-164, R-38); the confidence interval is obtained by similarly transforming the interval values for R_r. The attributable fraction for the population is calculated as AF $=$ AFE $\cdot a/M_1$ (KKM-161); no confidence interval is reported, but F-128 provides

$$\left\{ \frac{c + (a + d)\text{AFE}}{bT} \right\}^{1/2}$$

as the approximate standard error of $\ln(1 - \text{AF})$.

For $R_r < 1$, the prevented fraction among the exposed is calculated as PFE $= 1 - R_r$ (KKM-166, R-39); the confidence interval is obtained by similarly transforming the interval values for R_r. The prevented fraction for the population is calculated as PF $=$ PFE $\cdot N_1/T$; no confidence interval is reported.

The odds ratio is defined $\psi = (ad)/(bc)$ (R-165). The Woolf estimate (Woolf 1955) of the standard error of $\ln\psi$ is

$$s_{\ln\psi} = \left(\frac{1}{a} + \frac{1}{b} + \frac{1}{c} + \frac{1}{d} \right)^{1/2}$$

(R-173; Schlesselman 1982, 176), from which confidence intervals are calculated. Test-based confidence intervals are $\psi^{1 \pm z/\chi}$ (R-174). Alternatively, the Cornfield (1956) calculation is

$$\psi_l = a_l(M_0 - N_1 + a_l)\Big/\big\{(N_1 - a_l)(M_1 - a_l)\big\}$$

$$\psi_u = a_u(M_0 - N_1 + a_u)\Big/\big\{(N_1 - a_u)(M_1 - a_u)\big\}$$

where a_u and a_l are determined iteratively from

$$a_{i+1} = a \pm z_\alpha \left(\frac{1}{a_i} + \frac{1}{N_1 - a_i} + \frac{1}{M_1 - a_i} + \frac{1}{M_0 - N_1 + a_i}\right)^{-1/2}$$

where z_α is the index from the normal distribution for an α significance level (Schlesselman 1982, 177, but without the continuity correction). a_{i+1} converges to a_u using the plus signs and a_l using the minus signs. a_0 is taken as a. With small numbers, the iterative technique may fail. It is then restarted by decrementing (a_l) or incrementing (a_u) a_0. If that fails, a_0 is again decremented or incremented and iterations restarted, and so on, until a terminal condition is met ($a_0 < 0$ or $a_0 > M_1$), at which point the value is not calculated.

The χ^2 is defined

$$\chi^2 = \sum_{i=1}^{2} \sum_{j=1}^{2} \frac{(p_{ij} - p_{i\cdot}p_{\cdot j})^2}{p_{i\cdot}p_{\cdot j}}$$

(F-53, but without the continuity correction) where $p_{11} = a/T$, $p_{12} = b/T$, etc.

Fisher's exact p is calculated as described in [R] **tabulate twoway**.

Unstratified case–control data

Calculation of the odds ratio ψ and χ^2 is as described for unstratified cumulative incidence data. The other calculations described there are inappropriate.

The odds ratio ψ is used as an estimate of the risk ratio in calculating attributable or prevented fractions. For $\psi \geq 1$, the attributable fraction among the exposed is calculated as $\text{AFE} = (\psi - 1)/\psi$ (KKM-164); the confidence interval is obtained by similarly transforming the interval values for ψ. The attributable fraction for the population is calculated as $\text{AF} = \text{AFE} \cdot a/M_1$ (KKM-161). No confidence interval is reported; however, F-152 provides

$$\left(\frac{a}{M_1 b} + \frac{c}{M_0 d}\right)^{1/2}$$

as the standard error of $\ln(1 - \text{AF})$.

For $\psi < 1$, the prevented fraction among the exposed is calculated as $\text{PFE} = 1 - \psi$ (KKM-166); the confidence interval is obtained by similarly transforming the interval values for ψ. The prevented fraction for the population is calculated as $\text{PF} = \{(a/M_1)\text{PFE}\}/\{(a/M_1)\text{PFE} + \psi\}$ (KKM-164); no confidence interval is reported.

Unstratified matched case–control data

The columns of the 2×2 table indicate controls; the rows are cases. Each entry in the table reflects a pair of a matched case and a control.

McNemar's χ^2 (McNemar 1947) is defined as

$$\chi^2 = \frac{(b-c)^2}{b+c}$$

(R-259).

The proportion of controls with the factor is $p_1 = N_1/T$, and the proportion of cases with the factor is $p_2 = M_1/T$.

The difference in the proportions is $P_d = p_2 - p_1$. An estimate of its standard error when the two underlying proportions are *not* hypothesized to be equal is

$$s_{P_d} \approx \frac{\{(a+d)(b+c) + 4bc\}^{1/2}}{T^{3/2}}$$

(F-378), from which confidence intervals are calculated.

The ratio of the proportions is $P_r = p_2/p_1$ (R-276, R-278). The standard error of $\ln P_r$ is

$$s_{\ln P_r} \approx \left(\frac{b+c}{M_1 N_1}\right)^{1/2}$$

(R-276), from which confidence intervals are calculated.

The relative difference in the proportions $P_e = (b-c)/(b+d)$ (F-379) is a measure of the relative value of the factor assuming that the factor can affect only those patients who are unexposed controls. Its standard error is

$$s_{P_e} \approx (b+d)^{-2} \{(b+c+d)(bc + bd + cd) - bcd\}^{-1/2}$$

(F-379), from which confidence intervals are calculated.

The odds ratio is $\psi = b/c$ (F-376), and the exact Fisher confidence interval is obtained by transforming into odds ratios the exact binomial confidence interval for the binomial parameter from observing b successes in $b+c$ trials (R-264). Binomial confidence limits are obtained from cii (see [R] ci) and are transformed by $p/(1-p)$. Test-based confidence intervals are $\psi^{1 \pm z/\chi}$ (R-267), where χ is the square root of McNemar's χ^2, $(b-c)/\sqrt{b+c}$.

Stratified incidence-rate data

Statistics presented for each stratum are calculated independently according to the formulas in *Unstratified incidence-rate data* above. Within strata, the Mantel–Haenszel style weight is $W_i = b_i N_{1i}/T_i$, and the combined incidence-rate ratio (Rothman and Boice 1982) is

$$I_{\mathrm{mh}} = \frac{\sum_i a_i N_{0i}/T_i}{\sum_i W_i}$$

(R-196). The standard error is obtained by considering each a_i to be an independent binomial variate conditional on N_{1i} (Greenland and Robins 1985)

$$s_{\ln I_{\mathrm{mh}}} \approx \left\{ \frac{\sum_i M_{1i} N_{1i} N_{0i}/T_i^2}{\left(\sum_i a_i N_{0i}/T_i\right)\left(\sum_i b_i N_{1i}/T_i\right)} \right\}^{1/2}$$

(R-213), from which confidence intervals are calculated.

For standardized rates, let w_i be the user-specified weight within category i. The standardized rate difference and rate ratio are defined as

$$\text{SRD} = \frac{\sum_i w_i(R_{1i} - R_{0i})}{\sum_i w_i}$$

$$\text{SRR} = \frac{\sum_i w_i R_{1i}}{\sum_i w_i R_{0i}}$$

(R-229). The standard error of SRD is

$$s_{\text{SRD}} \approx \left\{ \frac{1}{(\sum_i w_i)^2} \sum_i w_i^2 \left(\frac{a_i}{N_{1i}^2} + \frac{b_i}{N_{0i}^2} \right) \right\}^{1/2}$$

(R-231), from which confidence intervals are calculated. The standard error of $\ln(\text{SRR})$ is

$$s_{\ln(\text{SRR})} \approx \left\{ \frac{\sum_i w_i^2 a_i / N_{1i}^2}{(\sum_i w_i R_{1i})^2} + \frac{\sum_i w_i^2 b_i / N_{0i}^2}{(\sum_i w_i R_{0i})^2} \right\}^{1/2}$$

(R-231), from which confidence intervals are calculated.

Internally and externally standardized measures are calculated using $w_i = N_{1i}$ and $w_i = N_{0i}$, respectively.

For directly pooled estimates of risk differences and risk ratios, stratum-specific point estimates and variances are calculated as given in *Unstratified incidence-rate data*. (For the risk ratio, this calculation is performed in the logs.) Inverse variance weights $w_i = 1/s^2$ are then used to sum the stratum-specific values (which are then exponentiated for the risk ratio). The overall variance of the pooled estimate is calculated as $1/\sum w_i$, from which confidence intervals are calculated (R-183–188).

For risk differences, the χ^2 test of homogeneity is calculated as $\sum (R_{di} - \widehat{R}_d)^2 / \text{var}(R_{di})$, where R_{di} are the stratum-specific rate differences and $\widehat{R}_d$ is the pooled estimate (Mantel–Haenszel or directly pooled). The number of degrees of freedom is one less than the number of strata (R-222).

For risk ratios, the same calculation is made, except that it is made on a logarithmic scale using $\ln(R_{ri})$ (R-222).

Stratified cumulative incidence data

Statistics presented for each stratum are calculated independently according to the formulas in *Unstratified cumulative incidence data* above. The Mantel–Haenszel χ^2 test (Mantel and Haenszel 1959) is

$$\chi^2_{\text{mh}} = \frac{\left(|\sum_i a_i - N_{1i} M_{1i} / T_i| \right)^2}{\sum_i (N_{1i} N_{0i} M_{1i} M_{0i}) / \{T_i^2 (T_i - 1)\}}$$

(R-206).

For the odds ratio, the Mantel–Haenszel weight is $W_i = b_i c_i / T_i$, and the combined odds ratio (Mantel and Haenszel 1959) is

$$\psi_{\text{mh}} = \frac{\sum_i a_i d_i / T_i}{\sum_i W_i}$$

(R-195). The standard error (Robins, Breslow, and Greenland 1986) is

$$s_{\ln\psi_{\mathrm{mh}}} \approx \left\{ \frac{\sum_i P_i R_i}{2\left(\sum_i R_i\right)^2} + \frac{\sum_i P_i S_i + Q_i R_i}{2\sum_i R_i \sum_i S_i} + \frac{\sum_i Q_i S_i}{2\left(\sum_i S_i\right)^2} \right\}^{1/2}$$

where

$$P_i = (a_i + d_i)/T_i$$
$$Q_i = (b_i + c_i)/T_i$$
$$R_i = a_i d_i/T_i$$
$$S_i = b_i c_i/T_i$$

(R-220). Alternatively, test-based confidence intervals are calculated as $\psi_{\mathrm{mh}}^{1 \pm z/\chi}$ (R-220).

For the risk ratio, the Mantel–Haenszel style weight is $W_i = b_i N_{1i}/T_i$, and the combined risk ratio (Rothman and Boice 1982) is

$$R_{\mathrm{mh}} = \frac{\sum_i a_i N_{0i}/T_i}{\sum_i W_i}$$

(R-196). The standard error (Greenland and Robins 1985) is

$$s_{\ln R_{\mathrm{mh}}} \approx \frac{\sum_i (M_{1i} N_{1i} N_{0i} - a_i b_i T_i)/T_i^2}{\left(\sum_i a_i N_{0i}/T_i\right)\left(\sum_i b_i N_{1i}/T_i\right)}$$

(R-216), from which confidence intervals are calculated.

For standardized rates, let w_i be the user-specified weight within category. The standardized rate difference (SRD) and rate ratios (SRR) are defined as in *Stratified incidence-rate data*, where the individual risks are defined $R_{1i} = a_i/N_{1i}$ and $R_{0i} = b_i/N_{0i}$. The standard error of SRD is

$$s_{\mathrm{SRD}} \approx \left[\frac{1}{\left(\sum_i w_i\right)^2} \sum_i w_i^2 \left\{ \frac{a_i(N_{1i} - a_i)}{N_{1i}^3} + \frac{b_i(N_{0i} - b_i)}{N_{0i}^3} \right\} \right]^{1/2}$$

(R-231), from which confidence intervals are calculated. The standard error of ln(SRR) is

$$s_{\ln(\mathrm{SRR})} \approx \left\{ \frac{\sum_i w_i^2 a_i(N_{1i} - a_i)/N_{1i}^3}{\left(\sum_i w_i R_{1i}\right)^2} + \frac{\sum_i w_i^2 b_i(N_{0i} - b_i)/N_{0i}^3}{\left(\sum_i w_i R_{0i}\right)^2} \right\}^{1/2}$$

(R-231), from which confidence intervals are calculated.

Internally and externally standardized measures are calculated using $w_i = N_{1i}$ and $w_i = N_{0i}$, respectively.

For directly pooled estimates of the odds ratio, stratum-specific odds ratios are summed with stratum-specific inverse variance weights with the calculation performed in the logs and the point estimate and variances being as given in *Unstratified cumulative incidence data*. The overall variance of the pooled estimate is calculated as the sum of the inverse weights, from which confidence intervals are calculated (R-189–190).

For pooled estimates of risk differences and risk ratios, stratum-specific point estimates and variances are calculated as given in *Unstratified cumulative incidence data*. (For the risk ratio, this calculation is performed in the logs.) Inverse variance weights $w_i = 1/s^2$ are then used to sum the stratum-specific values (which are then exponentiated for the risk ratio). The overall variance of the pooled estimate is calculated as $1/\sum w_i$, from which confidence intervals are calculated (R-183–188).

For risk differences, the χ^2 test of homogeneity is calculated as $\sum (R_{di} - \widehat{R}_d)^2 / \mathrm{var}(R_{di})$, where R_{di} are the stratum-specific rate differences and $\widehat{R}_d$ is the pooled estimate (Mantel–Haenszel or directly pooled). The number of degrees of freedom is one less than the number of strata (R-222).

For risk and odds ratios, the same calculation is made, except that it is made in the logs using $\ln(R_{ri})$ or $\ln(\psi_i)$ (R-222).

Stratified case–control data

Statistics presented for each stratum are calculated independently according to the formulas in *Unstratified cumulative incidence data* above. The combined odds ratio ψ_{mh} and the test that $\psi_{\mathrm{mh}} = 1$ (χ^2_{mh}) are calculated as described in *Stratified cumulative incidence data* above.

For standardized weights, let w_i be the user-specified weight within category. The standardized odds ratio is calculated as

$$\mathrm{SOR} = \frac{\sum_i w_i a_i / c_i}{\sum_i w_i b_i / d_i}$$

(Greenland 1987a). The standard error of $\ln(\mathrm{SOR})$ is

$$s_{\ln(\mathrm{SOR})} = \frac{\sum_i (w_j a_j / c_j)^2 (\frac{1}{a_i} + \frac{1}{b_i} + \frac{1}{c_i} + \frac{1}{d_i})}{\left(\sum_i w_i a_i / c_i \right)^2}$$

(Greenland 1987a), from which confidence intervals are calculated. The internally and externally standardized odds ratios are calculated using $w_i = c_i$ and $w_i = d_i$, respectively.

The directly pooled estimate of the odds ratio is calculated as described in *Stratified cumulative incidence data* above.

The direct and Mantel–Haenszel χ^2 tests of homogeneity are calculated as $\sum \left\{ \ln(R_{ri}) - \ln(\widehat{R}_r) \right\}^2 / \mathrm{var}\{\ln(R_{ri})\}$, where R_{ri} are the stratum-specific odds ratios and $\widehat{R}_r$ is the pooled estimate (Mantel–Haenszel or directly pooled). The number of degrees of freedom is one less than the number of strata (R-222).

The Breslow–Day χ^2 test of homogeneity is calculated as the sum over all strata of the stratum-specific squared deviations of the observed and fitted values on the basis of the overall odds ratio, divided by the variance of the fitted values:

$$\sum_i \frac{\{a_i - A_i(\widehat{\psi})\}^2}{\mathrm{Var}(a_i; \widehat{\psi})}$$

where $A_i(\widehat{\psi})$ is the fitted count for cell a determined as the root of the quadratic equation

$$A(M_0 - N_1 + A) = (\widehat{\psi})(M_1 - A)(N_1 - A)$$

which makes all cell values of the 2×2 table for the ith stratum positive; $\mathrm{Var}(a_i; \widehat{\psi})$ is the variance of the fitted table for the ith stratum; and $\widehat{\psi}$ is the Mantel–Haenszel estimate of the common odds ratio.

The Tarone χ^2 test of homogeneity is calculated as

$$\sum_i \frac{\{a_i - A_i(\widehat{\psi})\}^2}{\mathrm{Var}(a_i; \widehat{\psi})} - \frac{\{\sum_i a_i - \sum_i A_i(\widehat{\psi})\}^2}{\sum_i \mathrm{Var}(a_i; \widehat{\psi})}$$

Tarone (1985) provides this correction to the Breslow–Day statistic to ensure that its distribution is asymptotically chi-squared. Without the correction, the Breslow–Day statistic does not necessarily follow a chi-squared distribution because it is based on the Mantel–Haenszel estimate, $\widehat{\psi}$, which is an inefficient estimator of the common odds ratio.

When the exposure variable has multiple levels, `mhodds` calculates an approximate estimate of the rate ratio for a one-unit increase in exposure as the ratio of the score statistic, U, to its variance, V (Clayton and Hills 1993, 103), which are defined below. This is a one-step Newton-Raphson approximation to the maximum likelihood estimate.

By default, both `tabodds` and `mhodds` produce test statistics and confidence intervals based on score statistics (Clayton and Hills, 1993). Using the notation for $2 \times k$ tables, we find that the confidence interval for the odds of the ith exposure level, $odds_i$, $i = 1, \ldots, k$, is given by

$$odds_i \cdot \exp\left(\pm z \sqrt{1/a_i + 1/c_i}\right)$$

The score χ^2 test of homogeneity of odds is calculated as

$$\chi^2_{k-1} = \frac{T(T-1)}{M_1 M_0} \sum_{i=1}^{k} \frac{(a_i - E_i)^2}{N_i}$$

where $E_i = (M_1 N_i)/T$.

Let l_i denote the value of the exposure at the ith level. The score χ^2 test for trend of odds is calculated as

$$\chi^2_1 = \frac{U^2}{V}$$

where

$$U = \frac{M_1 M_0}{T} \left(\sum_{i=1}^{k} \frac{a_i l_i}{M_1} - \sum_{i=1}^{k} \frac{c_i l_i}{M_0} \right)$$

and

$$V = \frac{M_1 M_0}{T} \left\{ \frac{\sum_{i=1}^{k} N_i l_i^2 - (\sum_{i=1}^{k} N_i l_i)^2 / T}{T - 1} \right\}$$

Acknowledgments

We thank Hal Morgenstern, Department of Epidemiology, University of Michigan; Ardythe Morrow, Center for Pediatric Research, Norfolk, Virginia; and the late Stewart West, Baylor College of Medicine, for their assistance in designing these commands. We also thank Jonathan Freeman, Department of Epidemiology, Harvard School of Public Health, for encouraging us to extend these commands to include tests for homogeneity, for helpful comments on the default behavior of the commands, and for his comments on an early draft of this section. We also thank David Clayton, Cambridge Institute for Medical Research, and Michael Hills, London School of Hygiene and Tropical Medicine (retired); they wrote the original versions of `mhodds` and `tabodds`. Finally, we thank William Dupont and Dale Plummer for their contribution to the implementation of exact confidence intervals for the odds ratios for `cc` and `cci`.

Jerome Cornfield (1912–1979) was born in New York City. He majored in history at New York University and took courses in statistics at the U.S. Department of Agriculture Graduate School but otherwise had little formal training. Cornfield held positions at the Bureau of Labor Statistics, the National Cancer Institute, the National Institutes of Health, Johns Hopkins University, the University of Pittsburgh, and George Washington University. He worked on many problems in biomedical statistics, including the analysis of clinical trials, epidemiology (especially case–control studies), and Bayesian approaches.

Quinn McNemar (1900–1986) was born in West Virginia and attended college there and in Pennsylvania. After a brief spell of high school teaching, he began graduate study of psychology at Stanford and then joined the faculty. McNemar's text *Psychological statistics*, first published in 1949, was widely influential, and he made many substantive and methodological contributions to the application of statistics in psychology.

Barnet Woolf (1902–1983) was born in London. His parents were immigrants from Lithuania. Woolf was educated at Cambridge, where he studied physiology and biochemistry, and proposed methods for linearizing plots in enzyme chemistry that were later rediscovered by others (Haldane 1957). His later career in London, Birmingham, Rothamsted, and Edinburgh included lasting contributions to nutrition, epidemiology, public health, genetics, and statistics. He was also active in left-wing causes and wrote witty poems, songs, and revues.

References

Abramson, J. H., and Z. H. Abramson. 2001. *Making Sense of Data: A Self-Instruction Manual on the Interpretation of Epidemiological Data*. 3rd ed. New York: Oxford University Press.

Boice, J. D., and R. R. Monson. 1977. Breast cancer in women after repeated fluoroscopic examinations of the chest. *Journal of the National Cancer Institute* 59: 823–832.

Breslow, N. E. 1996. Statistics in Epidemiology: The Case-Control Study. *Journal of the American Statistical Association* 91: 14–28.

Breslow, N. E., and N. E. Day. 1980. *Statistical Methods in Cancer Research: The Analysis of Case–Control Studies, Vol. 1*. Lyon: IARC.

Carlin, J., and S. Vidmar. 2000. sbe35: Menus for epidemiological statistics. *Stata Technical Bulletin* 56: 15–16. Reprinted in *Stata Technical Bulletin Reprints*, vol. 10, pp. 86–87.

Clayton, D. G., and M. Hills. 1993. *Statistical Models in Epidemiology*. Oxford: Oxford University Press.

——. 1995. ssa8: Analysis of case–control and prevalence studies. *Stata Technical Bulletin* 27: 26–31. Reprinted in *Stata Technical Bulletin Reprints*, vol. 5, pp. 227–233.

Cornfield, J. 1956. A statistical problem arising from retrospective studies. In *Proceedings of the Third Berkeley Symposium*, vol. 4, ed. J. Neyman, 135–148. Berkeley, CA: University of California Press.

Dohoo, I., W. Martin, and H. Stryhn. 2003. *Veterinary Epidemiologic Research*. Charlottetown, Prince Edward Island: AVC.

Doll, R., and A. B. Hill. 1966. Mortality of British doctors in relation to smoking: Observations on coronary thrombosis. In *Epidemiological Approaches to the Study of Cancer and Other Chronic Diseases*, ed. W. Haenszel, *National Cancer Institute Monograph* 19: 205–268.

Dupont, W. D. 2002. *Statistical Modeling for Biomedical Researchers: A Simple Introduction to the Analysis of Complex Data*. Cambridge: Cambridge University Press.

Dupont, W. D., and D. Plummer. 1999. sbe31: Exact confidence intervals for odds ratios from case–control studies. *Stata Technical Bulletin* 52: 12–16. Reprinted in *Stata Technical Bulletin Reprints*, vol. 9, pp. 150–154.

Fleiss, J. L., B. Levin, and M. C. Paik. 2003. *Statistical Methods for Rates and Proportions*. 3rd ed. New York: Wiley.

Gini, R., and J. Pasquini. 2006. Automatic generation of documents. *Stata Journal* 6: 22–39.

Glass, R. I., A. M. Svennerholm, B. J. Stoll, M. R. Khan, K. M. B. Hossain, M. I. Huq, and J. Holmgren. 1983. Protection against cholera in breast-fed children by antibodies in breast milk. *New England Journal of Medicine* 308: 1389–1392.

Gleason, J. R. 1999. sbe30: Improved confidence intervals for odds ratios. *Stata Technical Bulletin* 51: 24–27. Reprinted in *Stata Technical Bulletin Reprints*, vol. 9, pp. 146–150.

Greenhouse, S. W., and J. B. Greenhouse. 1998. Cornfield, Jerome. In *Encyclopedia of Biostatistics*, vol. 1, ed. P. Armitage and T. Colton, 955–959. Chichester, UK: Wiley.

Greenland, S. 1987a. Interpretation and choice of effect measures in epidemiologic analysis. *American Journal of Epidemiology* 125: 761–768.

——. ed. 1987b. *Evolution of Epidemiologic Ideas: Annotated Readings on Concepts and Methods.* Newton Lower Falls, MA: Epidemiology Resources.

Greenland, S., and J. M. Robins. 1985. Estimation of a common effect parameter from sparse follow-up data. *Biometrics* 41: 55–68.

——. 1988. Conceptual problems in the definition and interpretation of attributable fractions. *American Journal of Epidemiology* 128: 1185–1197.

Haldane, J. B. S. 1957. Graphical methods in enzyme chemistry. *Nature* 179: 832.

Hastorf, A. H., E. R. Hilgard, and R. R. Sears. 1988. Quinn McNemar (1900–1986). *American Psychologist* 43: 196–197.

Hill, W. G. 1984. Barnet Woolf. *Year Book, Royal Society of Edinburgh 1984* 214–219.

Jewell, N. P. 2004. *Statistics for Epidemiology.* Boca Raton, FL: Chapman & Hall/CRC.

Jick, H., O. S. Miettinen, R. K. Neff, S. Shapiro, O. P. Heinonen, and D. Slone. 1973. Coffee and myocardial infarction. *New England Journal of Medicine* 289: 63–67.

Kleinbaum, D. G. 2004. *ActivEpi Multimedia CD.* New York: Springer.

Kleinbaum, D. G., L. L. Kupper, and H. Morgenstern. 1982. *Epidemiologic Research: Principles and Quantitative Methods (Industrial Health and Safety).* New York: Wiley.

Lilienfeld, D. E., and P. D. Stolley. 1994. *Foundations of Epidemiology.* 3rd ed. New York: Oxford University Press.

López-Vizcaíno, M. E., S. Pérez-Hoyos, and L. Abraira-García. 2000a. sbe32: Automated outbreak detection from public health surveillance data. *Stata Technical Bulletin* 54: 23–25. Reprinted in *Stata Technical Bulletin Reprints*, vol. 9, pp. 154–157.

——. 2000b. sbe32.1: Automated outbreak detection from public health surveillance data: Errata. *Stata Technical Bulletin* 55: 2.

MacMahon, B., S. Yen, D. Trichopoulos, K. Warren, and G. Nardi. 1981. Coffee and cancer of the pancreas. *New England Journal of Medicine* 11: 630–633.

Mantel, N., and W. Haenszel. 1959. Statistical aspects of the analysis of data from retrospective studies of disease. *Journal of the National Cancer Institute* 22: 719–748. Reprinted in *Evolution of Epidemiologic Ideas*, ed. S. Greenland, 112–141. Newton Lower Falls, MA: Epidemiology Resources.

McNemar, Q. 1947. Note on the sampling error of the difference between correlated proportions or percentages. *Psychometrika* 12: 153–157.

Miettinen, O. S. 1976. Estimability and estimation in case-referent studies. *American Journal of Epidemiology* 103: 226–235. Reprinted in *Evolution of Epidemiologic Ideas*, ed. S. Greenland, 181–190. Newton Lower Falls, MA: Epidemiology Resources.

Pearce, M. S., and R. Feltbower. 2000. sg149: Tests for seasonal data via the Edwards and Walter & Elwood tests. *Stata Technical Bulletin* 56: 47–49. Reprinted in *Stata Technical Bulletin Reprints*, vol. 10, pp. 214–217.

Reilly, M., and A. Salim. 2000. sxd2: Computing optimal sampling designs for two-stage studies. *Stata Technical Bulletin* 58: 37–41. Reprinted in *Stata Technical Bulletin Reprints*, vol. 10, pp. 376–382.

Robins, J. M., N. E. Breslow, and S. Greenland. 1986. Estimators of the Mantel–Haenszel variance consistent in both sparse data and large-strata limiting models. *Biometrics* 42: 311–323.

Rothman, K. J. 1982. Spermicide use and Down's syndrome. *American Journal of Public Health* 72: 399–401.

——. 1986. *Modern Epidemiology.* Boston: Little, Brown.

——. 2002. *Epidemiology: An Introduction.* New York: Oxford University Press.

Rothman, K. J., and J. D. Boice. 1982. *Epidemiologic Analysis with a Programmable Calculator*. Brookline, MA: Epidemiology Resources. (First edition published June 1979 by U.S. Government Printing Office, Washington D.C., NIH Publication No. 79-1649.)

Rothman, K. J., D. C. Fyler, A. Goldblatt, and M. B. Kreidberg. 1979. Exogenous hormones and other drug exposures of children with congenital heart disease. *American Journal of Epidemiology* 109: 433–439.

Rothman, K. J., and S. Greenland. 1998. *Modern Epidemiology*. 2nd ed. Philadelphia: Lippincott–Raven.

Rothman, K. J., and R. R. Monson. 1973. Survival in trigeminal neuralgia. *Journal of Chronic Diseases* 26: 303–309.

Royston, P., and A. Babiker. 2002. A menu-driven facility for complex sample size calculation in randomized controlled trials with a survival or a binary outcome. *Stata Journal* 2: 151–163.

Schlesselman, J. J. 1982. *Case–Control Studies: Design, Conduct, Analysis*. New York: Oxford University Press.

Tarone, R. E. 1985. On heterogeneity tests based on efficient scores. *Biometrika* 72: 91–95.

University Group Diabetes Program. 1970. A study of the effects of hypoglycemic agents on vascular complications in patients with adult onset diabetes. *Diabetes* 19, supplement 2: 747–830.

van Belle, G., L. D. Fisher, P. J. Heagerty, and T. Lumley. 2004. *Biostatistics: A Methodology for the Health Sciences*. 2nd ed. New York: Wiley.

Walker, A. M. 1991. *Observation and Inference: An Introduction to the Methods of Epidemiology*. Newton Lower Falls, MA: Epidemiology Resources.

Wang, Z. 1999. sbe27: Assessing confounding effects in epidemiological studies. *Stata Technical Bulletin* 49: 12–15. Reprinted in *Stata Technical Bulletin Reprints*, vol. 9, pp. 134–138.

Woolf, B. 1955. On estimating the relation between blood group and disease. *Annals of Human Genetics* 19: 251–253. Reprinted in *Evolution of Epidemiologic Ideas*, ed. S. Greenland, 108–110. Newton Lower Falls, MA: Epidemiology Resources.

Also See

[ST] **stcox** — Fit Cox proportional hazards model

[R] **bitest** — Binomial probability test

[R] **ci** — Confidence intervals for means, proportions, and counts

[R] **clogit** — Conditional (fixed-effects) logistic regression

[R] **dstdize** — Direct and indirect standardization

[R] **glogit** — Logit and probit regression for grouped data

[R] **logistic** — Logistic regression, reporting odds ratios

[R] **poisson** — Poisson regression

[R] **symmetry** — Symmetry and marginal homogeneity tests

[R] **tabulate twoway** — Two-way tables of frequencies

[ST] **glossary** — Glossary of terms

Title

> **estimation options** — Estimation options

Description

This entry describes the options common to many st estimation commands. Not all the options documented below work with all estimation commands; see the documentation for the particular estimation command. If an option is listed there, it is applicable.

Options

Model

noconstant suppresses the constant term (intercept) in the model.

offset(*varname*) specifies that *varname* be included in the model with the coefficient constrained to be 1.

constraints(*numlist* | *matname*) specifies the linear constraints to be applied during estimation. The default is to perform unconstrained estimation. See [R] **reg3** for the use of constraints in multiple-equation contexts.

constraints(*numlist*) specifies the constraints by number after they have been defined by using the constraint command; see [R] **constraint**.

constraints(*matname*) specifies a matrix containing the constraints; see [P] **makecns**.

collinear specifies that the estimation command not remove collinear variables. Usually there is no reason to leave collinear variables in place and in fact doing so usually causes the estimation to fail because of the matrix singularity caused by the collinearity. However, with certain models, the variables may be collinear, yet the model is fully identified because of constraints or other features of the model. In such cases, using option collinear allows the estimation to take place, leaving the equations with collinear variables intact. This option is seldom used.

Reporting

level(*#*) specifies the confidence level, as a percentage, for confidence intervals. The default is level(95) or as set by set level; see [U] **20.7 Specifying the width of confidence intervals**.

Also See

[U] **20 Estimation and postestimation commands**

[ST] **st** — Survival-time data

Title

> **ltable** — Life tables for survival data

Syntax

ltable *timevar* [*deadvar*] [*if*] [*in*] [*weight*] [, *options*]

options	description
Main	
<u>n</u>otable	display graph only; suppress display of table
<u>g</u>raph	present the table graphically as well as in tabular form
by(*groupvar*)	produce separate tables (or graphs) for each value of *groupvar*;
<u>t</u>est	report χ^2 measure of differences between groups (2 tests)
overlay	overlay plots on the same graph
<u>s</u>urvival	display survival table; the default
<u>f</u>ailure	display cumulative failure table
<u>h</u>azard	display hazard table
ci	graph confidence interval
<u>l</u>evel(*#*)	set confidence level; default is level(95)
<u>noa</u>djust	suppress actuarial adjustment for deaths and censored observations
<u>tv</u>id(*varname*)	subject ID variable to use with time-varying parameters
<u>i</u>ntervals(w | *numlist*)	time intervals in which data are to be aggregated for tables
<u>sav</u>ing(*filename*[, replace])	save the life-table data to *filename*; use replace to overwrite existing *filename*
Plot	
<u>p</u>lotopts(*plot_options*)	affect rendition of the plotted line and plotted points
plot#opts(*plot_options*)	affect rendition of the #th plotted line and plotted points; available only with overlay
CI plot	
<u>c</u>iopts(*rspike_options*)	affect rendition of the confidence intervals
ci#opts(*rspike_options*)	affect rendition of the #th confidence interval; available only with overlay
Add plots	
addplot(*plot*)	add other plots to the generated graph
Y axis, X axis, Titles, Legend, Overall	
twoway_options	any options other than by() documented in [G] *twoway_options*
<u>byop</u>ts(*byopts*)	how subgraphs are combined, labeled, etc.

plot_options	description
connect_options	change look of lines or connecting method
marker_options	change look of markers (color, size, etc.)

fweights are allowed; see [U] **11.1.6 weight**.

Description

ltable displays and graphs life tables for individual-level or aggregate data and optionally presents the likelihood-ratio and log-rank tests for equivalence of groups. ltable also allows you to examine the empirical hazard function through aggregation. See also [ST] **sts** for alternative commands.

timevar specifies the time of failure or censoring. If *deadvar* is not specified, all values of *timevar* are interpreted as failure times; otherwise, *timevar* is interpreted as a failure time, where *deadvar* $\neq$ 0, and as a censoring time otherwise. Observations with *timevar* or *deadvar* equal to missing are ignored.

deadvar does not specify the *number* of failures. An observation with *deadvar* equal to 1 or 50 has the same interpretation—the observation records one failure. Specify frequency weights for aggregated data (e.g., ltable time [freq=number]).

Options

___ Main ___

notable suppresses displaying the table. This option is often used with graph.

graph requests that the table be presented graphically, as well as in tabular form; when notable is also specified, only the graph is presented. When you specify graph, only one table can be calculated and graphed at a time; see survival, failure, and hazard below.

graph may not be specified with hazard. Use sts graph to graph estimates of the hazard function.

by(*groupvar*) creates separate tables (or graphs within the same image) for each value of *groupvar*. *groupvar* may be string or numeric.

test presents two χ^2 measures of the differences between groups, the likelihood-ratio test of homogeneity and the log-rank test for equality of survivor functions. The two groups are identified by the by() option, so by() must also be specified.

overlay causes the plot from each group identified in the by() option to be overlaid on the same graph. The default is to generate a separate graph (within the same image) for each group. This option requires the by() option.

survival, failure, and hazard indicate the table to be displayed. If none is specified, the default is the survival table. Specifying failure displays the cumulative failure table. Specifying survival failure would display both the survival and the cumulative failure table. If graph is specified, multiple tables may not be requested.

ci graph the confidence intervals around survival, failure, or hazard.

level(#) specifies the confidence level, as a percentage, for confidence intervals. The default is level(95) or as set by set level; see [R] **level**.

noadjust suppresses the actuarial adjustment for deaths and censored observations. The default is to consider the adjusted number at risk at the start of the interval as the total at the start minus (the number dead or censored)/2. If noadjust is specified, the number at risk is simply the total at the start, corresponding to the standard Kaplan–Meier assumption. noadjust should be specified when using ltable to list results corresponding to those produced by sts list; see [ST] **sts list**.

tvid(*varname*) is for use with longitudinal data with time-varying parameters. Each subject appears in the data more than once, and equal values of *varname* identify observations referring to the same subject. When tvid() is specified, only the last observation on each subject is used in making the table. The order of the data does not matter, and *last* here means the last observation chronologically.

intervals(w | *numlist*) specifies the intervals into which the data are to be aggregated for tabular presentation. A numeric argument is interpreted as the width of the interval. For instance, interval(2) aggregates data into the intervals $0 \le t < 2$, $2 \le t < 4$, and so on. Not specifying interval() is equivalent to specifying interval(1). Since in most data failure times are recorded as integers, this amounts to no aggregation except that implied by the recording of the time variable, and so it produces Kaplan–Meier product-limit estimates of the survival curve (with an actuarial adjustment; see the noadjust option below). Also see [ST] **sts list**. Although it is possible to examine survival and failure without aggregation, some form of aggregation is almost always required to examine the hazard.

When more than one argument is specified, intervals are aggregated as specified. For instance, interval(0,2,8,16) aggregates data into the intervals $0 \le t < 2$, $2 \le t < 8$, and $8 \le t < 16$, and (if necessary) the open-ended interval $t \ge 16$.

interval(w) is equivalent to interval(0,7,15,30,60,90,180,360,540,720), corresponding to 1 week, (roughly) 2 weeks, 1 month, 2 months, 3 months, 6 months, 1 year, 1.5 years, and 2 years when failure times are recorded in days. The w suggests widening intervals.

saving(*filename*[, replace]) creates a Stata data file (.dta file) containing the life table. This option will not save the graph to disk; see [G] **graph save** to save the resulting graph to disk.

replace indicates that *filename* be overwritten, if it exists. This option is not shown in the dialog box.

⌐___ Plot ⌐_____

plotopts(*plot_options*) affects the rendition of the plotted line and plotted points; see [G] **connect_options** and [G] **marker_options**.

plot#opts(*plot_options*) affects the rendition of the #th plotted line and plotted points; see [G] **connect_options** and [G] **marker_options**. This option is valid only if overlay is specified.

⌐___ CI plot ⌐_____

ciopts(*rspike_options*) affects the rendition of the confidence intervals for the graphed survival, failure, or hazard; see [G] **rspike_options**.

ci#opts(*rspike_options*) affects the rendition of the #th confidence interval for the graphed survival, failure, or hazard; see [G] **rspike_options**. This option is valid only if overlay is specified.

⌐___ Add plots ⌐_____

addplot(*plot*) provides a way to add other plots to the generated graph; see [G] **addplot_option**.

Y axis, X axis, Titles, Legend, and Overall

twoway_options are any of the options documented in [G] ***twoway_options***, excluding by(). These include options for titling the graph (see [G] ***title_options***) and for saving the graph to disk (see [G] ***saving_option***).

byopts(*byopts*) affects the appearance of the combined graph when by() is specified, including the overall graph title and the organization of subgraphs. See [G] ***by_option***.

Remarks

Life tables describe death rates in a given population over time. Such tables date back to the 17th century, Edmund Halley (1693) is often credited with their development. ltable is for use with "cohort" data, and, although one often thinks of such tables as monitoring a population from the "birth" of the first member to the "death" of the last, more generally, such tables can be thought of as a reasonable way to list any kind of survival data. For an introductory discussion of life tables, see Pagano and Gauvreau (2000, 489–495); for an intermediate discussion, see Selvin (2004, 335–377); and for a more complete discussion, see Chiang (1984).

▷ Example 1

In Pike (1966), two groups of rats were exposed to a carcinogen, and the number of days to death from vaginal cancer was recorded (reprinted in Kalbfleisch and Prentice 2002, 2):

Group 1	143	164	188	188	190	192	206	209	213	216
	220	227	230	234	246	265	304	216*	244*	
Group 2	142	156	163	198	205	232	232	233	233	233
	233	239	240	261	280	280	296	296	323	204*
	344*									

The '*' on a few of the entries indicates that the observation was censored—as of the recorded day, the rat had still not died because of vaginal cancer but was withdrawn from the experiment for other reasons.

Having entered these data into Stata, we see the first few observations are

```
. use http://www.stata-press.com/data/r10/rat
. list in 1/5
```

	group	t	died
1.	1	143	1
2.	1	164	1
3.	1	188	1
4.	1	188	1
5.	1	190	1

That is, the first observation records a rat from group 1 that died on the 143rd day. The variable died records whether that rat died or was withdrawn (censored):

(Continued on next page)

```
. list if died==0
```

	group	t	died
18.	1	216	0
19.	1	244	0
39.	2	204	0
40.	2	344	0

Four rats, two from each group, did not die but were withdrawn.

The life table for group 1 is

```
. ltable t died if group==1
```

Interval		Beg. Total	Deaths	Lost	Survival	Std. Error	[95% Conf. Int.]	
143	144	19	1	0	0.9474	0.0512	0.6812	0.9924
164	165	18	1	0	0.8947	0.0704	0.6408	0.9726
188	189	17	2	0	0.7895	0.0935	0.5319	0.9153
190	191	15	1	0	0.7368	0.1010	0.4789	0.8810
192	193	14	1	0	0.6842	0.1066	0.4279	0.8439
206	207	13	1	0	0.6316	0.1107	0.3790	0.8044
209	210	12	1	0	0.5789	0.1133	0.3321	0.7626
213	214	11	1	0	0.5263	0.1145	0.2872	0.7188
216	217	10	1	1	0.4709	0.1151	0.2410	0.6713
220	221	8	1	0	0.4120	0.1148	0.1937	0.6194
227	228	7	1	0	0.3532	0.1125	0.1502	0.5648
230	231	6	1	0	0.2943	0.1080	0.1105	0.5070
234	235	5	1	0	0.2355	0.1012	0.0751	0.4459
244	245	4	0	1	0.2355	0.1012	0.0751	0.4459
246	247	3	1	0	0.1570	0.0931	0.0312	0.3721
265	266	2	1	0	0.0785	0.0724	0.0056	0.2864
304	305	1	1	0	0.0000	.	.	.

The reported survival rates are the survival rates at the end of the interval. Thus, 94.7% of rats survived 144 days or more.

◁

❑ Technical Note

If you compare the table just printed with the corresponding table in Kalbfleisch and Prentice (2002, 16), you will notice that the survival estimates differ beginning with the interval 216–217, which is the first interval containing a censored observation. ltable treats censored observations as if they were withdrawn halfway through the interval. The table printed in Kalbfleisch and Prentice treated censored observations as if they were withdrawn at the end of the interval, even though Kalbfleisch and Prentice (2002, 19) mention how results could be adjusted for censoring.

Here the same results as those printed in Kalbfleisch and Prentice could be obtained by incrementing the time of withdrawal by 1 for the four censored observations. We say "here" because there were no deaths on the incremented dates. For instance, one of the rats was withdrawn on the 216th day, a day on which there was also a real death. There were no deaths on day 217, however, so moving the withdrawal forward 1 day is equivalent to assuming that the withdrawal occurred at the end of the day 216–217 interval. If the adjustments are made and ltable is used to calculate survival in both groups, the results are the same as those printed in Kalbfleisch and Prentice, except that for group 2 in the interval 240–241, they report the survival as .345 when they mean .354.

In any case, the one-half adjustment for withdrawals is generally accepted, but it is only a crude adjustment that becomes cruder the wider the intervals.

❏

▷ Example 2: ltable with aggregated intervals

When you do not specify the intervals, ltable uses unit intervals. The only aggregation performed on the data was aggregation due to deaths or withdrawals occurring on the same "day". If we wanted to see the table aggregated into 30-day intervals, we would type

```
. ltable t died if group==1, interval(30)
```

	Interval	Beg. Total	Deaths	Lost	Survival	Std. Error	[95% Conf. Int.]	
120	150	19	1	0	0.9474	0.0512	0.6812	0.9924
150	180	18	1	0	0.8947	0.0704	0.6408	0.9726
180	210	17	6	0	0.5789	0.1133	0.3321	0.7626
210	240	11	6	1	0.2481	0.1009	0.0847	0.4552
240	270	4	2	1	0.1063	0.0786	0.0139	0.3090
300	330	1	1	0	0.0000	.	.	.

The interval displayed as 120 150 indicates the interval including 120 and up to, but not including, 150. The reported survival rate is the survival rate just after the close of the interval.

When you specify more than one number as the argument to interval(), you specify the cutoff points, not the widths.

```
. ltable t died if group==1, interval(120,180,210,240,330)
```

	Interval	Beg. Total	Deaths	Lost	Survival	Std. Error	[95% Conf. Int.]	
120	180	19	2	0	0.8947	0.0704	0.6408	0.9726
180	210	17	6	0	0.5789	0.1133	0.3321	0.7626
210	240	11	6	1	0.2481	0.1009	0.0847	0.4552
240	330	4	3	1	0.0354	0.0486	0.0006	0.2245

If any of the underlying failure or censoring times are larger than the last cutoff specified, they are treated as being in the open ended interval:

```
. ltable t died if group==1, interval(120,180,210,240)
```

	Interval	Beg. Total	Deaths	Lost	Survival	Std. Error	[95% Conf. Int.]	
120	180	19	2	0	0.8947	0.0704	0.6408	0.9726
180	210	17	6	0	0.5789	0.1133	0.3321	0.7626
210	240	11	6	1	0.2481	0.1009	0.0847	0.4552
240	.	4	3	1	0.0354	0.0486	0.0006	0.2245

Whether the last interval is treated as open ended or not makes no difference for survival and failure tables, but it does affect hazard tables. If the interval is open-ended, the hazard is not calculated for it.

◁

▷ Example 3: ltable with separate tables for each group

The by(*varname*) option specifies that separate tables be presented for each value of *varname*. Remember that our rat dataset contains two groups:

. ltable t died, by(group) interval(30)

Interval		Beg. Total	Deaths	Lost	Survival	Std. Error	[95% Conf. Int.]	
group = 1								
120	150	19	1	0	0.9474	0.0512	0.6812	0.9924
150	180	18	1	0	0.8947	0.0704	0.6408	0.9726
180	210	17	6	0	0.5789	0.1133	0.3321	0.7626
210	240	11	6	1	0.2481	0.1009	0.0847	0.4552
240	270	4	2	1	0.1063	0.0786	0.0139	0.3090
300	330	1	1	0	0.0000	.	.	.
group = 2								
120	150	21	1	0	0.9524	0.0465	0.7072	0.9932
150	180	20	2	0	0.8571	0.0764	0.6197	0.9516
180	210	18	2	1	0.7592	0.0939	0.5146	0.8920
210	240	15	7	0	0.4049	0.1099	0.1963	0.6053
240	270	8	2	0	0.3037	0.1031	0.1245	0.5057
270	300	6	4	0	0.1012	0.0678	0.0172	0.2749
300	330	2	1	0	0.0506	0.0493	0.0035	0.2073
330	360	1	0	1	0.0506	0.0493	0.0035	0.2073

◁

▷ Example 4: ltable for failure tables

A failure table is simply a different way of looking at a survival table; failure is 1 − survival:

. ltable t died if group==1, interval(30) failure

Interval		Beg. Total	Deaths	Lost	Cum. Failure	Std. Error	[95% Conf. Int.]	
120	150	19	1	0	0.0526	0.0512	0.0076	0.3188
150	180	18	1	0	0.1053	0.0704	0.0274	0.3592
180	210	17	6	0	0.4211	0.1133	0.2374	0.6679
210	240	11	6	1	0.7519	0.1009	0.5448	0.9153
240	270	4	2	1	0.8937	0.0786	0.6910	0.9861
300	330	1	1	0	1.0000	.	.	.

◁

▷ Example 5: Survival rate at start of interval versus end of interval

Selvin (2004, 357) presents follow-up data from Cutler and Ederer (1958) on six cohorts of kidney cancer patients. The goal is to estimate the 5-year survival probability.

Year	Interval	Alive	Deaths	Lost	With- drawn	Year	Interval	Alive	Deaths	Lost	With- drawn
1946	0–1	9	4	1		1948	0–1	21	11	0	
	1–2	4	0	0			1–2	10	1	2	
	2–3	4	0	0			2–3	7	0	0	
	3–4	4	0	0			3–4	7	0	0	7
	4–5	4	0	0		1949	0–1	34	12	0	
	5–6	4	0	0	4		1–2	22	3	3	
1947	0–1	18	7	0			2–3	16	1	0	15
	1–2	11	0	0		1950	0–1	19	5	1	
	2–3	11	1	0			1–2	13	1	1	11
	3–4	10	2	2		1951	0–1	25	8	2	15
	4–5	6	0	0	6						

The following is the Stata dataset corresponding to the table:

```
. use http://www.stata-press.com/data/r10/selvin

. list
```

	year	t	died	pop
1.	1946	.5	1	4
2.	1946	.5	0	1
3.	1946	5.5	0	4
4.	1947	.5	1	7
5.	1947	2.5	1	1
	(output omitted)			

As summary data may often come in the form shown above, it is worth understanding exactly how the data were translated for use with ltable. t records the time of death or censoring (lost to follow-up or withdrawal). died contains 1 if the observation records a death and 0 if it instead records lost or withdrawn patients. pop records the number of patients in the category. The first line of the original table stated that, in the 1946 cohort, there were nine patients at the start of the interval 0–1, and during the interval, four died and one was lost to follow-up. Thus we entered in observation 1 that at t = .5, four patients died and in observation 2 that at t = .5, one patient was censored. We ignored the information on the total population because ltable will figure that out for itself.

The second line of the table indicated that in the interval 1–2, four patients were still alive at the beginning of the interval, and, during the interval, 0 died or were lost to follow-up. Since no patients died or were censored, we entered nothing into our data. Similarly, we entered nothing for lines 3, 4, and 5 of the table. The last line for 1946 stated that, in the interval 5–6, four patients were alive at the beginning of the interval and that those four patients were withdrawn. In observation 3, we entered that there were four censorings at t = 5.5.

It does not matter that we chose to record the times of deaths or censoring as midpoints of intervals; we could just as well have recorded the times as 0.8 and 5.8. By default, ltable will form intervals 0–1, 1–2, and so on, and place observations into the intervals to which they belong. We suggest using 0.5 and 5.5 because those numbers correspond to the underlying assumptions made by ltable in making its calculations. Using midpoints reminds you of these assumptions.

(Continued on next page)

To obtain the survival rates, we type

```
. ltable t died [freq=pop]
```

Interval		Beg. Total	Deaths	Lost	Survival	Std. Error	[95% Conf. Int.]	
0	1	126	47	19	0.5966	0.0455	0.5017	0.6792
1	2	60	5	17	0.5386	0.0479	0.4405	0.6269
2	3	38	2	15	0.5033	0.0508	0.4002	0.5977
3	4	21	2	9	0.4423	0.0602	0.3225	0.5554
4	5	10	0	6	0.4423	0.0602	0.3225	0.5554
5	6	4	0	4	0.4423	0.0602	0.3225	0.5554

We estimate the 5-year survival rate as .4423 and the 95% confidence interval as .3225 to .5554.

Selvin (2004, 361), in presenting these results, lists the survival in the interval 0–1 as 1, in 1–2 as .597, in 2–3 as .539, and so on. That is, relative to us, he shifted the rates down one row and inserted a 1 in the first row. In his table, the survival rate is the survival rate at the *start* of the interval. In our table, the survival rate is the survival rate at the *end* of the interval (or, equivalently, at the start of the next interval). This is, of course, simply a difference in the way the numbers are presented and not in the numbers themselves.

                                                             ◁

▷ Example 6: ltable for hazard tables

The discrete hazard function is the rate of failure—the number of failures occurring within a time interval divided by the width of the interval (assuming that there are no censored observations). Although the survival and failure tables are meaningful at the "individual" level—with intervals so narrow that each contains only one failure—that is not true for the discrete hazard. If all intervals contained one death and if all intervals were of equal width, the hazard function would be $1/\Delta t$ and so appear to be a constant!

The empirically determined discrete hazard function can be revealed only by aggregation. Gross and Clark (1975, 37) print data on malignant melanoma at the University of Texas M. D. Anderson Tumor Clinic between 1944 and 1960. The interval is the time from initial diagnosis:

Interval (years)	Number lost to follow-up	Number with- drawn alive	Number dying
0–1	19	77	312
1–2	3	71	96
2–3	4	58	45
3–4	3	27	29
4–5	5	35	7
5–6	1	36	9
6–7	0	17	3
7–8	2	10	1
8–9	0	8	3
9+	0	0	32

For our statistical purposes, there is no difference between the number lost to follow-up (patients who disappeared) and the number withdrawn alive (patients dropped by the researchers)—both are censored. We have entered the data into Stata; here are a few of the data:

```
. use http://www.stata-press.com/data/r10/tumor
. list in 1/6, separator(0)
```

	t	d	pop
1.	.5	1	312
2.	.5	0	19
3.	.5	0	77
4.	1.5	1	96
5.	1.5	0	3
6.	1.5	0	71

We entered each group's time of death or censoring as the midpoint of the intervals and entered the numbers of the table, recording d as 1 for deaths and 0 for censoring. The hazard table is

```
. ltable t d [freq=pop], hazard interval(0(1)9)
```

Interval		Beg. Total	Cum. Failure	Std. Error	Hazard	Std. Error	[95% Conf. Int.]	
0	1	913	0.3607	0.0163	0.4401	0.0243	0.3924	0.4877
1	2	505	0.4918	0.0176	0.2286	0.0232	0.1831	0.2740
2	3	335	0.5671	0.0182	0.1599	0.0238	0.1133	0.2064
3	4	228	0.6260	0.0188	0.1461	0.0271	0.0931	0.1991
4	5	169	0.6436	0.0190	0.0481	0.0182	0.0125	0.0837
5	6	122	0.6746	0.0200	0.0909	0.0303	0.0316	0.1502
6	7	76	0.6890	0.0208	0.0455	0.0262	0.0000	0.0969
7	8	56	0.6952	0.0213	0.0202	0.0202	0.0000	0.0598
8	9	43	0.7187	0.0235	0.0800	0.0462	0.0000	0.1705
9	.	32	1.0000	.	.	.	.	.

We specified the interval() option as we did—and not as interval(1) or omitting the option altogether—to force the last interval to be open ended. Had we not, and if we had recorded t as 9.5 for observations in that interval (as we did), ltable would have calculated a hazard rate for the "interval". Here the result of that calculation would have been 2, but no matter the result, it would have been meaningless since we do not know the width of the interval.

When dealing with the survivor or failure function, you are not limited to merely examining a column of numbers. With the graph option, you can see the result graphically:

(Continued on next page)

```
. ltable t d [freq=pop], i(0(1)9) graph notable ci xlab(0(2)10)
```

The vertical lines in the graph represent the 95% confidence intervals for the survivor function. Among the options we specified, although it is not required, is `notable`, which suppressed printing the table, saving us some paper. `xlab()` was passed through to the `graph` command (see [G] *twoway_options*) and was unnecessary but made the graph look better.

◁

❑ Technical Note

Because many intervals can exist during which no failures occur (in which case the hazard estimate is zero), the estimated hazard is best graphically represented using a kernel smooth. Such an estimate is available in `sts graph`; see [ST] **sts graph**.

❑

Methods and Formulas

`ltable` is implemented as an ado-file.

Let τ_i be the individual failure or censoring times. The data are aggregated into intervals given by t_j, $j = 1, \ldots, J$, and $t_{J+1} = \infty$ with each interval containing counts for $t_j \leq \tau < t_{j+1}$. Let d_j and m_j be the number of failures and censored observations during the interval and N_j the number alive at the start of the interval. Define $n_j = N_j - m_j/2$ as the adjusted number at risk at the start of the interval. If the `noadjust` option is specified, $n_j = N_j$.

The product-limit estimate of the survivor function is

$$S_j = \prod_{k=1}^{j} \frac{n_k - d_k}{n_k}$$

(Kalbfleisch and Prentice 2002, 10, 15). Greenwood's formula for the asymptotic standard error of S_j is

$$s_j = S_j \sqrt{\sum_{k=1}^{j} \frac{d_k}{n_k(n_k - d_k)}}$$

(Greenwood 1926; Kalbfleisch and Prentice 2002, 17). s_j is reported as the standard deviation of survival but is not used in generating the confidence intervals since it can produce intervals outside 0 and 1. The "natural" units for the survivor function are $\log(-\log S_j)$, and the asymptotic standard error of that quantity is

$$\widehat{s}_j = \sqrt{\frac{\sum d_k/\{n_k(n_k - d_k)\}}{\left[\sum \log\{(n_k - d_k)/n_k\}\right]^2}}$$

(Kalbfleisch and Prentice 2002, 18). The corresponding confidence intervals are $S_j^{\exp(\pm z_{1-\alpha/2}\widehat{s}_j)}$.

The cumulative failure time is defined as $G_j = 1 - S_j$, and thus the variance is the same as for S_j and the confidence intervals are $1 - S_j^{\exp(\pm z_{1-\alpha/2}\widehat{s}_j)}$.

Both S_j and G_j are graphed against t_{j+1}.

Define the within-interval failure rate as $f_j = d_j/n_j$. The maximum likelihood estimate of the (within interval) hazard is then

$$\lambda_j = \frac{f_j}{(1 - f_j/2)(t_{j+1} - t_j)}$$

The standard error of λ_j is

$$s_{\lambda_j} = \lambda_j \sqrt{\frac{1 - \{(t_{j+1} - t_j)\lambda_j/2\}^2}{d_j}}$$

from which a confidence interval is calculated.

If the `noadjust` option is specified, the estimate of the hazard is

$$\lambda_j = \frac{f_j}{t_{j+1} - t_j}$$

and its standard error is

$$s_{\lambda_j} = \frac{\lambda_j}{\sqrt{d_j}}$$

The confidence interval is

$$\left[\frac{\lambda_j}{2d_j}\chi^2_{2d_j,\alpha/2}, \; \frac{\lambda_j}{2d_j}\chi^2_{2d_j,1-\alpha/2}\right]$$

where $\chi^2_{2d_j,q}$ is the qth quantile of the χ^2 distribution with $2d_j$ degrees of freedom (Cox and Oakes 1984, 53–54, 38–40).

For the likelihood-ratio test for homogeneity, let d_g be the total number of deaths in the gth group. Define $T_g = \sum_{i \in g} \tau_i$, where i indexes the individual failure or censoring times. The χ^2 value with $G - 1$ degrees of freedom (where G is the total number of groups) is

$$\chi^2 = 2\left\{ \left(\sum d_g\right) \log\left(\frac{\sum T_g}{\sum d_g}\right) - \sum d_g \log\left(\frac{T_g}{d_g}\right) \right\}$$

(Lawless 2003, 155).

The log-rank test for homogeneity is the test presented by `sts test`; see [ST] **sts**.

Acknowledgments

`ltable` is based on the `lftbl` command by Henry Krakauer and John Stewart (1991). We also thank Michel Henry-Amar, Centre Regional François Baclesse, Caen, France, for his comments.

References

Chiang, C. L. 1984. *The Life Table and Its Applications*. Malabar, FL: Krieger.

Cox, D. R., and D. Oakes. 1984. *Analysis of Survival Data*. London: Chapman & Hall/CRC.

Cutler, S. J., and E. Ederer. 1958. Maximum utilization of the life table method in analyzing survival. *Journal of Chronic Diseases* 8: 699–712.

Greenwood, M. 1926. The natural duration of cancer. *Reports on Public Health and Medical Subjects* 33: 1–26.

Gross, A. J., and V. A. Clark. 1975. *Survival Distributions: Reliability Applications in the Biomedical Sciences*. New York: Wiley.

Halley, E. 1693. An estimate of the degrees of the mortality of mankind, drawn from curious tables of the births and funerals at the city of Breslaw; with an attempt to ascertain the price of annuities upon lives. *Philosophical Transactions* 17: 596–610.

Kahn, H. A., and C. T. Sempos. 1989. *Statistical Methods in Epidemiology*. New York: Oxford University Press.

Kalbfleisch, J. D., and R. L. Prentice. 2002. *The Statistical Analysis of Failure Time Data*. 2nd ed. New York: Wiley.

Krakauer, H., and J. Stewart. 1991. ssa1: Actuarial or life-table analysis of time-to-event data. *Stata Technical Bulletin* 1: 23–25. Reprinted in *Stata Technical Bulletin Reprints*, vol. 1, pp. 200–202.

Lawless, J. F. 2003. *Statistical Models and Methods for Lifetime Data*. 2nd ed. New York: Wiley.

Pagano, M., and K. Gauvreau. 2000. *Principles of Biostatistics*. 2nd ed. Belmont, CA: Duxbury.

Pike, M. C. 1966. A method of analysis of a certain class of experiments in carcinogenesis. *Biometrics* 22: 142–161.

Ramalheira, C. 2001. ssa14: Global and multiple causes-of-death life tables from complete or aggregated vital data. *Stata Technical Bulletin* 59: 29–45. Reprinted in *Stata Technical Bulletin Reprints*, vol. 10, pp. 333–355.

Selvin, S. 2004. *Statistical Analysis of Epidemiologic Data*. 3rd ed. New York: Oxford University Press.

Also See

[ST] **stcox** — Fit Cox proportional hazards model

Title

> **snapspan** — Convert snapshot data to time-span data

Syntax

snapspan *idvar timevar varlist* [, <u>g</u>enerate(*newt0var*) replace]

Description

snapspan converts snapshot data to time-span data. See *Remarks* below for a description of snapshot and time-span data. Time-span data are required for use with survival analysis commands, such as stcox, streg, and stset.

idvar records the subject ID and may be string or numeric.

timevar records the time of the snapshot; it must be numeric and may be recorded on any scale: date, hour, minute, second, etc.

varlist are the "event" variables, meaning that they occur at the instant of *timevar*. *varlist* can also include retrospective variables that are to apply to the time span ending at the time of the current snapshot. The other variables are assumed to be measured at the time of the snapshot and thus apply from the time of the snapshot forward. See *Specifying varlist* below.

Options

<u>g</u>enerate(*newt0var*) adds *newt0var* to the dataset containing the entry time for each converted time-span record.

replace specifies that it is okay to change the data in memory, even though the dataset has not been saved on disk in its current form.

Remarks

Remarks are presented under the following headings:

> *Snapshot and time-span datasets*
> *Specifying varlist*

Snapshot and time-span datasets

snapspan converts a snapshot dataset to a time-span dataset. A snapshot dataset records a subject *id*, a *time*, and then other variables measured at the *time*:

```
Snapshot datasets:

    idvar     timevar     x1     x2    ...
  ─────────────────────────────────────────
       47          12       5     27    ...
       47          42       5     18    ...
       47          55       5     19    ...

    idvar     datevar     x1     x2    ...
  ─────────────────────────────────────────
      122   14jul1998      5     27    ...
      122   12aug1998      5     18    ...
      122   08sep1998      5     19    ...

    idvar        year     x1     x2    ...
  ─────────────────────────────────────────
      122        1994      5     27    ...
      122        1995      5     18    ...
      122        1997      5     19    ...
```

A time-span dataset records a span of time (*time0*, *time1*):

```
                                      some variables assumed
                                       to occur at time1

          |<─ other variables assumed constant over span ─>|
          _____> time
        time0                                             time1
```

Time-span data are required, for instance, by stset and the st system. The variables assumed to occur at time1 are the failure or event variables. All the other variables are assumed to be constant over the span.

```
Time-span datasets:

    idvar       time0      time1     x1     x2    ...   event
  ──────────────────────────────────────────────────────────────
       47           0         12      5     13    ...       0
       47          12         42      5     27    ...       0
       47          42         55      5     18    ...       1

    idvar       time0      time1     x1     x2    ...   event
  ──────────────────────────────────────────────────────────────
      122   01jan1998   14jul1998     5     13    ...       0
      122   14jul1998   12aug1998     5     27    ...       0
      122   12aug1998   08sep1998     5     18    ...       1

    idvar       time0      time1     x1     x2    ...   event
  ──────────────────────────────────────────────────────────────
      122        1993       1994      5     13    ...       0
      122        1994       1995      5     27    ...       0
      122        1995       1997      5     18    ...       1
```

To convert snapshot data to time-span data, you need to distinguish between event and nonevent variables. Event variables happen at an instant.

Say that you have a snapshot dataset containing variable e recording an event (e = 1 might record surgery, death, or becoming unemployed, etc.) and the rest of the variables—call them x1, x2, etc.—recording characteristics (such as sex, birth date, blood pressure, or weekly wage). The same data, in snapshot and time-span form, would be

In snapshot form:						In time-span form:					
id	time	x1	x2	e		id	time0	time	x1	x2	e
1	5	a1	b1	e1		1	.	5	.	.	e1
1	7	a2	b2	e2		1	5	7	a1	b1	e2
1	9	a3	b3	e3		1	7	9	a2	b2	e3
1	11	a4	b4	e4		1	9	11	a3	b3	e4

snapspan converts data from the form on the left to the form on the right:

```
. snapspan id time e, generate(time0) replace
```

The form on the right is suitable for use by stcox and stset and the other survival analysis commands.

Specifying varlist

The *varlist*—the third variable on—specifies the "event" variables.

In fact, the *varlist* specifies the variables that apply to the time span ending at the time of the current snapshot. The other variables are assumed to be measured at the time of the snapshot and thus apply from the time of the snapshot forward.

Thus *varlist* should include retrospective variables.

For instance, say that the snapshot recorded bp, blood pressure; smokes, the answer to the question whether the patient smoked in the last 2 weeks; and event, a variable recording examination, surgery, etc. Then *varlist* should include smokes and event. The remaining variables, bp and the rest, would be assumed to apply from the time of snapshot forward.

Suppose that the snapshot recorded ecs, employment change status (hired, fired, promoted, etc.); wage, the current hourly wage; and ms, current marital status. Then *varlist* should include esc and ms (assuming snapshot records are not generated for reason of ms change). The remaining variables, wage and the rest, would be assumed to apply from the time of the snapshot forward.

Methods and Formulas

snapspan is implemented as an ado-file.

Also See

[ST] **stset** — Declare data to be survival-time data

Title

> **st** — Survival-time data

Description

The term st refers to survival-time data and the commands—most of which begin with the letters st—for analyzing these data. If you have data on individual subjects with observations recording that this subject came under observation at time t_0 and that later, at t_1, a failure or censoring was observed, you have what we call survival-time data.

If you have subject-specific data, with observations recording not a span of time, but measurements taken on the subject at that point in time, you have what we call a snapshot dataset; see [ST] **snapspan**.

If you have data on populations, with observations recording the number of units under test at time t (subjects alive) and the number of subjects that failed or were lost because of censoring, you have what we call count-time data; see [ST] **ct**.

The st commands are

stset	[ST] **stset**	Declare data to be survival-time data
stdescribe	[ST] **stdescribe**	Describe survival-time data
stsum	[ST] **stsum**	Summarize survival-time data
stvary	[ST] **stvary**	Report whether variables vary over time
stfill	[ST] **stfill**	Fill in by carrying forward values of covariates
stgen	[ST] **stgen**	Generate variables reflecting entire histories
stsplit	[ST] **stsplit**	Split time-span records
stjoin	[ST] **stsplit**	Join time-span records
stbase	[ST] **stbase**	Form baseline dataset
sts	[ST] **sts**	Generate, graph, list, and test the survivor and cumulative hazard functions
stir	[ST] **stir**	Report incidence-rate comparison
stci	[ST] **stci**	Confidence intervals for means and percentiles of survival time
strate	[ST] **strate**	Tabulate failure rate
stptime	[ST] **stptime**	Calculate person-time
stmh	[ST] **strate**	Calculate rate ratios with the Mantel–Haenszel method
stmc	[ST] **strate**	Calculate rate ratios with the Mantel–Cox method
stcox	[ST] **stcox**	Fit Cox proportional hazards model
estat concordance	[ST] **stcox postestimation**	Calculate Harrell's C
estat phtest	[ST] **stcox postestimation**	Test Cox proportional-hazards assumption
stphplot	[ST] **stcox diagnostics**	Graphically assess the Cox proportional-hazards assumption
stcoxkm	[ST] **stcox diagnostics**	Graphically assess the Cox proportional-hazards assumption

streg	[ST] **streg**	Fit parametric survival models
stcurve	[ST] **stcurve**	Plot survivor, hazard, or cumulative hazard function
stpower	[ST] **stpower**	Sample-size, power, and effect-size determination for survival studies
stpower cox	[ST] **stpower cox**	Sample size, power, and effect size for the Cox proportional hazards model
stpower exponential	[ST] **stpower exponential**	Sample size and power for the exponential test
stpower logrank	[ST] **stpower logrank**	Sample size, power, and effect size for the log-rank test
sttocc	[ST] **sttocc**	Convert survival-time data to case–control data
sttoct	[ST] **sttoct**	Convert survival-time data to count-time data
st_*	[ST] **st_is**	Survival analysis subroutines for programmers

The st commands are used for analyzing time-to-absorbing-event (single failure) data and for analyzing time-to-repeated-event (multiple failure) data.

You begin an analysis by stsetting your data, which tells Stata the key survival-time variables; see [ST] **stset**. Once you have stset your data, you can use the other st commands. If you save your data after stsetting it, you will not have to stset it again in the future; Stata will remember.

The subsequent st entries are printed in this manual in alphabetical order. You can skip around, but if you want to be an expert on all Stata's survival analysis capabilities, we suggest the above reading order.

Reference

Cleves, M. A. 1999. ssa13: Analysis of multiple failure-time data with Stata. *Stata Technical Bulletin* 49: 30–39. Reprinted in *Stata Technical Bulletin Reprints*, vol. 9, pp. 338–349.

Also See

[ST] **stset** — Declare data to be survival-time data

[ST] **ct** — Count-time data

[ST] **snapspan** — Convert snapshot data to time-span data

[ST] **survival analysis** — Introduction to survival analysis & epidemiological tables commands

[ST] **glossary** — Glossary of terms

Title

> **st_is** — Survival analysis subroutines for programmers

Syntax

Verify data in memory are survival-time data

> st_is 2 {full | analysis}

Display or do not display summary of survival-time variables

> st_show [noshow]

Risk-group summaries

> st_ct "[byvars]" -> newtvar newpopvar newfailvar [newcensvar [newentvar]]

You must have stset your data before using st_is, st_show, and st_ct; see [ST] **stset**.

Description

These commands are provided for programmers wishing to write new st commands.

st_is verifies that the data in memory are survival-time (st) data. If not, it issues the error message "data not st", r(119).

st is currently "release 2", meaning that this is the second design of the system. Programs written for the previous release continue to work. (The previous release of st corresponds to Stata 5.)

Modern programs code st_is 2 full or st_is 2 analysis. st_is 2 verifies that the dataset in memory is in release 2 format; if it is in the earlier format, it is converted to release 2 format. (Older programs simply code st_is. This verifies that no new features are stset about the data that would cause the old program to break.)

The full and analysis parts indicate whether the dataset may include past, future, or past and future data. Code st_is 2 full if the command is suitable for running on the analysis sample and the past and future data (many data-management commands fall into this category). Code st_is 2 analysis if the command is suitable for use only with the analysis sample (most statistical commands fall into this category). See [ST] **stset** for the definitions of past and future.

st_show displays the summary of the survival-time variables or does nothing, depending on what you specify when stsetting the data. noshow requests that st_show display nothing.

st_ct is a low-level utility that provides risk-group summaries from survival-time data.

Remarks

Remarks are presented under the following headings:

> *Definitions of characteristics and st variables*
> *Outline of an st command*
> *Using the st_ct utility*
> *Comparison of st_ct with sttoct*
> *Verifying data*
> *Converting data*

Definitions of characteristics and st variables

From a programmer's perspective, st is a set of conventions that specify where certain pieces of information are stored and how that information should be interpreted, together with a few subroutines that make it easier to follow the conventions.

At the lowest level, st is nothing more than a set of Stata characteristics that programmers may access:

char _dta[_dta]	st (marks that the data is st)
char _dta[st_ver]	2 (version number)
char _dta[st_id]	*varname* or nothing; id() variable
char _dta[st_bt0]	*varname* or nothing; t0() variable
char _dta[st_bt]	*varname*; *t* variable from stset t, ...
char _dta[st_bd]	*varname* or nothing; failure() variable
char _dta[st_ev]	list of numbers or nothing; *numlist* from failure(*varname*[==*numlist*])
char _dta[st_enter]	contents of enter() or nothing; *numlist* expanded
char _dta[st_exit]	contents of exit() or nothing; *numlist* expanded
char _dta[st_orig]	contents of origin() or nothing; *numlist* expanded
char _dta[st_bs]	# or 1; scale() value
char _dta[st_o]	_origin or #
char _dta[st_s]	_scale or #
char _dta[st_ifexp]	*exp* or nothing; from stset ... if exp ...
char _dta[st_if]	*exp* or nothing; contents of if()
char _dta[st_ever]	*exp* or nothing; contents of ever()
char _dta[st_never]	*exp* or nothing; contents of never()
char _dta[st_after]	*exp* or nothing; contents of after()
char _dta[st_befor]	*exp* or nothing; contents of before()
char _dta[st_wt]	weight type or nothing; user-specified weight
char _dta[st_wv]	*varname* or nothing; user-specified weighting variable
char _dta[st_w]	[*weighttype=weightvar*] or nothing
char _dta[st_show]	noshow or nothing
char _dta[st_t]	_t (for compatibility with release 1)
char _dta[st_t0]	_t0 (for compatibility with release 1)
char _dta[st_d]	_d (for compatibility with release 1)
char _dta[st_n0]	# or nothing; number of st notes
char _dta[st_n1]	text of first note or nothing
char _dta[st_n2]	text of second note or nothing
char _dta[st_set]	text or nothing. If filled in, streset will refuse to execute and present this text as the reason

All st datasets also have the following four variables:

_t0	time of entry (in t units) into risk pool
_t	time of exit (in t units) from risk pool
_d	contains 1 if failure, 0 if censoring
_st	contains 1 if observation is to be used and 0 otherwise

Thus, in a program you might code

```
display "the failure/censoring base time variable is _t"
display "and its mean in the uncensored subsample is"
summarize _t if _d
```

No matter how simple or complicated the data, these four variables exist and are filled in. For instance, in simple data, _t0 might contain 0 for every observation, and _d might always contain 1.

Some st datasets also contain the variables

_origin	evaluated value of origin()
_scale	evaluated value of scale()

The characteristic _dta[st_o] contains either the name _origin or a number, often 0. It contains a number when the origin does not vary across observations. _dta[st_s] works the same way with the scale() value. Thus the origin and scale are _dta[st_o] and _dta[st_s]. In fact, these characteristics are seldom used because variables _t and _t0 are already adjusted.

Some st datasets have an id() variable that clusters together records on the same subject. The name of the variable varies, and the name can be obtained from the characteristic _dta[st_id]. If there is no id() variable, the characteristic contains nothing.

Outline of an st command

If you are writing a new st command, place st_is near the top of your code to ensure that your command does not execute on inappropriate data. Also place st_show following the parsing of your command's syntax to display the key st variables. The minimal outline for an st command is

```
program st name
        version 10
        st_is 2 ...
        ... syntax command ...
        ... determined there are no syntax errors ...
        st_show
        ... guts of program ...
end
```

st_is 2 appears even before the input is parsed. This is to avoid irritating users when they type a command, get a syntax error, work hard to eliminate the error, and then learn that "data not st".

A fuller outline for an st command, particularly one that performs analysis on the data, is

```
program st name
        version 10
        st_is 2 ...
        syntax ... [, ... noSHow ... ]
        st_show 'show'
        marksample touse
        quietly replace 'touse' = 0 if _st==0
        ... guts of program ...
end
```

All calculations and actions are to be restricted, at the least, to observations for which _st ≠ 0. Observations with _st = 0 are to be ignored.

Using the st_ct utility

st_ct converts the data in memory to observations containing summaries of risk groups. Consider the code

```
st_is 2 analysis
preserve
st_ct "" -> t pop die
```

Typing this would change the data in memory to contain something akin to count-time data. The transformed data would have observations containing

t	time
pop	population at risk at time t
die	number who fail at time t

There would be one record per time t, and the data would be sorted by t. The original data are discarded, which is why you should code preserve; see [P] **preserve**.

The above three lines could be used as the basis for calculating the Kaplan–Meier product-limit survivor function estimate. The rest of the code is

```
keep if die
gen double hazard = die/pop
gen double km      = 1-hazard  if _n==1
replace     km     = (1-hazard)*km[_n-1] if _n>1
```

st_ct can be used to obtain risk groups separately for subgroups of the population. The code

```
st_is 2 analysis
preserve
st_ct "race sex" -> t pop die
```

would change the data in memory to contain

race	
sex	
t	time
pop	population at risk at time t
die	number who fail at time t

There would be one observation for each race–sex–t combination, and the data would be sorted by race sex t.

With this dataset, you could calculate the Kaplan–Meier product-limit survivor function estimate for each race–sex group by coding

```
keep if die
gen double hazard = die/pop
by race sex: gen double km      = 1-hazard  if _n==1
by race sex: replace     km     = (1-hazard)*km[_n-1] if _n>1
```

st_ct is a convenient subroutine. The above code fragment works regardless of the complexity of the underlying survival-time data. It does not matter whether there is one record per subject, no censoring, and one failure per subject, or multiple records per subject, gaps, and recurring failures for the same subject. st_ct forms risk groups that summarize the events recorded by the data.

st_ct can provide the number of censored records and the number who enter the risk group. The code

```
st_ct "" -> t pop die cens ent
```

creates records containing

t	time
pop	population at risk at time t
die	number who fail at time t
cens	number who are censored at t (after the failures)
ent	number who enter at t (after the censorings)

As before,

```
st_ct "race sex" -> t pop die cens ent
```

would create a similar dataset with records for each race–sex group.

Comparison of st_ct with sttoct

sttoct—see [ST] **sttoct**—is related to st_ct, and in fact, sttoct is implemented in terms of st_ct. The differences between them are that

1. sttoct creates ct data, meaning that the dataset is marked as being ct. st_ct merely creates a useful dataset; it does not ctset the data.

2. st_ct creates a total population at risk variable—which is useful in programming—but sttoct creates no such variable.

3. sttoct eliminates thrashings—censorings and reentries of the same subject as covariates change—if there are no gaps, strata shifting, etc. st_ct does not do this. Thus, at a particular time, sttoct might show that there are two lost to censoring and none entered, whereas st_ct might show 12 censorings and 10 entries. This makes no difference in calculating the number at risk and the number who fail, which are the major ingredients in survival calculations.

4. st_ct is faster.

Verifying data

As long as you code st_is at the top of your program, you need not verify the consistency of the data. That is, you need not verify that subjects do not fail before they enter, etc.

The dataset is verified when you stset it. If you make a substantive change to the data, you must rerun stset (which can be done by typing stset or streset without arguments) to reverify that all is well.

Converting data

If you write a program that converts the data from one form of st data to another, or from st data to something else, be sure to issue the appropriate stset command. For instance, a command we have written, stbase, converts the data from st to a simple cross-section in one instance. In our program, we coded stset, clear so that all other st commands would know that these are no longer st data and that making st calculations on them would be inappropriate.

Even if we had forgotten, other st programs would have found many of the key st variables missing and would have ended with a "[such-and-such] not found" error.

Also See

[ST] **stset** — Declare data to be survival-time data

[ST] **sttoct** — Convert survival-time data to count-time data

[ST] **st** — Survival-time data

[ST] **survival analysis** — Introduction to survival analysis & epidemiological tables commands

Title

stbase — Form baseline dataset

Syntax

stbase $\begin{bmatrix} if \end{bmatrix}$ $\begin{bmatrix} in \end{bmatrix}$ $\begin{bmatrix} , & options \end{bmatrix}$

options	description
Main	
at(#)	convert single/multiple-record st data to cross-sectional dataset at time #
gap(newvar)	name of variable containing gap time; default is gap or gaptime
replace	overwrite current data in memory
noshow	do not show st setting information
† nopreserve	programmer's option; see Options below

† nopreserve is not shown in the dialog box.

You must stset your data before using stbase; see [ST] **stset**.

fweights, iweights, and pweights may be specified using stset; see [ST] **stset**.

Description

stbase without the at() option converts multiple-record st data to st data with every variable set to its value at baseline, defined as the earliest time at which each subject was observed. stbase without at() does nothing to single-record st data.

stbase, at() converts single- or multiple-record st data to a cross-sectional dataset (not st data), recording the number of failures at the specified time. All variables are given their values at baseline—the earliest time at which each subject was observed. In this form, single-failure data could be analyzed by logistic regression and multiple-failure data by Poisson regression, for instance.

stbase can be used with single- or multiple-record or single- or multiple-failure st data.

Options

Main

at(#) changes what stbase does. Without the at() option, stbase produces another related st dataset. With the at() option, stbase produces a related cross-sectional dataset.

gap(newvar) is allowed only with at(); it specifies the name of a new variable to be added to the data containing the amount of time the subject was not at risk after entering and before # as specified in at(). If gap() is not specified, the new variable will be named gap or gaptime, depending on which name does not already exist in the data.

replace specifies that it is okay to change the data in memory, even though the dataset has not been saved to disk in its current form.

noshow prevents stbase from showing the key st variables. This option is rarely used since most people type stset, show or stset, noshow to set once and for all whether they want to see these variables mentioned at the top of the output of every st command; see [ST] **stset**.

103

The following option is available with `stbase` but is not shown in the dialog box:

`nopreserve` is for use by programmers using `stbase` as a subroutine. It specifies that `stbase` not preserve the original dataset so that it can be restored should an error be detected or should the user press *Break*. Programmers would specify this option if, in their program, they had already preserved the original data.

Remarks

Remarks are presented under the following headings:

> *stbase without the at() option*
> *stbase with the at() option*
> *Single-failure st data where all subjects enter at 0*
> *Single-failure st data where all subjects enter after time 0*
> *Single-failure st data with gaps and perhaps delayed entry*
> *Multiple-failure st data*

stbase without the at() option

Once you type `stbase`, you may not `streset` your data, even though the data are st. `streset` will refuse to run because the data have changed, and if the original rules were reapplied, they might produce different, incorrect results. The st commands use four key variables:

_t0	the time at which the record came under observation
_t	the time at which the record left observation
_d	1 if the record left under failure, 0 otherwise
_st	whether the observation is to be used (contains 1 or 0)

These variables are adjusted by `stbase`. The variables _t0 and _t, in particular, are derived from your variables according to options you specified at the time you `stset` the data, which might include an `origin()` rule, an `entry()` rule, and the like. Once intervening observations are eliminated, those rules will not necessarily produce the same results that they did previously.

To illustrate how `stbase` works, consider multiple-record, time-varying st data, on which you have performed some analysis. You now wish to compare your results with a simpler, non–time-varying analysis. For instance, suppose that the variables `x1` and `x2` measure blood pressure and weight, respectively, and that readings were taken at various times. Perhaps you fitted the model

```
. use http://www.stata-press.com/data/r10/mfail
. stset
-> stset t, id(id) failure(d) exit(time .) noshow
                id:  id
     failure event:  d != 0 & d < .
obs. time interval:  (t[_n-1], t]
 exit on or before:  time .

    1734  total obs.
       0  exclusions

    1734  obs. remaining, representing
     926  subjects
     808  failures in multiple failure-per-subject data
  435855  total analysis time at risk, at risk from t =         0
                               earliest observed entry t =         0
                                last observed exit t =         960
```

```
. stcox x1 x2

Iteration 0:   log likelihood = -5034.9569
Iteration 1:   log likelihood = -4978.4198
Iteration 2:   log likelihood = -4978.1915
Iteration 3:   log likelihood = -4978.1914
Refining estimates:
Iteration 0:   log likelihood = -4978.1914

Cox regression -- Breslow method for ties

No. of subjects =          926            Number of obs   =       1734
No. of failures =          808
Time at risk    =       435855
                                          LR chi2(2)      =     113.53
Log likelihood  =    -4978.1914           Prob > chi2     =     0.0000
```

_t	Haz. Ratio	Std. Err.	z	P>|z|	[95% Conf. Interval]	
x1	2.273456	.216537	8.62	0.000	1.886311	2.740059
x2	.329011	.0685638	-5.33	0.000	.2186883	.4949888

with these data. You now wish to fit that same model but this time use the values of x1 and x2 at baseline. You do this by typing

```
. stbase, replace
notes:
    1.  no gaps
    2.  there were multiple failures or reentries after failures
    3.  baseline data has multiple records per id(id)
    4.  all records have covariate values at baseline

. stcox x1 x2

Iteration 0:   log likelihood = -7886.9779
Iteration 1:   log likelihood = -7863.9974
Iteration 2:   log likelihood = -7863.9295
Iteration 3:   log likelihood = -7863.9295
Refining estimates:
Iteration 0:   log likelihood = -7863.9295

Cox regression -- Breslow method for ties

No. of subjects =          926            Number of obs   =       1734
No. of failures =         1337
Time at risk    =       435855
                                          LR chi2(2)      =      46.10
Log likelihood  =    -7863.9295           Prob > chi2     =     0.0000
```

_t	Haz. Ratio	Std. Err.	z	P>|z|	[95% Conf. Interval]	
x1	1.413195	.1107945	4.41	0.000	1.211903	1.647921
x2	.4566673	.0765272	-4.68	0.000	.3288196	.6342233

Another way you could perform the analysis is to type

```
. generate x1_0 = x1

. generate x2_0 = x2

. stfill x1_0 x2_0, baseline

. stcox x1 x2
```

See [ST] **stfill**. The method you use makes no difference, but if there were many explanatory variables, stbase would be easier.

stbase changes the data to record the same events but changes the values of all other variables to their values at the earliest time the subject was observed.

stbase also simplifies the st data where possible. Say that one of your subjects has three records in the original data and ends in a failure:

After running stbase, this subject would have one record in the data:

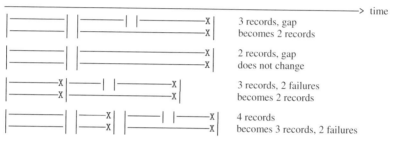

Here are some other examples of how stbase would process records with gaps and multiple failure events:

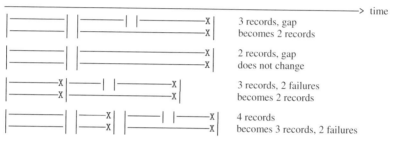

The following example shows numerically what is shown in the diagram above.

```
. use http://www.stata-press.com/data/r10/stbasexmpl, clear
. list id time0 time wgt death, sepby(id)
```

	id	time0	time	wgt	death
1.	1	0	2	114	0
2.	1	3	5	110	0
3.	1	5	11	118	1
4.	2	0	2	120	0
5.	2	3	11	111	1
6.	3	0	2	108	1
7.	3	2	4	105	0
8.	3	4	7	113	1
9.	4	0	2	98	0
10.	4	3	4	101	1
11.	4	5	6	106	0
12.	4	6	11	104	1

```
. stset time, id(id) fail(death) time0(time0) exit(time .)
                id:  id
     failure event:  death != 0 & death < .
obs. time interval:  (time0, time]
 exit on or before:  time .
```

```
        12  total obs.
         0  exclusions
```

```
        12  obs. remaining, representing
         4  subjects
         6  failures in multiple failure-per-subject data
        36  total analysis time at risk, at risk from t =          0
                            earliest observed entry t =            0
                               last observed exit t =             11
```

```
. list, sepby(id)
```

	id	time0	time	wgt	death	_st	_d	_t	_t0
1.	1	0	2	114	0	1	0	2	0
2.	1	3	5	110	0	1	0	5	3
3.	1	5	11	118	1	1	1	11	5
4.	2	0	2	120	0	1	0	2	0
5.	2	3	11	111	1	1	1	11	3
6.	3	0	2	108	1	1	1	2	0
7.	3	2	4	105	0	1	0	4	2
8.	3	4	7	113	1	1	1	7	4
9.	4	0	2	98	0	1	0	2	0
10.	4	3	4	101	1	1	1	4	3
11.	4	5	6	106	0	1	0	6	5
12.	4	6	11	104	1	1	1	11	6

```
. stbase, replace
        failure _d:  death
  analysis time _t:  time
 exit on or before:  time .
                id:  id
notes:
    1.  there were gaps
    2.  there were multiple failures or reentries after failures
    3.  baseline data has multiple records per id(id)
    4.  all records have covariate values at baseline
```

(Continued on next page)

```
. list, sepby(id)
```

	id	time0	time	wgt	death	_st	_d	_t	_t0
1.	1	0	2	114	0	1	0	2	0
2.	1	3	11	114	1	1	1	11	3
3.	2	0	2	120	0	1	0	2	0
4.	2	3	11	120	1	1	1	11	3
5.	3	0	2	108	1	1	1	2	0
6.	3	2	7	108	1	1	1	7	2
7.	4	0	2	98	0	1	0	2	0
8.	4	3	4	98	1	1	1	4	3
9.	4	5	11	98	1	1	1	11	5

stbase with the at() option

stbase, at() produces a cross-sectional dataset recording the status of each subject at the specified time. This new dataset is not st. Four "new" variables are created:

- the first entry time for the subject,
- the time on gap,
- the time at risk, and
- the number of failures during the time at risk.

The names given to those variables depend on how your data are stset. Pretend that your stset command was

```
. stset var1, failure(var2) time0(var3) ...
```

Then

the first entry time	will be named	*var3* or time0 or _t0
the time on gap	will be named	gap() or gap or gaptime
the time at risk	will be named	*var1*
the number of (or whether) failures	will be named	*var2* or failure or _d

The names may vary because, for instance, if you did not specify a *var2* variable when you stset your data, stbase, at() looks around for a name.

You need not memorize this; the names are obvious from the output produced by stbase, at().

Consider the actions of stbase, at() with some particular st datasets. Pretend that the command given is

```
. use http://www.stata-press.com/data/r10/stbasexmpl2, clear
. list id time0 time wgt death, sepby(id)
```

	id	time0	time	wgt	death
1.	1	0	2	114	0
2.	1	2	8	110	0
3.	1	8	11	118	1
4.	2	0	1	120	0
5.	2	1	3	111	0
6.	2	3	8	108	0
7.	2	8	10	98	1

```
. stset time, id(id) fail(death) time0(time0)
                 id:  id
      failure event:  death != 0 & death < .
obs. time interval:  (time0, time]
 exit on or before:  failure
```

```
        7  total obs.
        0  exclusions
```

```
        7  obs. remaining, representing
        2  subjects
        2  failures in single failure-per-subject data
       21  total analysis time at risk, at risk from t =          0
                               earliest observed entry t =          0
                                   last observed exit t =         11
```

```
. list, sepby(id)
```

	id	time0	time	wgt	death	_st	_d	_t	_t0
1.	1	0	2	114	0	1	0	2	0
2.	1	2	8	110	0	1	0	8	2
3.	1	8	11	118	1	1	1	11	8
4.	2	0	1	120	0	1	0	1	0
5.	2	1	3	111	0	1	0	3	1
6.	2	3	8	108	0	1	0	8	3
7.	2	8	10	98	1	1	1	10	8

(Continued on next page)

```
. stbase, at(5) replace
            failure _d:  death
    analysis time _t:  time
                 id:  id
```

        data now cross-section at time 5

Variable	description
id	subject identifier
time0	first entry time
gap	time on gap
time	time at risk
death	number of failures during interval time

Variable	Obs	Mean	Std. Dev.	Min	Max
time0	2	0	0	0	0
gap	2	0	0	0	0
time	2	5	0	5	5
death	2	0	0	0	0

```
. list
```

	id	wgt	death	time	time0	gap
1.	1	114	0	5	0	0
2.	2	120	0	5	0	0

thus producing a cross-section at analysis time 5.

Note that the value of time specified with the at() option must correspond to time in the analysis scale, i.e., *t*. See [ST] **stset** for a definition of analysis time.

Single-failure st data where all subjects enter at 0

The result of stbase, at(5) would be one record per subject. Any subject who was censored before time 5 would not appear in the data; the rest would. Those that failed after time 5 will be recorded as having been censored at time 5 (*failvar* = 0); those that failed at time 5 or earlier will have *failvar* = 1.

timevar will contain

for the failures:		
	time of failure	if failed on or before time 5 or
	5	if the subject has not failed yet
for the censored:		
	5	if the subject has not failed yet

With such data, you could perform

1. logistic regression of *failvar* on any of the characteristics or

2. incidence-rate analysis, summing the failures (perhaps within strata) and the time at risk *timevar*.

With these data, you could examine 5-year survival probabilities.

Single-failure st data, some subjects enter after time 0

The data produced by stbase, at(5) would be similar to the above, except

1. persons who enter on or after time 5 would not be included in the data (because they have not entered yet) and

2. the time at risk *timevar* would properly account for the time at which each patient entered.

timevar (the time at risk) will contain

for the failures:
: time of failure or less — if failed on or before time 5 (or less because the subject may not have entered at 0); or

: 5 or less — if the subject has not failed yet (or less because subject may not have entered at time 0)

for the censored:
: 5 or less — if the subject has not failed yet (or less because the subject may not have entered at time 0)

Depending on the analysis you are performing, you may have to discard those that enter late. This is easy to do because t0 contains the first time of entry.

With these data, you could perform

1. Logistic regression of *failvar* on any of the characteristics, but only if you restricted the sample to if t0 == 0 because those who entered after time 0 have a lesser risk of failing over the fixed interval and

2. Incidence-rate analysis, summing the failures (perhaps within stratum) and the time at risk *timevar*. Here you would have to do nothing differently from what you did in the previous example. The time-at-risk variable already includes the time of entry for each patient.

Single-failure st data with gaps and perhaps delayed entry

These data will be similar to the delayed-entry, no-gap data, but gap will contain 0 only for those observations that have no gap.

If analyzing these data, you could perform

1. logistic regression, but the sample must be restricted to if t0 == 0 & gap == 0 or

2. incidence-rate analysis, and nothing would need to be done differently; the time at risk *timevar* accounts for late entry and gaps.

Multiple-failure st data

The multiple-failure case parallels the single-failure case, except that fail will not solely contain 0 and 1; it will contain 0, 1, 2, ..., depending on the number of failures observed. Regardless of late entry, gaps, etc., you could perform

1. Poisson regression of fail, the number of events, but remember to specify exposure(*timevar*) and

2. incidence-rate analysis.

Methods and Formulas

stbase is implemented as an ado-file.

Also See

[ST] **stfill** — Fill in by carrying forward values of covariates

[ST] **stset** — Declare data to be survival-time data

Title

> **stci** — Confidence intervals for means and percentiles of survival time

Syntax

> stci [*if*] [*in*] [, *options*]

options	description
Main	
by(*varlist*)	report separate summaries by grouping variables
<u>med</u>ian	calculate median survival times; the default
<u>r</u>mean	calculate mean survival time restricted to longest follow-up time
<u>e</u>mean	calculate the mean survival time by exponentially extending the survival curve to zero
p(*#*)	compute the *#* percentile of survival times
<u>cc</u>orr	calculate the standard error for **rmean** using a continuity correction
<u>nos</u>how	do not show st setting information
dd(*#*)	set maximum number of decimal digits to report
<u>l</u>evel(*#*)	set confidence level; default is level(95)
<u>g</u>raph	plot exponentially extended survivor function
<u>t</u>max(*#*)	set maximum analysis time of *#* to be plotted
Plot	
cline_options	affect rendition of the plotted lines
Add plots	
addplot(*plot*)	add other plots to the generated graph
Y axis, X axis, Titles, Legend, Overall	
twoway_options	any options other than by() documented in [G] *twoway_options*

You must stset your data before using stci; see [ST] **stset**.
by is allowed; see [D] **by**.

Description

stci computes means and percentiles of survival time, standard errors, and confidence intervals. For multiple-event data, survival time is the time until a failure.

stci can be used with single- or multiple-record or single- or multiple-failure st data.

Options

> ⌐ Main ⌐

by(*varlist*) requests separate summaries for each group, along with an overall total. Observations are in the same group if they have equal values of the variables in *varlist*. *varlist* may contain any number of variables, each of which may be string or numeric.

113

median specifies median survival times. This is the default.

rmean and emean specify mean survival times. If the longest follow-up time is censored, emean (extended mean) computes the mean survival by exponentially extending the survival curve to zero, and rmean (restricted mean) computes the mean survival time restricted to the longest follow-up time. If the longest follow-up time is a failure, the restricted mean survival time and the extended mean survival time are equal.

p(#) specifies the percentile of survival time to be computed. For example, p(25) will compute the 25th percentile of survival times, and p(75) will compute the 75th percentile of survival times. Specifying p(50) is the same as specifying the median option.

ccorr specifies that the standard error for the restricted mean survival time be computed using a continuity correction. ccorr is valid only with option rmean.

noshow prevents stci from showing the key st variables. This option is seldom used since most people type stset, show or stset, noshow to set whether they want to see these variables mentioned at the top of the output of every st command; see [ST] **stset**.

dd(#) specifies the maximum number of decimal digits to be reported for standard errors and confidence intervals. This option affects only how values are reported and not how they are calculated.

level(#) specifies the confidence level, as a percentage, for confidence intervals. The default is level(95) or as set by set level; see [U] **20.7 Specifying the width of confidence intervals**.

graph specifies that the exponentially extended survivor function be plotted. This option is valid only when option emean is also specified and is not valid in conjunction with the by() option.

tmax(#) is for use with the graph option. It specifies the maximum analysis time to be plotted.

⎡ Plot ⎤
_____

cline_options affect the rendition of the plotted lines; see [G] *cline_options*.

⎡ Add plots ⎤
_____

addplot(*plot*) provides a way to add other plots to the generated graph. See [G] *addplot_option*.

⎡ Y axis, X axis, Titles, Legend, Overall ⎤
_____

twoway_options are any of the options documented in [G] *twoway_options*, excluding by(). These include options for titling the graph (see [G] *title_options*) and for saving the graph to disk (see [G] *saving_option*).

Remarks

Remarks are presented under the following headings:

> *Single-failure data*
> *Multiple-failure data*

Single-failure data

Here is an example of stci with single-record survival data:

```
. use http://www.stata-press.com/data/r10/page2
. stset, noshow
. stci
```

	no. of subjects	50%	Std. Err.	[95% Conf. Interval]	
total	40	232	2.562933	213	239

```
. stci, by(group)
```

group	no. of subjects	50%	Std. Err.	[95% Conf. Interval]	
1	19	216	5.171042	190	234
2	21	233	2.179595	232	280
total	40	232	2.562933	213	239

In the example above, we obtained the median survival time, by default.

To obtain the 25th or any other percentile of survival time, specify the p(#) option.

```
. stci, p(25)
```

	no. of subjects	25%	Std. Err.	[95% Conf. Interval]	
total	40	198	10.76878	164	220

```
. stci, p(25) by(group)
```

group	no. of subjects	25%	Std. Err.	[95% Conf. Interval]	
1	19	190	8.411659	143	213
2	21	232	14.88531	142	233
total	40	198	10.76878	164	220

The p-percentile of survival time is the analysis time at which $p\%$ of subjects have failed and $1 - p\%$ have not. In the table above, 25% of subjects in group 1 failed by time 190, whereas 25% of subjects in group 2 failed by time 232, indicating a better survival experience for this group.

(Continued on next page)

We can verify the quantities reported by `stci` by plotting and examining the Kaplan–Meier survival curves.

```
. sts graph, by(group)
```

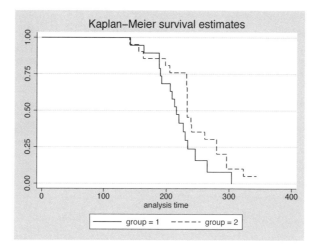

The mean survival time reported by `rmean` is calculated as the area under the Kaplan–Meier survivor function. If the observation with the largest analysis time is censored, the survivor function does not go to zero. Consequently, the area under the curve underestimates the mean survival time.

In the graph above, the survival probability for `group = 1` goes to 0 at analysis time 344, but the survivor function for `group = 2` never goes to 0. For these data, the mean survival time for `group = 1` will be properly estimated, but it will be underestimated for `group = 2`. When we specify the `rmean` option, Stata informs us if any of the mean survival times is underestimated.

```
. stci, rmean by(group)
```

group	no. of subjects	restricted mean	Std. Err.	[95% Conf. Interval]	
1	19	218.7566	9.122424	200.877	236.636
2	21	241.8571(*)	11.34728	219.617	264.097
total	40	231.3522(*)	7.700819	216.259	246.446

(*) largest observed analysis time is censored, mean is underestimated.

Stata flagged the mean for `group = 2` and the overall mean as being underestimated.

If the largest observed analysis time is censored, `stci`'s `emean` option extends the survivor function from the last observed time to zero by using an exponential function and computes the area under the entire curve.

```
. stci, emean
```

	no. of subjects	extended mean
total	40	234.2557

The resulting area must be evaluated with care because it is an ad hoc approximation that can at times be misleading. We recommend that you plot and examine the extended survivor function. This is facilitated by the use of `stci`'s `graph` option.

. stci, emean graph

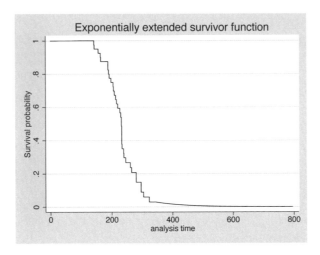

stci also works with multiple-record survival data. Here is a summary of the multiple-record Stanford heart transplant data introduced in [ST] **stset**:

. use http://www.stata-press.com/data/r10/stan3
(Heart transplant data)
. stset, noshow
. stci

	no. of subjects	50%	Std. Err.	[95% Conf. Interval]	
total	103	100	38.64425	69	219

stci with the by() option may produce results with multiple-record data that you might think are in error:

. stci, by(posttran)

posttran	no. of subjects	50%	Std. Err.	[95% Conf. Interval]	
0	103	149	22.16591	69	340
1	69	96	38.01968	45	285
total	103	100	38.64425	69	219

For the number of subjects, $103 + 69 \neq 103$. Variable posttran is not constant for the subjects in this dataset:

. stvary posttran

	subjects for whom the variable is				
variable	constant	varying	never missing	always missing	sometimes missing
posttran	34	69	103	0	0

In this dataset, subjects have one or two records. All subjects were eligible for heart transplantation. They have one record if they die or are lost because of censoring before transplantation, and they have two records if the operation was performed. Then the first record records their survival up to transplantation, and the second records their subsequent survival. `posttran` is 0 in the first record and 1 in the second.

Therefore, all 103 subjects have records with `posttran = 0`, and when `stci` reported results for this group, it summarized the pretransplantation survival. The median survival time was 149 days.

The `posttran = 1` line of `stci`'s output summarizes the posttransplantation survival: 69 patients underwent transplantation, and the median survival time was 96 days. For these data, this is not 96 more days, but 96 days in total. That is, the clock was not reset on transplantation. Thus, without attributing cause, we can describe the differences between the groups as an increased hazard of death at early times followed by a decreased hazard later.

Multiple-failure data

If you simply type `stci` with multiple-failure data, the reported survival time is the survival time to the first failure, assuming that the hazard function is not indexed by number of failures.

Here we have some multiple-failure data:

```
. use http://www.stata-press.com/data/r10/mfail2

. st
-> stset t, id(id) failure(d) time0(t0) exit(time .) noshow
                id:  id
     failure event:  d != 0 & d < .
  obs. time interval:  (t0, t]
   exit on or before:  time .

. stci
```

	no. of subjects	50%	Std. Err.	[95% Conf. Interval]	
total	926	420	13.42537	394	451

To understand this output, let's also obtain output for each failure separately:

```
. stgen nf = nfailures()

. stci, by(nf)
```

nf	no. of subjects	50%	Std. Err.	[95% Conf. Interval]	
0	926	399	11.50173	381	430
1	529	503	13.68105	425	543
2	221	687	16.83127	549	817
3	58	.	.	.	.
total	926	420	13.42537	394	451

The `stgen` command added, for each subject, a variable containing the number of previous failures. `nf` is 0 for a subject, up to and including the first failure. Then `nf` is 1 up to and including the second failure, and then it is 2, and so on; see [ST] **stgen**.

The first line, corresponding to `nf = 0`, states that among those who had experienced no failures yet, the median time to first failure is 399.

Similarly, the second line, corresponding to `nf = 1`, is for those who have already experienced one failure. The median time of second failures is 503.

When we simply typed `stci`, we obtained the same information shown as the total line of the more detailed output. The total survival time distribution is an estimate of the distribution of the time to first failure, assuming that the hazard function $h(t)$ is the same across failures—that the second failure is no different from the first failure. This is an odd definition of *same* because the clock t is not reset in $h(t)$ upon failure. The hazard of a failure—any failure—at time t is $h(t)$.

Another definition of *same* would have it that the hazard of a failure is given by $h(\tau)$, where τ is the time since the last failure—that the process resets itself. These definitions are different unless $h()$ is a constant function of t.

Let's examine this multiple-failure data, assuming that the process repeats itself. The key variables in this st data are `id`, `t0`, `t`, and `d`:

```
. st
-> stset t, id(id) failure(d) time0(t0) exit(time .) noshow
                 id:  id
      failure event:  d != 0 & d < .
  obs. time interval:  (t0, t]
   exit on or before:  time .
```

Our goal, for each subject, is to reset `t0` and `t` to 0 after every failure event. We must trick Stata, or at least trick `stset` because it will not let us set data where the same subject has multiple records summarizing the overlapping periods. The trick is create a new `id` variable that is different for every `id`–`nf` combination (remember, `nf` is the variable we previously created that records the number of prior failures). Then each of the "new" subjects can have their clock start at time 0:

```
. egen newid = group(id nf)

. sort newid t

. by newid: replace t = t - t0[1]
(808 real changes made)

. by newid: generate newt0 = t0 - t0[1]

. stset t, failure(d) id(newid) time0(newt0)
                 id:  newid
      failure event:  d != 0 & d < .
  obs. time interval:  (newt0, t]
   exit on or before:  failure

      1734  total obs.
         0  exclusions

      1734  obs. remaining, representing
      1734  subjects
       808  failures in single failure-per-subject data
    435444  total analysis time at risk, at risk from t =         0
                             earliest observed entry t =         0
                               last observed exit t =          797
```

`stset` no longer thinks that we have multiple-failure data. Whereas with `id`, subjects had multiple failures, `newid` gives a unique identity to each `id`–`nf` combination. Each "new" subject has at most one failure.

```
. stci, by(nf)
          failure _d:  d
    analysis time _t:  t
                 id:  newid
```

nf	no. of subjects	50%	Std. Err.	[95% Conf. Interval]	
0	926	399	11.22457	381	430
1	529	384	9.16775	359	431
2	221	444	7.406977	325	515
3	58	.	.	.	.
total	1734	404	10.29992	386	430

Compare this table with the one we previously obtained. The number of subjects is the same, but the survival times differ because now we measure the times from one failure to the next, whereas previously we measured the time from a fixed point. The time between events in these data appears to be independent of event number.

Similarly, we can obtain the mean survival time for these data restricted to the longest follow-up time:

```
. stci, rmean by(nf)
        failure _d:  d
   analysis time _t:  t
                id:  newid
```

nf	no. of subjects	restricted mean	Std. Err.	[95% Conf. Interval]	
0	926	399.1802	8.872794	381.79	416.571
1	529	397.0077(*)	13.36058	370.821	423.194
2	221	397.8051(*)	25.78559	347.266	448.344
3	58	471(*)	0	471	471
total	1734	404.7006	7.021657	390.938	418.463

(*) largest observed analysis time is censored, mean is underestimated.

Saved Results

stci saves the following in r():

Scalars

r(N_sub)	number of subjects	r(se)	standard error
r(p#)	#th percentile	r(lb)	lower bound of CI
r(rmean)	restricted mean	r(ub)	upper bound of CI
r(emean)	extended mean		

Methods and Formulas

stci is implemented as an ado-file.

The percentiles of survival times are obtained from $S(t)$, the Kaplan–Meier product-limit estimate of the survivor function. The 25th percentile, for instance, is obtained as the minimum value of t such that $S(t) \leq .75$. The restricted mean is obtained as the area under the Kaplan–Meier product-limit survivor curve. The extended mean is obtained by extending the Kaplan–Meier product-limit survivor curve to zero by using an exponentially fitted curve and then computing the area under the entire curve. If the longest follow-up time ends in failure, the Kaplan–Meier product-limit survivor curve goes to zero, and the restricted mean and extended mean are identical.

The large-sample standard error for the pth percentile of the distribution is given by Collett (2003, 35) and Klein and Moeschberger (2003, 122) as

$$\frac{\sqrt{\widehat{g}}}{\widehat{f}(t_p)}$$

where $\widehat{g}$ is the Greenwood pointwise standard error estimate for $\widehat{S}(t_p)$ and $\widehat{f}(t_p)$ is the estimated density function at the pth percentile.

Confidence intervals, however, are not calculated based on this standard error. For a given confidence level, the upper confidence limit for the pth percentile is defined as the first time at which the upper confidence limit for $S(t)$ (based on a $\ln\{-\ln S(t)\}$ transformation) is less than or equal to $1 - p/100$, and similarly, the lower confidence limit is defined as the first time at which the lower confidence limit of $S(t)$ is less than or equal to $1 - p/100$.

The restricted mean is obtained as the area under the Kaplan–Meier product-limit survivor curve. The extended mean is obtained by extending the Kaplan–Meier product-limit survivor curve to zero by using an exponentially fitted curve and then computing the area under the entire curve. If the longest follow-up time ends in failure, the Kaplan–Meier product-limit survivor curve goes to zero, and the restricted mean and the extended mean are identical.

The standard error for the estimated restricted mean is computed as given by Klein and Moeschberger (2003, 118) and Collett (2003, 340):

$$\widehat{SE} = \sum_{i=1}^{D} \widehat{A}_i \sqrt{\frac{d_i}{R_i(R_i - d_i)}}$$

where the sum is over all distinct failure times, $\widehat{A}_i$ is the estimated area under the curve from time i to the maximum follow-up time, R_i is the number of subjects at risk at time i, and d_i is the number of failures at time i.

The $100(1 - \alpha)\%$ confidence interval for the estimated restricted mean is computed as

$$\widehat{A}_i \pm Z_{1-\alpha/2}\widehat{SE}$$

References

Collett, D. 2003. *Modelling Survival Data in Medical Research.* 2nd ed. London: Chapman & Hall/CRC.

Klein, J. P., and M. L. Moeschberger. 2003. *Survival Analysis: Techniques for Censored and Truncated Data.* 2nd ed. New York: Springer.

Also See

[ST] **stdescribe** — Describe survival-time data

[ST] **stir** — Report incidence-rate comparison

[ST] **sts** — Generate, graph, list, and test the survivor and cumulative hazard functions

[ST] **stset** — Declare data to be survival-time data

[ST] **stvary** — Report whether variables vary over time

[ST] **stptime** — Calculate person-time, incidence rates, and SMR

Title

> **stcox** — Fit Cox proportional hazards model

Syntax

stcox [*varlist*] [*if*] [*in*] [, *options*]

options	description
Model	
<u>esti</u>mate	fit model without covariates
<u>stra</u>ta(*varnames*)	strata ID variables
<u>shar</u>ed(*varname*)	shared-frailty ID variable
<u>off</u>set(*varname*)	include *varname* in model with coefficient constrained to 1
<u>bres</u>low	use Breslow method to handle tied failures; the default
<u>efr</u>on	use Efron method to handle tied failures
exactm	use exact marginal-likelihood method to handle tied failures
exactp	use exact partial-likelihood method to handle tied failures
Time varying	
tvc(*varlist*)	time-varying covariates
texp(*exp*)	multiplier for time-varying covariates; default is texp(_t)
SE/Robust	
vce(*vcetype*)	*vcetype* may be oim, <u>r</u>obust, <u>cl</u>uster *clustvar*, <u>boot</u>strap, or <u>jack</u>knife
<u>noadj</u>ust	do not use standard degree-of-freedom adjustment
Reporting	
<u>l</u>evel(*#*)	set confidence level; default is level(95)
nohr	report coefficients, not hazard ratios
<u>nosh</u>ow	do not show st setting information
Reporting 2	
<u>mga</u>le(*newvar*)	create *newvar* containing partial martingale residuals
<u>basech</u>azard(*newvar*)	create *newvar* containing cumulative baseline hazard
basehc(*newvar*)	create *newvar* containing baseline hazard contributions
<u>basesur</u>v(*newvar*)	create *newvar* containing baseline survivor function
<u>eff</u>ects(*newvar*)	create *newvar* containing estimated log-frailties
esr(*newvars*)	create *newvars* containing partial efficient score residuals
<u>schoenf</u>eld(*newvars*)	create *newvars* containing Schoenfeld residuals
<u>scaledsch</u>(*newvars*)	create *newvars* containing scaled Schoenfeld residuals
Max options	
maximize_options	control the maximization process; seldom used

You must stset your data before using stcox; see [ST] **stset**.

bootstrap, by, jackknife, nestreg, statsby, stepwise, svy, and xi are allowed; see [U] **11.1.10 Prefix commands**.

estimate, shared(), efron, exactm, exactp, vce(), and noadjust are not allowed with the svy prefix.

fweights, iweights, and pweights may be specified using stset; see [ST] **stset**. However, weights may not be specified if you are using the bootstrap prefix with the stcox command.

See [U] **20 Estimation and postestimation commands** for more capabilities of estimation commands.

Description

stcox fits, via maximum likelihood, proportional hazards models on st data. stcox can be used with single- or multiple-record or single- or multiple-failure st data.

Options for stcox

    | Model |

estimate forces fitting of the null model. All Stata estimation commands redisplay results when the command name is typed without arguments. So does stcox. What if you wish to fit a Cox model on $x_j b$, where $x_j b$ is defined as 0? Logic says that you would type stcox. There are no explanatory variables, so there is nothing to type after the command. Unfortunately, stcox looks the same as stcox typed without arguments, which is a request to redisplay results.

To fit the null model, type stcox, estimate.

strata(*varnames*) specifies up to five strata variables. Observations with equal values of the strata variables are assumed to be in the same stratum. Stratified estimates (equal coefficients across strata but with baseline hazard unique to each stratum) are then obtained.

shared(*varname*) specifies that a Cox model with shared frailty be fitted. Observations with equal value of *varname* are assumed to have shared (the same) frailty. Across groups, the frailties are assumed to be gamma-distributed latent random effects that affect the hazard multiplicatively, or, equivalently, the logarithm of the frailty enters the linear predictor as a random offset. Think of a shared-frailty model as a Cox model for panel data. *varname* is a variable in the data that identifies the groups.

Shared-frailty models are discussed more in *Cox regression with shared frailty*.

offset(*varname*); see [ST] **estimation options**.

breslow, efron, exactm, and exactp specify the method for handling tied failures in the calculation of the log partial likelihood (and residuals). breslow is the default. Each method is described in the *Methods and Formulas* section below. efron and the exact methods require substantially more computer time than the default breslow option. exactm and exactp may not be specified with tvc(), vce(robust), or vce(cluster *clustvar*).

    | Time varying |

tvc(*varlist*) specifies those variables that vary continuously with respect to time, i.e., time-varying covariates. This is a convenience option used to speed up calculations and to avoid having to stsplit the data over many failure times.

texp(*exp*) is used in conjunction with tvc(*varlist*) to specify the function of analysis time that should be multiplied by the time-varying covariates. For example, specifying texp(ln(_t)) would cause the time-varying covariates to be multiplied by the logarithm of analysis time. If tvc(*varlist*) is used without texp(*exp*), Stata understands that you mean texp(_t) and thus multiplies the time-varying covariates by the analysis time.

Both tvc(*varlist*) and texp(*exp*) are explained more in the section on *Cox regression with continuously time-varying covariates* below.

┌─ SE/Robust ──

vce(*vcetype*) specifies the type of standard error reported, which includes types that are derived from asymptotic theory, that are robust to some kinds of misspecification, that allow for intragroup correlation, and that use bootstrap or jackknife methods; see [R] *vce_option*.

noadjust is for use with vce(robust) or vce(cluster *clustvar*). noadjust prevents the estimated variance matrix from being multiplied by $N/(N-1)$ or $g/(g-1)$, where g is the number of clusters. The default adjustment is somewhat arbitrary because it is not always clear how to count observations or clusters. In such cases, however, the adjustment is likely to be biased toward 1, so we would still recommend making it.

┌─ Reporting ──

level(*#*); see [ST] **estimation options**.

nohr specifies that coefficients be displayed rather than exponentiated coefficients or hazard ratios. This option affects only how results are displayed and not how they are estimated. nohr may be specified at estimation time or when redisplaying previously estimated results (which you do by typing stcox without a variable list).

noshow prevents stcox from showing the key st variables. This option is seldom used since most people type stset, show or stset, noshow to set whether they want to see these variables mentioned at the top of the output of every st command; see [ST] **stset**.

┌─ Reporting 2 ──

mgale(*newvar*) adds *newvar* containing the partial martingale residuals, which are fully described in *Methods and Formulas*. If each observation in your data represents a different subject (single-record-per-subject data), the partial martingale residuals are the martingale residuals.

If you have data with multiple records per subject, the value that mgale() stores in each observation is the observation's contribution to the martingale residual, and these partial residuals can be summed within id() to obtain the subject's martingale residual. Say that you specify mgale(pmr) and that you have previously stset, id(patid). Then egen mr = total(pmr), by(patid) would create the martingale residuals.

basechazard(*newvar*) adds *newvar* to the data containing the estimated cumulative baseline hazard. If strata() is also specified, cumulative baseline estimates for each stratum are provided.

basehc(*newvar*) adds *newvar* to the data containing the estimated baseline hazard contributions as described by Kalbfleisch and Prentice (2002, 115). These are used to construct the product-limit type estimator for the baseline survivor function generated by basesurv(). If strata() is also specified, baseline estimates for each stratum are provided.

basesurv(*newvar*) adds *newvar* to the data containing the estimated baseline survivor function. In the null model, this is equivalent to the Kaplan–Meier product-limit estimate. If strata() is also specified, baseline estimates for each stratum are provided.

effects(*newvar*) is for use with shared() and creates *newvar* containing estimates of the log-frailty for each group. The log-frailties are random group-specific offsets to the linear predictor that measure the group effect on the log-relative hazard.

esr(*newvars*) adds *newvars* containing the partial efficient score residuals; see *Methods and Formulas*. If each observation in your data represents a different subject (single-record-per-subject data), the partial efficient score residuals are the efficient score residuals.

If you have data with multiple records per subject, the values esr() stores are each observation's contribution to the score residuals, and these partial residuals can be summed within id() to form the subject's efficient score residuals. This could be accomplished as noted under mgale() above.

One efficient score residual variable is created for each regressor in the model; the first new variable corresponds to the first regressor, the second to the second, and so on.

schoenfeld(*newvars*) adds *newvars* containing the Schoenfeld residuals; see *Methods and Formulas*. This option may not be used with the exactm and exactp options. Schoenfeld residuals are calculated and reported only at failure times.

One Schoenfeld residual variable is created for each regressor in the model; the first new variable corresponds to the first regressor, the second to the second, and so on.

scaledsch(*newvars*) adds *newvars* containing the scaled Schoenfeld residuals; see *Methods and Formulas*. This option may not be used with the exactm or exactp options. Scaled Schoenfeld residuals are calculated and reported only at failure times.

One scaled Schoenfeld residual variable is created for each regressor in the model; the first new variable corresponds to the first regressor, the second to the second, and so on.

Note: the easiest way to specify the preceding three options is, for example, esr(*stub**), where *stub* is a short name of your choosing. Stata then creates variables *stub*1, *stub*2, etc. You may also specify each variable explicitly, in which case there must be as many (and no more) variables specified in esr() as regressors in the model.

However, be aware that stcox will drop variables from the model because of collinearity. This is a desirable feature. A side effect is that the score residual variable, the Schoenfeld residual variable, and the scaled Schoenfeld residual variable may not align with the regressors in the way you expect. Say that you fit a model by typing

    . stcox x1 x2 x3, esr(r1 r2 r3)

Usually, r1 will contain the residual associated with x1, r2 the residual associated with x2, etc.

Now assume that x2 is dropped because of collinearity. Then r1 will correspond to x1, r2 to x3, and r3 will contain 0. This happens because, after the collinear variables are omitted, there are only two variables in the model: x1 and x3.

⌐ Max options ⌐

maximize_options: <u>iter</u>ate(*#*), [<u>no</u>]<u>log</u>, <u>tr</u>ace, <u>tol</u>erance(*#*), <u>ltol</u>erance(*#*), see [R] **maximize**. These options are seldom used.

(Continued on next page)

Remarks

Remarks are presented under the following headings:

Cox regression with uncensored data
Cox regression with censored data
Treatment of tied failure times
Cox regression with discrete time-varying covariates
Cox regression with continuous time-varying covariates
Robust estimate of variance
Cox regression with multiple-failure data
Stratified estimation
Cox regression with shared frailty
Obtaining baseline function estimates

What follows is a summary of what can be done with `stcox`. For a complete tutorial, see Cleves, Gould, and Gutierrez (2004), which devotes three chapters to this topic.

In the Cox proportional hazards model, the hazard is assumed to be

$$h(t) = h_0(t) \exp(\beta_1 x_1 + \cdots + \beta_k x_k)$$

The Cox model provides estimates of $\beta_1, \ldots, \beta_k$ but provides no direct estimate of $h_0(t)$—the baseline hazard. Formally, the function $h_0(t)$ is not directly estimated, but it is possible to recover an estimate of the cumulative hazard $H_0(t)$ and, from that, an estimate of the baseline survivor function $S_0(t)$.

`stcox` fits the Cox proportional hazards model; that is, it provides estimates of β and its variance–covariance matrix.

`stcox, basehc(`*newvar*`)` fits the Cox proportional hazards model and calculates the set of baseline hazard contributions used to estimate the baseline survivor function $S_0(t)$.

`stcox, basechazard(`*newvar*`)` fits the Cox proportional hazards model and estimates the cumulative baseline hazard function $H_0(t)$.

`stcox, basesurv(`*newvar*`)` fits the Cox model and estimates the baseline survivor function $S_0(t)$.

The three baseline options may also be used in combination to concurrently produce estimates of their respective functions. Also, `stcox` with the `strata()` option will produce stratified Cox regression estimates. In the stratified estimator, the hazard at time t for a subject in group i is assumed to be

$$h_i(t) = h_{0i}(t) \exp(\beta_1 x_1 + \cdots + \beta_k x_k)$$

That is, the coefficients are assumed to be the same, regardless of group, but the baseline hazard can be group specific. If you specify the `strata()` option, the baseline options produce the group-specific estimates of the baseline functions.

Whether or not you specify `strata()`, `stcox` can produce either of two variance estimators for β. The default is to calculate the conventional, inverse matrix of negative second derivatives. The theoretical justification for this estimator is based on likelihood theory.

The `vce(robust)` option instead switches to the robust measure developed by Lin and Wei (1989). This variance estimator is a variant of the estimator discussed in [U] **20.15 Obtaining robust variance estimates**.

Finally, `stcox`, with the `shared()` option, fits a Cox model with shared frailty. A *frailty* is a group-specific latent random effect that multiplies into the hazard function. The distribution of the frailties is gamma with mean one and variance to be estimated by the data. Shared-frailty models are used to model within-group correlation (observations within a group are correlated because they share the same frailty).

We give examples below with uncensored, censored, time-varying, and recurring failure data, but it does not matter in terms of what you type. Once you have `stset` your data, to fit a model you type `stcox` followed by the names of the explanatory variables. You do this whether your dataset has single or multiple records, includes censored observations or delayed entry, or even has single or multiple failures. You use `stset` to describe the properties of the data, and then that information is available to `stcox`—and all the other st commands—so that you do not have to specify it again.

Cox regression with uncensored data

▷ Example 1

We wish to analyze an experiment testing the ability of emergency generators with a new-style bearing to withstand overloads. For this experiment, the overload protection circuit was disabled, and the generators were run overloaded until they burned up. Here are our data:

```
. use http://www.stata-press.com/data/r10/kva
(Generator experiment)

. list
```

	failtime	load	bearings
1.	100	15	0
2.	140	15	1
3.	97	20	0
4.	122	20	1
5.	84	25	0
6.	100	25	1
7.	54	30	0
8.	52	30	1
9.	40	35	0
10.	55	35	1
11.	22	40	0
12.	30	40	1

Twelve generators, half with the new-style bearings and half with the old, were allocated to this destructive test. The first observation reflects an old-style generator (`bearings = 0`) under a 15-kVA overload. It stopped functioning after 100 hours. The second generator had new-style bearings (`bearings = 1`) and, under the same overload condition, lasted 140 hours. Paired experiments were also performed under overloads of 20, 25, 30, 35, and 40 kVA.

We wish to fit a Cox proportional hazards model in which the failure rate depends on the amount of overload and the style of the bearings. That is, we assume that `bearings` and `load` do not affect the shape of the overall hazard function, but they do affect the relative risk of failure. To fit this model, we type

(Continued on next page)

```
. stset failtime
 (output omitted )
. stcox load bearings
         failure _d:  1 (meaning all fail)
   analysis time _t:  failtime
Iteration 0:   log likelihood = -20.274897
Iteration 1:   log likelihood = -10.515114
Iteration 2:   log likelihood = -8.8700259
Iteration 3:   log likelihood = -8.5915211
Iteration 4:   log likelihood = -8.5778991
Iteration 5:   log likelihood =  -8.577853
Refining estimates:
Iteration 0:   log likelihood =  -8.577853
Cox regression -- Breslow method for ties
No. of subjects =             12                 Number of obs   =          12
No. of failures =             12
Time at risk    =            896
                                                 LR chi2(2)      =       23.39
Log likelihood  =    -8.577853                   Prob > chi2     =      0.0000
```

_t	Haz. Ratio	Std. Err.	z	P>|z|	[95% Conf. Interval]	
load	1.52647	.2188172	2.95	0.003	1.152576	2.021653
bearings	.0636433	.0746609	-2.35	0.019	.0063855	.6343223

We find that after controlling for overload, the new-style bearings result in a lower hazard and therefore a longer survivor time.

Once an `stcox` model has been fitted, typing `stcox` without arguments redisplays the previous results. Options that affect the display, such as `nohr`—which requests that coefficients rather than hazard ratios be displayed—can be specified upon estimation or when results are redisplayed:

```
. stcox, nohr
Cox regression -- Breslow method for ties
No. of subjects =             12                 Number of obs   =          12
No. of failures =             12
Time at risk    =            896
                                                 LR chi2(2)      =       23.39
Log likelihood  =    -8.577853                   Prob > chi2     =      0.0000
```

_t	Coef.	Std. Err.	z	P>|z|	[95% Conf. Interval]	
load	.4229578	.1433485	2.95	0.003	.1419999	.7039157
bearings	-2.754461	1.173115	-2.35	0.019	-5.053723	-.4551981

◁

❑ Technical Note

   `stcox`'s iteration log looks like a standard Stata iteration log right up to the point where it says "Refining estimates". The Cox proportional hazards likelihood function is indeed a difficult function, both conceptually and numerically. Until Stata says "Refining estimates", it maximizes the Cox likelihood in the standard way using double-precision arithmetic. Then just to be sure that the answers are accurate, Stata switches to quad-precision routines (double double precision) and completes the maximization procedure from its current location on the likelihood.

❑

Cox regression with censored data

▷ Example 2

We have data on 48 participants in a cancer drug trial. Of these 48, 28 receive treatment (drug = 1) and 20 receive a placebo (drug = 0). The participants range in age from 47 to 67 years. We wish to analyze time until death, measured in months. Our data include 1 observation for each patient. The variable studytime records either the month of their death or the last month that they were known to be alive. Some of the patients still live, so together with studytime is died, indicating their health status. Persons known to have died—"noncensored" in the jargon—have died = 1, whereas the patients who are still alive—"right-censored" in the jargon—have died = 0.

Here is an overview of our data:

```
. use http://www.stata-press.com/data/r10/drugtr
(Patient Survival in Drug Trial)

. st
-> stset studytime, failure(died)

      failure event:  died != 0 & died < .
  obs. time interval:  (0, studytime]
 exit on or before:  failure

. summarize
```

Variable	Obs	Mean	Std. Dev.	Min	Max
studytime	48	15.5	10.25629	1	39
died	48	.6458333	.4833211	0	1
drug	48	.5833333	.4982238	0	1
age	48	55.875	5.659205	47	67
_st	48	1	0	1	1
_d	48	.6458333	.4833211	0	1
_t	48	15.5	10.25629	1	39
_t0	48	0	0	0	0

We typed stset studytime, failure(died) previously; that is how st knew about this dataset. To fit the Cox model, we type

```
. stcox drug age

        failure _d:  died
   analysis time _t:  studytime

Iteration 0:   log likelihood = -99.911448
Iteration 1:   log likelihood = -83.551879
Iteration 2:   log likelihood = -83.324009
Iteration 3:   log likelihood = -83.323546
Refining estimates:
Iteration 0:   log likelihood = -83.323546

Cox regression -- Breslow method for ties

No. of subjects =          48          Number of obs   =          48
No. of failures =          31
Time at risk    =         744
                                        LR chi2(2)      =       33.18
Log likelihood  =    -83.323546         Prob > chi2     =      0.0000
```

_t	Haz. Ratio	Std. Err.	z	P>|z|	[95% Conf. Interval]
drug	.1048772	.0477017	-4.96	0.000	.0430057	.2557622
age	1.120325	.0417711	3.05	0.002	1.041375	1.20526

We find that the drug results in a lower hazard—and therefore a longer survivor time—controlling for age. Older patients are more likely to die. The model as a whole is statistically significant.

The hazard ratios reported correspond to a one-unit change in the corresponding variable. It is more typical to report relative risk for 5-year changes in age. To obtain such a hazard ratio, we create a new age variable such that a one-unit change indicates a 5-year change:

```
. replace age = age/5
age was int now float
(48 real changes made)

. stcox drug age, nolog

        failure _d:  died
    analysis time _t:  studytime

Cox regression -- Breslow method for ties

No. of subjects =           48                  Number of obs   =         48
No. of failures =           31
Time at risk    =          744
                                                LR chi2(2)      =      33.18
Log likelihood  =    -83.323544                 Prob > chi2     =     0.0000
```

_t	Haz. Ratio	Std. Err.	z	P>|z|	[95% Conf. Interval]	
drug	.1048772	.0477017	-4.96	0.000	.0430057	.2557622
age	1.764898	.3290196	3.05	0.002	1.224715	2.543338

◁

Treatment of tied failure times

The proportional hazards model assumes that the hazard function is continuous and, thus, that there are no tied survival times. Because of the way that time is recorded, however, tied events do occur in survival data. In such cases, the partial likelihood must be modified. See *Methods and Formulas* for more details on the methods described below.

Stata provides four methods for handling tied failures in calculating the Cox partial likelihood through the options breslow, efron, exactm, and exactp. If there are no ties in the data, the results are identical, regardless of the method selected.

When there are tied failure times, we must decide how to calculate the risk pools for these tied observations. Assume that there are 2 observations that fail in succession. In the calculation involving the second observation, the first observation is not in the risk pool since failure has already occurred. If the 2 observations have the same failure time, we must decide how to calculate the risk pool for the second observation and in which order to calculate the two observations.

There are two views of time. In the first, time is continuous, so ties should not occur. If they have occurred, the likelihood reflects the marginal probability that the tied-failure events occurred before the nonfailure events in the risk pool (the order that they occurred is not important). This is called the exact marginal likelihood (option exactm).

In the second view, time is discrete, so ties are expected. The likelihood is changed to reflect this discreteness and calculates the conditional probability that the observed failures are those that fail in the risk pool given the observed number of failures. This is called the exact partial likelihood (option exactp).

Let's assume that there are five subjects—e_1, e_2, e_3, e_4, e_5—in the risk pool and that subjects e_1 and e_2 fail. Had we been able to observe the events at a better resolution, we might have seen that e_1 failed from risk pool $e_1 + e_2 + e_3 + e_4 + e_5$ and then e_2 failed from risk pool $e_2 + e_3 + e_4 + e_5$. Alternatively, e_2 might have failed first from risk pool $e_1 + e_2 + e_3 + e_4 + e_5$, and then e_1 failed from risk pool $e_1 + e_3 + e_4 + e_5$.

The Breslow method (option `breslow`) for handling tied values simply says that since we do not know the order, we will use the largest risk pool for each tied failure event. This method assumes that both e_1 and e_2 failed from risk pool $e_1 + e_2 + e_3 + e_4 + e_5$. This approximation is fast and is the default method for handling ties. If there are many ties in the dataset, this approximation will not be accurate since the risk pools include too many observations. The Breslow method is an approximation of the exact marginal likelihood.

The Efron method (option `efron`) for handling tied values assumes that the first risk pool is $e_1 + e_2 + e_3 + e_4 + e_5$ and the second risk pool is either $e_2 + e_3 + e_4 + e_5$ or $e_1 + e_3 + e_4 + e_5$. From this, Efron noted that the e_1 and e_2 terms were in the second risk pool with probability 1/2 and so used for the second risk pool $.5(e_1 + e_2) + e_3 + e_4 + e_5$. Efron's approximation is a more accurate approximation of the exact marginal likelihood than Breslow's but takes longer to calculate.

The exact marginal method (option `exactm`) is a misnomer in that the calculation performed is also an *approximation* of the exact marginal likelihood. It is an approximation because it evaluates the likelihood (and derivatives) by using 15-point Gauss–Laguerre quadrature. For small-to-moderate samples, this is slower than the Efron approximation, but the difference in execution time diminishes when samples become larger. You may want to consider the quadrature when deciding to use this method. If the number of tied deaths is large (on average), the quadrature approximation of the function is not well behaved. A little empirical checking suggests that if the number of tied deaths is larger (on average) than 30, the quadrature does not approximate the function well.

When we view time as discrete, the exact partial method (option `exactp`) is the final method available. This approach is equivalent to computing conditional logistic regression where the groups are defined by the risk sets and the outcome is given by the death variable. This is the slowest method to use and can take a significant amount of time if the risk sets and the number of tied failures are large.

Cox regression with discrete time-varying covariates

In [ST] **stset**, we introduce the Stanford heart transplant data in which there are one or two records per patient depending on whether they received a new heart.

This dataset (Crowley and Hu 1977) consists of 103 patients admitted to the Stanford Heart Transplantation Program. Patients were admitted into the program after review by a committee and then waited for an available donor heart. While waiting, some patients died or were transferred out of the program, but 67% received a transplant. The dataset includes the year the patient was accepted into the program along with the patient's age, whether the patient had other heart surgery previously, and whether the patient received a transplant.

In the data, `posttran` becomes 1 when a patient receives a new heart, so it is a time-varying covariate. That does not affect what we type to fit the model:

```
. use http://www.stata-press.com/data/r10/stan3, clear
(Heart transplant data)
. stset t1, failure(died) id(id)
 (output omitted )
```

```
. stcox age posttran surg year
        failure _d:  died
   analysis time _t:  t1
              id:  id
Iteration 0:   log likelihood = -298.31514
Iteration 1:   log likelihood =  -289.7344
Iteration 2:   log likelihood = -289.53498
Iteration 3:   log likelihood = -289.53378
Iteration 4:   log likelihood = -289.53378
Refining estimates:
Iteration 0:   log likelihood = -289.53378
Cox regression -- Breslow method for ties
No. of subjects =          103              Number of obs    =         172
No. of failures =           75
Time at risk    =      31938.1
                                            LR chi2(4)       =       17.56
Log likelihood  =    -289.53378             Prob > chi2      =      0.0015
```

_t	Haz. Ratio	Std. Err.	z	P>|z|	[95% Conf. Interval]	
age	1.030224	.0143201	2.14	0.032	1.002536	1.058677
posttran	.9787243	.3032597	-0.07	0.945	.5332291	1.796416
surgery	.3738278	.163204	-2.25	0.024	.1588759	.8796
year	.8873107	.059808	-1.77	0.076	.7775022	1.012628

We find that older patients have higher hazards, that patients tend to do better over time, and that patients with prior surgery do better. Whether a patient ultimately receives a transplant does not seem to make much difference.

Cox regression with continuous time-varying covariates

The basic proportional hazards regression assumes the relationship

$$h(t) = h_0(t) \exp(\beta_1 x_1 + \cdots + \beta_k x_k)$$

where $h_0(t)$ is the baseline hazard function. For most purposes this model is sufficient, but sometimes we may wish to introduce variables of the form $z_i(t) = z_i g(t)$, which vary continuously with time so that

$$h(t) = h_0(t) \exp \{\beta_1 x_1 + \cdots + \beta_k x_k + g(t)(\gamma_1 z_1 + \cdots + \gamma_m z_m)\}$$

where $(z_1, \ldots, z_m)$ are the time-varying covariates and where estimation has the net effect of estimating, say, a regression coefficient γ_i for a covariate $g(t)z_i$, which is a function of the current time.

The time-varying covariates $(z_1, \ldots, z_m)$ are specified using the tvc(*varlist*) option, and $g(t)$ is specified using the texp(*exp*) option, where t in $g(t)$ is analysis time. For example, if we want $g(t) = \ln(t)$, we would use texp(ln(_t)) since _t stores the analysis time once the data are stset.

Since the calculations in Cox regression concern themselves only with the times at which failures occur, the above results could also be achieved by stsplitting the data at the observed failure times and manually generating the time-varying covariates. When this is feasible, stsplit merely represents a more convenient way to accomplish this. However, for large datasets with many distinct failure times, using stsplit may produce datasets that are too large to fit in memory, and even if this were not so, the estimation would take far longer to complete. For these reasons, the options described above were introduced.

▷ Example 3

Consider a dataset consisting of 45 observations on recovery time from walking pneumonia. Recovery time (in days) is recorded in the variable time, and there are measurements on the covariates age, drug1, and drug2, where drug1 and drug2 interact a choice of treatment with initial dosage level. The study was terminated after 30 days, so those who had not recovered by that time were censored (cured = 0).

```
. use http://www.stata-press.com/data/r10/drugtr2
. list age drug1 drug2 time cured in 1/12, sep(0)
```

	age	drug1	drug2	time	cured
1.	36	0	50	20.6	1
2.	14	0	50	6.8	1
3.	43	0	125	8.6	1
4.	25	100	0	10	1
5.	50	100	0	30	0
6.	26	0	100	13.6	1
7.	21	150	0	5.4	1
8.	25	0	100	15.4	1
9.	32	125	0	8.6	1
10.	28	150	0	8.5	1
11.	34	0	100	30	0
12.	40	0	50	30	0

Patient 1 took 50 mg of drug number 2 and was cured after 20.6 days, whereas patient 5 took 100 mg of drug number 1 and had yet to recover when the study ended and so was censored at 30 days.

We run a standard Cox regression after stsetting the data.

```
. stset time, failure(cured)

     failure event:  cured != 0 & cured < .
obs. time interval:  (0, time]
 exit on or before:  failure
```
_____

```
    45  total obs.
     0  exclusions
```
_____

```
    45  obs. remaining, representing
    36  failures in single record/single failure data
 677.9  total analysis time at risk, at risk from t =          0
                            earliest observed entry t =        0
                             last observed exit t =           30
```

(Continued on next page)

```
. stcox age drug1 drug2

        failure _d:  cured
  analysis time _t:  time

Iteration 0:   log likelihood = -116.54385
Iteration 1:   log likelihood = -102.77311
Iteration 2:   log likelihood = -101.92794
Iteration 3:   log likelihood = -101.92504
Iteration 4:   log likelihood = -101.92504
Refining estimates:
Iteration 0:   log likelihood = -101.92504

Cox regression -- Breslow method for ties

No. of subjects =           45                    Number of obs   =          45
No. of failures =           36
Time at risk    =  677.9000034
                                                  LR chi2(3)      =       29.24
Log likelihood  =   -101.92504                    Prob > chi2     =      0.0000
```

_t	Haz. Ratio	Std. Err.	z	P>|z|	[95% Conf. Interval]	
age	.8759449	.0253259	-4.58	0.000	.8276873	.9270162
drug1	1.008482	.0043249	1.97	0.049	1.000041	1.016994
drug2	1.00189	.0047971	0.39	0.693	.9925323	1.011337

The output includes p-values for the tests of the null hypotheses that each regression coefficient is zero or, equivalently, that each hazard ratio is one. That all hazard ratios are apparently close to one is a matter of scale; however, we can see that drug number 1 significantly increases the risk of being cured and so is an effective drug, whereas drug number 2 is ineffective (given the presence of age and drug number 1 in the model).

Suppose now that we wish to fit a model in which we account for the effect that as time goes by, the actual level of the drug remaining in the body diminishes, say, at an exponential rate. If it is known that the half-life of both drugs is close to 2 days, we can say that the actual concentration level of the drug in the patient's blood is proportional to the initial dosage times $\exp(-0.35t)$, where t is analysis time. We now fit a model that reflects this change.

```
. stcox age, tvc(drug1 drug2) texp(exp(-0.35*_t)) nolog

        failure _d:  cured
  analysis time _t:  time

Cox regression -- Breslow method for ties

No. of subjects =           45                    Number of obs   =          45
No. of failures =           36
Time at risk    =  677.9000034
                                                  LR chi2(3)      =       36.98
Log likelihood  =   -98.052763                    Prob > chi2     =      0.0000
```

_t	Haz. Ratio	Std. Err.	z	P>|z|	[95% Conf. Interval]	
rh						
age	.8614636	.028558	-4.50	0.000	.8072706	.9192948
t						
drug1	1.304744	.1135967	3.06	0.002	1.100059	1.547514
drug2	1.200613	.1113218	1.97	0.049	1.001103	1.439882

Note: second equation contains variables that continuously vary with respect
      to time; variables are interacted with current values of exp(-0.35*_t).

The first equation, rh, reports the results (hazard ratios) for the covariates that do not vary over time; the second equation, t, reports the results for the time-varying covariates.

As the level of drug in the blood system decreases, the drug's effectiveness diminishes. Accounting for this serves to unmask the effects of both drugs in that we now see increased effects on both. In fact, the effect on recovery time of drug number 2 now becomes significant.

❏ Technical Note

The interpretation of hazard ratios requires careful consideration here. For the first model, the hazard ratio for, say, drug1 is interpreted as the proportional change in hazard when the dosage level of drug1 is increased by one unit. For the second model, the hazard ratio for drug1 is the proportional change in hazard when the blood concentration level—i.e., $drug1*\exp(-0.35t)$—increases by one.

❏

Since the number of observations in our data is relatively small, for illustrative purposes we can stsplit the data at each recovery time, manually generate the blood concentration levels, and refit the second model.

```
. generate id=_n
. streset, id(id)
 (output omitted )
. stsplit, at(failures)
(31 failure times)
(812 observations (episodes) created)
. generate drug1emt = drug1*exp(-0.35*_t)
. generate drug2emt = drug2*exp(-0.35*_t)
. stcox age drug1emt drug2emt
         failure _d:  cured
   analysis time _t:  time
                 id:  id
Iteration 0:   log likelihood = -116.54385
Iteration 1:   log likelihood = -99.321912
Iteration 2:   log likelihood =  -98.07369
Iteration 3:   log likelihood =  -98.05277
Iteration 4:   log likelihood = -98.052763
Refining estimates:
Iteration 0:   log likelihood = -98.052763

Cox regression -- Breslow method for ties

No. of subjects =           45                  Number of obs   =        857
No. of failures =           36
Time at risk    =  677.9000034
                                                LR chi2(3)      =      36.98
Log likelihood  =   -98.052763                  Prob > chi2     =     0.0000
```

_t	Haz. Ratio	Std. Err.	z	P>|z|	[95% Conf. Interval]	
age	.8614636	.028558	-4.50	0.000	.8072706	.9192948
drug1emt	1.304744	.1135967	3.06	0.002	1.100059	1.547514
drug2emt	1.200613	.1113218	1.97	0.049	1.001103	1.439882

We get the same answer. However, this required more work both for Stata and for you.

◁

The full functionality of stcox is available with time-varying covariates, including the ability to generate residuals and baseline functions. The only exception is when the exactm or exactp options is specified for handling ties, in which case the tvc(*varlist*) option is currently not supported. You must then use the stsplit approach outlined above.

❏ Technical Note

Finally, specifying $g(t)$ via the texp(*exp*) option is intended for functions of analysis time, _t only, with the default being texp(_t) if left unspecified. However, specifying any other valid Stata expression will not produce a syntax error, yet usually will not yield the anticipated output. For example, specifying texp(*varname*) will not generate interaction terms. This has to do mainly with how the calculations are carried out—by careful summations over risk pools at each failure time.

❏

Robust estimate of variance

By default, stcox produces the conventional estimate for the variance–covariance matrix of the coefficients (and hence the reported standard errors). If, however, you specify the vce(robust) option, stcox switches to the robust variance estimator (Lin and Wei 1989).

The key to the robust calculation is using the efficient score residual for each subject in the data for the variance calculation. Even in simple single-record, single-failure survival data, the same subjects appear repeatedly in the risk pools, and the robust calculation tries to account for that.

▷ Example 4

Refitting the Stanford heart transplant data model with robust standard errors, we obtain

```
. use http://www.stata-press.com/data/r10/stan3, clear
(Heart transplant data)

. stset t1, failure(died) id(id)

                id:  id
     failure event:  died != 0 & died < .
obs. time interval:  (t1[_n-1], t1]
 exit on or before:  failure


       172  total obs.
         0  exclusions


       172  obs. remaining, representing
       103  subjects
        75  failures in single failure-per-subject data
   31938.1  total analysis time at risk, at risk from t =         0
                             earliest observed entry t =         0
                                  last observed exit t =      1799
```

```
. stcox age posttran surg year, vce(robust)

          failure _d:  died
    analysis time _t:  t1
                 id:  id

Iteration 0:   log pseudolikelihood = -298.31514
Iteration 1:   log pseudolikelihood =  -289.7344
Iteration 2:   log pseudolikelihood = -289.53498
Iteration 3:   log pseudolikelihood = -289.53378
Iteration 4:   log pseudolikelihood = -289.53378
Refining estimates:
Iteration 0:   log pseudolikelihood = -289.53378

Cox regression -- Breslow method for ties

No. of subjects    =          103            Number of obs   =        172
No. of failures    =           75
Time at risk       =      31938.1
                                             Wald chi2(4)    =      19.68
Log pseudolikelihood =   -289.53378          Prob > chi2     =     0.0006

                         (Std. Err. adjusted for 103 clusters in id)
```

_t	Haz. Ratio	Robust Std. Err.	z	P>|z|	[95% Conf. Interval]
age	1.030224	.0148771	2.06	0.039	1.001474 1.059799
posttran	.9787243	.2961736	-0.07	0.943	.5408498 1.771104
surgery	.3738278	.1304912	-2.82	0.005	.1886013 .7409665
year	.8873107	.0613176	-1.73	0.084	.7749139 1.01601

Note the word Robust above Std. Err. in the table and the phrase "Std. Err. adjusted for 103 clusters in id" above the table.

The hazard ratio estimates are the same as before, but the standard errors are slightly different.

◁

❑ Technical Note

In the previous example, stcox knew to specify vce(cluster id) for us when we specified vce(robust).

To see the importance of vce(cluster id), consider simple single-record, single-failure survival data, a piece of which is

```
   t0         t        died         x
    0         5          1          1
    0         9          0          1
    0         8          0          0
```

and then consider the absolutely equivalent multiple-record survival data:

```
   id        t0         t         died         x
    1         0         3          0          1
    1         3         5          1          1
    2         0         6          0          1
    2         6         9          0          1
    3         0         3          0          0
    3         3         8          0          0
```

Both datasets record the same underlying data, and so both should produce the same numerical results. This should be true whether or not vce(robust) is specified.

In the second dataset, were we to ignore id, it would appear that there are 6 observations on six subjects. The key ingredients in the robust calculation are the efficient score residuals, and viewing the data as 6 observations on six subjects produces different score residuals. Let us call the six score residuals $s_1, s_2, \ldots, s_6$ and the three score residuals that would be generated by the first dataset S_1, S_2, and S_3. $S_1 = s_1 + s_2$, $S_2 = s_3 + s_4$, and $S_3 = s_5 + s_6$.

That residuals sum is the key to understanding the vce(cluster *clustvar*) option. When you specify vce(cluster id), Stata makes the robust calculation based not on the overly detailed s_1, $s_2, \ldots, s_6$ but on $s_1 + s_2$, $s_3 + s_4$, and $s_5 + s_6$. That is, Stata sums residuals within clusters before entering them into subsequent calculations (where they are squared), so results estimated from the second dataset are equal to those estimated from the first. In more complicated datasets with time-varying regressors, delayed entry, and gaps, this action of summing within cluster, in effect, treats the cluster (which is typically a subject) as a unified whole.

Because we had stset an id() variable, stcox knew to specify vce(cluster id) for us when we specified vce(robust). You may, however, override the default clustering by specifying vce(cluster *clustvar*) with a different variable from the one you used in stset, id(). This is useful in analyzing multiple-failure data, where you need to stset a pseudo-ID establishing the time from the last failure as the onset of risk.

❑

Cox regression with multiple-failure data

In [ST] **stsum**, we introduce a multiple-failure dataset:

```
. use http://www.stata-press.com/data/r10/mfail
. stdescribe
```

Category	total		per subject		
		mean	min	median	max
no. of subjects	926				
no. of records	1734	1.87257	1	2	4
(first) entry time		0	0	0	0
(final) exit time		470.6857	1	477	960
subjects with gap	0				
time on gap if gap	0	.	.	.	.
time at risk	435855	470.6857	1	477	960
failures	808	.8725702	0	1	3

This dataset contains two variables—x1 and x2—which we believe affect the hazard of failure.

If we simply want to analyze these multiple-failure data as if the baseline hazard remains unchanged as events occur (that is, the hazard may change with time, but time is measured from 0 and is independent of when the last failure occurred), we can type

```
. stcox x1 x2, vce(robust)

Iteration 0:    log pseudolikelihood = -5034.9569
Iteration 1:    log pseudolikelihood = -4978.4198
Iteration 2:    log pseudolikelihood = -4978.1915
Iteration 3:    log pseudolikelihood = -4978.1914
Refining estimates:
Iteration 0:    log pseudolikelihood = -4978.1914

Cox regression -- Breslow method for ties

No. of subjects    =         926          Number of obs    =       1734
No. of failures    =         808
Time at risk       =      435855
                                          Wald chi2(2)     =     152.13
Log pseudolikelihood =   -4978.1914       Prob > chi2      =     0.0000

                           (Std. Err. adjusted for 926 clusters in id)
```

_t	Haz. Ratio	Robust Std. Err.	z	P>|z|	[95% Conf. Interval]	
x1	2.273456	.1868211	9.99	0.000	1.935259	2.670755
x2	.329011	.0523425	-6.99	0.000	.2408754	.4493951

We chose to fit this model with robust standard errors—we specified vce(robust)—but you can estimate conventional standard errors if you wish.

In [ST] **stsum**, we discuss analyzing this dataset as the time since last failure. We wished to assume that the hazard function remained unchanged with failure, except that one restarted the same hazard function. To that end, we made the following changes to our data:

```
. stgen nf = nfailures()

. egen newid = group(id nf)

. sort newid t

. by newid: replace t = t - t0[1]
(808 real changes made)

. by newid: gen newt0 = t0 - t0[1]

. stset t, id(newid) failure(d) time0(newt0) noshow
                id:  newid
     failure event:  d != 0 & d < .
obs. time interval:  (newt0, t]
 exit on or before:  failure


      1734  total obs.
         0  exclusions


      1734  obs. remaining, representing
      1734  subjects
       808  failures in single failure-per-subject data
    435444  total analysis time at risk, at risk from t =         0
                            earliest observed entry t =         0
                              last observed exit t =       797
```

That is, we took each subject and made many newid subjects out of each, with each subject entering at time 0 (now meaning the time of the last failure). id still identifies a real subject, but Stata thinks the identifier variable is newid because we stset, id(newid). If we were to fit a model with vce(robust), we would get

```
. stcox x1 x2, vce(robust) nolog

Cox regression -- Breslow method for ties

No. of subjects    =        1734          Number of obs    =        1734
No. of failures    =         808
Time at risk       =      435444
                                          Wald chi2(2)     =       88.51
Log pseudolikelihood =   -5062.5815       Prob > chi2      =      0.0000

                    (Std. Err. adjusted for 1734 clusters in newid)
```

		Robust				
_t	Haz. Ratio	Std. Err.	z	P>|z|	[95% Conf. Interval]	
x1	2.002547	.1936906	7.18	0.000	1.656733	2.420542
x2	.2946263	.0569167	-6.33	0.000	.2017595	.4302382

Note carefully the message concerning the clustering: standard errors have been adjusted for clustering on newid. We, however, want the standard errors adjusted for clustering on id, so we must specify the vce(cluster *clustvar*) option:

```
. stcox x1 x2, vce(cluster id) nolog

Cox regression -- Breslow method for ties

No. of subjects    =        1734          Number of obs    =        1734
No. of failures    =         808
Time at risk       =      435444
                                          Wald chi2(2)     =       93.66
Log pseudolikelihood =   -5062.5815       Prob > chi2      =      0.0000

                     (Std. Err. adjusted for 926 clusters in id)
```

		Robust				
_t	Haz. Ratio	Std. Err.	z	P>|z|	[95% Conf. Interval]	
x1	2.002547	.1920151	7.24	0.000	1.659452	2.416576
x2	.2946263	.0544625	-6.61	0.000	.2050806	.4232709

That is, if you are using vce(robust), you must remember to specify vce(cluster *clustvar*) for yourself when

1. you are analyzing multiple-failure data and

2. you have reset time to time since last failure, so what Stata considers the subjects are really subsubjects.

Stratified estimation

When you type

```
. stcox xvars, strata(svars)
```

you are allowing the baseline hazard functions to differ for the groups identified by *svars*. This is equivalent to fitting separate Cox proportional hazards models under the constraint that the coefficients are equal but not the baseline hazard functions.

▷ Example 5

Say that in the Stanford heart experiment data, there was a change in treatment for all patients, before and after transplant, in 1970 and then again in 1973. Further assume that the proportional-hazards assumption is not reasonable for these changes in treatment—perhaps the changes result in short-run benefit but little expected long-run benefit. Our interest in the data is not in the effect of these treatment changes but in the effect of transplantation, for which we still find the proportional-hazards assumption reasonable. We might fit our model to account for these fictional changes by typing

```
. use http://www.stata-press.com/data/r10/stan3, clear
(Heart transplant data)
. generate pgroup = year
. recode pgroup min/69=1 70/72=2 73/max=3
(pgroup: 172 changes made)
. stcox age posttran surg year, strata(pgroup) nolog
          failure _d:  died
    analysis time _t:  t1
                 id:  id
Stratified Cox regr. -- Breslow method for ties
No. of subjects =          103              Number of obs    =        172
No. of failures =           75
Time at risk     =      31938.1
                                            LR chi2(4)       =      20.67
Log likelihood   =    -213.35033            Prob > chi2      =     0.0004

         _t | Haz. Ratio   Std. Err.      z    P>|z|     [95% Conf. Interval]
------------+----------------------------------------------------------------
        age |  1.027406    .0150188     1.85   0.064     .9983874    1.057268
   posttran |  1.075476    .3354669     0.23   0.816      .583567    1.982034
    surgery |  .2222415    .1218386    -2.74   0.006     .0758882    .6508429
       year |  .5523966    .1132688    -2.89   0.004     .3695832     .825638

                                                    Stratified by pgroup
```

Of course, we could obtain the robust estimate of variance by also including the vce(robust) option.

◁

Cox regression with shared frailty

A shared-frailty model is the survival-data analog to regression models with random effects. A *frailty* is a latent random effect that enters multiplicatively on the hazard function. In a Cox model, the data are organized as $i = 1, \ldots, n$ groups with $j = 1, \ldots, n_i$ observations in group i. For the jth observation in the ith group, the hazard is

$$h_{ij}(t) = h_0(t)\alpha_i \exp(\mathbf{x}_{ij}\boldsymbol{\beta})$$

where α_i is the group-level frailty. The frailties are unobservable positive quantities and are assumed to have mean one and variance θ, to be estimated from the data. You can fit a Cox shared-frailty model by specifying shared(*varname*), where *varname* defines the groups over which frailties are shared. stcox, shared() treats the frailties as being gamma distributed, but this is mainly an issue of computational convenience; see *Methods and Formulas*. Theoretically, any distribution with positive support, mean one, and finite variance may be used to model frailty.

Shared-frailty models are used to model within-group correlation; observations within a group are correlated because they share the same frailty. The estimate of θ is used to measure the degree of within-group correlation, and the shared-frailty model reduces to standard Cox when $\theta = 0$.

For $\nu_i = \log\alpha_i$, the hazard can also be expressed as

$$h_{ij}(t) = h_0(t)\exp(\mathbf{x}_{ij}\boldsymbol{\beta} + \nu_i)$$

and thus the log-frailties, ν_i, are analogous to random effects in standard linear models. In fact, you can retrieve estimates of the ν_i by specifying effects(*newvar*).

▷ Example 6

Consider the data from a study of 38 kidney dialysis patients, as described in McGilchrist and Aisbett (1991). The study is concerned with the prevalence of infection at the catheter insertion point. Two recurrence times (in days) are measured for each patient, and each recorded time is the time from initial insertion (onset of risk) to infection or censoring.

```
. use http://www.stata-press.com/data/r10/catheter, clear
(Kidney data, McGilchrist and Aisbett, Biometrics, 1991)

. list patient time infect age female in 1/10
```

	patient	time	infect	age	female
1.	1	16	1	28	0
2.	1	8	1	28	0
3.	2	13	0	48	1
4.	2	23	1	48	1
5.	3	22	1	32	0
6.	3	28	1	32	0
7.	4	318	1	31.5	1
8.	4	447	1	31.5	1
9.	5	30	1	10	0
10.	5	12	1	10	0

Each patient (patient) has two recurrence times (time) recorded, with each catheter insertion resulting in either infection (infect==1) or right-censoring (infect==0). Among the covariates measured are age and sex (female==1 if female, female==0 if male).

One subtlety to note concerns the use of the generic term *subjects*. In this example, the subjects are taken to be the individual catheter insertions, not the patients themselves. This is a function of how the data were recorded—the onset of risk occurs at catheter insertion (of which there are two for each patient), and not (say) at the time of admission of the patient into the study. We therefore have two subjects (insertions) within each group (patient).

It is reasonable to assume independence of patients but unreasonable to assume that recurrence times within each patient are independent. One solution would be to fit a standard Cox model, adjusting the standard errors of the estimated hazard ratios to account for the possible correlation by specifying vce(cluster patient).

We could instead model the correlation by assuming that the correlation is the result of a latent patient-level effect, or frailty. That is, rather than fitting a standard model and specifying vce(cluster patient), we could fit a frailty model by specifying shared(patient).

```
. stset time, fail(infect)
(output omitted )
```

```
. stcox age female, shared(patient)

        failure _d:  infect
  analysis time _t:  time
```

Fitting comparison Cox model:

Estimating frailty variance:

```
Iteration 0:    log profile likelihood = -182.06713
Iteration 1:    log profile likelihood =  -181.9791
Iteration 2:    log profile likelihood = -181.97453
Iteration 3:    log profile likelihood = -181.97453
```

Fitting final Cox model:

```
Iteration 0:    log likelihood = -199.05599
Iteration 1:    log likelihood = -183.72296
Iteration 2:    log likelihood = -181.99509
Iteration 3:    log likelihood = -181.97455
Iteration 4:    log likelihood = -181.97453
Refining estimates:
Iteration 0:    log likelihood = -181.97453
```

```
Cox regression --
        Breslow method for ties          Number of obs     =       76
        Gamma shared frailty             Number of groups  =       38
Group variable: patient

No. of subjects =          76             Obs per group: min =        2
No. of failures =          58                            avg =        2
Time at risk    =        7424                            max =        2

                                          Wald chi2(2)      =    11.66
Log likelihood  =   -181.97453            Prob > chi2       =   0.0029
```

_t	Haz. Ratio	Std. Err.	z	P>|z|	[95% Conf. Interval]	
age	1.006202	.0120965	0.51	0.607	.9827701	1.030192
female	.2068678	.095708	-3.41	0.001	.0835376	.5122756
theta	.4754497	.2673108				

```
Likelihood-ratio test of theta=0: chibar2(01) =     6.27 Prob>=chibar2 = 0.006
Note: standard errors of hazard ratios are conditional on theta.
```

From the output, we obtain $\widehat{\theta} = 0.475$, and given the standard error of $\widehat{\theta}$ and likelihood-ratio test of H_0: $\theta = 0$, we find a significant frailty effect, meaning that the correlation within patient cannot be ignored. Contrast this with the analysis of the same data in [ST] **streg**, which considered both Weibull and lognormal shared-frailty models. For Weibull, there was significant frailty; for lognormal, there was not.

The estimated ν_i are not displayed in the coefficient table but may be retrieved at estimation by specifying effects(*newvar*).

```
. qui stcox age female, shared(patient) effects(nu)

. sort nu

. list patient nu in 1/2
```

	patient	nu
1.	21	-2.4487067
2.	21	-2.4487067

```
. list patient nu in 75/1
```

	patient	nu
75.	7	.51871587
76.	7	.51871587

From the results above, we estimate that the least frail patient is patient 21, with $\hat{\nu}_{21} = -2.45$, and that the frailest patient is patient 7, with $\hat{\nu}_7 = 0.52$.

◁

In shared-frailty Cox models, the estimation consists of two steps. In the first step, the optimization is in terms of θ only. For fixed θ, the second step consists of fitting a standard Cox model via penalized log likelihood, with the ν_i introduced as estimable coefficients of dummy variables identifying the groups. The penalty term in the penalized log likelihood is a function of θ; see *Methods and Formulas*. The final estimate of θ is taken to be the one that maximizes the penalized log likelihood. Once the optimal θ is obtained, it is held fixed, and a final penalized Cox model is fitted. As a result, the standard errors of the main regression parameters (or hazard ratios, if displayed as such) are treated as conditional on θ fixed at its optimal value.

❑ Technical Note

With gamma-distributed frailty, hazard ratios decay over time in favor of the *frailty effect* and thus the displayed "Haz. Ratio" in the above output is actually the hazard ratio only for $t = 0$. The degree of decay depends on θ. Should the estimated θ be close to zero, the hazard ratios do regain their usual interpretation; see Gutierrez (2002) for details.

❑

❑ Technical Note

The likelihood-ratio test of $\theta = 0$ is a boundary test and thus requires careful consideration concerning the calculation of its p-value. In particular, the null distribution of the likelihood-ratio test statistic is not the usual χ_1^2 but is rather a 50:50 mixture of a χ_0^2 (point mass at zero) and a χ_1^2, denoted as $\bar{\chi}_{01}^2$. See Gutierrez, Carter, and Drukker (2001) for more details.

❑

❑ Technical Note

In [ST] **streg**, shared-frailty models are compared and contrasted with *unshared* frailty models. Unshared-frailty models are used to model heterogeneity, and the frailties are integrated out of the conditional survivor function to produce an unconditional survivor function, which serves as a basis for all likelihood calculations.

Given the nature of Cox regression (the baseline hazard remains unspecified), there is no Cox regression analog to the unshared parametric frailty model as fitted using **streg**. That is not to say that you cannot fit a shared-frailty model with 1 observation per group; you can as long as you do not fit a null model. However, there are subtle differences in singleton-group data between shared- and unshared-frailty models; see Gutierrez (2002).

❑

Obtaining baseline function estimates

When you specify options basechazard(*newvar*) and basesurv(*newvar*) — which you may do together or separately — you obtain estimates of the baseline cumulative hazard and survivor functions. When you specify the option basehc(*newvar*), you obtain estimates of the baseline hazard contribution at each failure time, which are factors used to develop both the product-limit estimator for the survivor function generated by basesurv(*newvar*) and the estimator of the cumulative hazard function generated by basechazard(*newvar*).

Although in theory $S_0(t) = \exp\{-H_0(t)\}$, where $S_0(t)$ is the baseline survivor function and $H_0(t)$ is the baseline cumulative hazard, the estimates produced by basechazard() and basesurv() do not exactly correspond in this manner, although they closely do. The reason is that stcox uses different estimation schemes for each; the exact formulas are given in *Methods and Formulas*.

When the model is fitted with the strata() option, you obtain estimates of the baseline functions for each stratum.

Let us first understand how stcox stores the results.

Mathematically, the baseline hazard contribution $h_i = (1 - \alpha_i)$ (see Kalbfleisch and Prentice 2002, 115) is defined at every analytic time t_i at which a failure occurs and is undefined (or, if you prefer, 0) at other times. Stata stores h_i in observations where a failure occurred and missing values in the other observations. For instance, here are some data on which we have fitted a Cox model and specified the option basehc(h):

```
. use http://www.stata-press.com/data/r10/stan3, clear
(Heart transplant data)
. generate age40 = age - 40
. generate year70 = year - 70
. stcox age40 posttran surg year70, basehc(h)
(output omitted )
. list id _t0 _t _d h in 1/10
```

	id	_t0	_t	_d	h
1.	1	0	50	1	.01503465
2.	2	0	6	1	.02035303
3.	3	0	1	0	.
4.	3	1	16	1	.03339642
5.	4	0	36	0	.
6.	4	36	39	1	.01365406
7.	5	0	18	1	.01167142
8.	6	0	3	1	.02875689
9.	7	0	51	0	.
10.	7	51	675	1	.06215003

Here is the interpretation: At time $\_t = 50$, the hazard contribution h_1 is .0150. At time $\_t = 6$, the hazard contribution h_2 is .0204.

In observation 3, no hazard contribution is stored. Observation 3 contains a missing because observation 3 did not fail at time 1.

We see that values of the hazard contributions are stored only in observations that are marked as failing.

The baseline survivor function $S_0(t)$ is defined at all values of t: its estimate changes its value when failures occur, and at times when no failures occur, the estimated $S_0(t)$ is equal to its value at the time of the last failure.

Here are some data on which we have fitted a Cox model and specified both basehc(h) and basesurv(s):

```
. drop h

. stcox age40 posttran surg year70, basehc(h) bases(s)
  (output omitted )

. list id _t0 _t _d h s in 1/10
```

	id	_t0	_t	_d	h	s
1.	1	0	50	1	.01503465	.68100303
2.	2	0	6	1	.02035303	.89846438
3.	3	0	1	0	.	.99089681
4.	3	1	16	1	.03339642	.84087361
5.	4	0	36	0	.	.7527663
6.	4	36	39	1	.01365406	.73259264
7.	5	0	18	1	.01167142	.82144038
8.	6	0	3	1	.02875689	.93568733
9.	7	0	51	0	.	.6705895
10.	7	51	675	1	.06215003	.26115633

At time $\_t = 50$, the baseline survivor function is .6810, or more precisely, $S_0(50 + 0) = .6810$. What we mean by $S_0(t)$ is $S(t + 0)$, the probability of surviving just beyond time t. This is done to clarify that the probability does not include failure at precisely time t.

Understanding what is stored is easier if we sort by _t:

```
. gen notd = -_d

. sort _t notd

. drop notd

. sort _t

. list id _t0 _t _d h s in 1/18
```

	id	_t0	_t	_d	h	s
1.	15	0	1	1	.00910319	.99089681
2.	3	0	1	0	.	.99089681
3.	45	0	1	0	.	.99089681
4.	20	0	1	0	.	.99089681
5.	61	0	2	1	.02775802	.96339147
6.	75	0	2	1	.02775802	.96339147
7.	43	0	2	1	.02775802	.96339147
8.	39	0	2	0	.	.96339147
9.	46	0	2	0	.	.96339147
10.	95	0	2	0	.	.96339147
11.	54	0	3	1	.02875689	.93568733
12.	42	0	3	1	.02875689	.93568733
13.	6	0	3	1	.02875689	.93568733
14.	23	0	3	0	.	.93568733
15.	68	0	3	0	.	.93568733
16.	60	0	3	0	.	.93568733
17.	72	0	4	0	.	.93568733
18.	94	0	4	0	.	.93568733

The baseline hazard contribution is stored on every failure record—if multiple failures occur at a time, the value of the hazard contribution is repeated—and the baseline survivor is stored on every record. (More correctly, baseline values are stored on records that meet the criterion and that were used in estimation. If some observations are explicitly or implicitly excluded from the estimation, their baseline values will be set to missing, no matter what.)

With this listing, we can better understand how the hazard contributions are used to calculate the survivor function. Since the patient with $id = 15$ died at time $t_1 = 1$, the hazard contribution for that patient is $h_{15} = .00910319$. Since that was the only death at $t_1 = 1$, the estimated survivor function at this time is $S_0(1) = 1 - h_{15} = 1 - .00910319 = .99089681$. The next death occurs at time $t_1 = 2$, and the hazard contribution at this time for patient 61 is $h_{61} = .02775802$. Multiplying the previous survivor function value by $1 - h_{61}$ gives the new survivor function at $t_1 = 2$ as $S_0(2) = .96339147$. The other survivor function values are then calculated in succession, using this method at each failure time. At times when no failures occur, the survivor function remains unchanged.

If we had fitted a stratified model by using the `strata()` option, the recorded baseline hazard contribution and survivor on each record would be for the stratum of the record.

❏ Technical Note

If you want to store the baseline hazard contribution on every record for which it is defined and not just on the failure records, you would do the following:

```
. sort _t _d
. by _t: replace h = h[_N]
```

The above assumes that you specified `basehc(h)` when fitting the Cox model. If you also specified the `strata()` option, say, `strata(group)`, the instructions would be

```
. sort group _t _d
. by group _t: replace h = h[_N]
```

In both examples, we placed the data in time order: we put the failures at the end of each time group and then copied the last value of `h` within each time to all the observations for that time.

Consider obtaining the estimate of $S_0(t)$ from the h_is:

```
. sort _t _d
. by _t: keep if _d & _n==_N
. generate s = 1-h
. replace s = s[_n-1]*s if _n>1
```

If you had obtained stratified estimates, the equivalent code would be

```
. sort group _t _d
. by group _t: keep if _d & _n==_N
. generate s = 1-h
. by group: replace s = s[_n-1]*s if _n>1
```

❏

▷ Example 7

Baseline functions refer to the values of the functions when all covariates are set to 0. Let's graph the survival curve for the heart transplant model that we have been fitting, and to make the baseline curve reasonable, let us do that at $age = 40$ and $year = 70$. (We did so previously without explanation, but the following technical note provides important information on why baseline values should be chosen to be reasonable, meaning that they are in the range of the data.)

Thus we will begin by creating variables that, when 0, correspond to the baseline values we desire, and then we will refit our model, specifying the `basesurv()` option:

```
. use http://www.stata-press.com/data/r10/stan3, clear
(Heart transplant data)
. generate age40 = age-40
. generate year70 = year-70
. stcox age40 posttran surg year70, bases(s) nolog
        failure _d: died
   analysis time _t: t1
             id: id
Cox regression -- Breslow method for ties
No. of subjects =          103                 Number of obs    =         172
No. of failures =           75
Time at risk    =      31938.1
                                               LR chi2(4)       =       17.56
Log likelihood  =   -289.53378                 Prob > chi2      =      0.0015
```

_t	Haz. Ratio	Std. Err.	z	P>|z|	[95% Conf. Interval]	
age40	1.030224	.0143201	2.14	0.032	1.002536	1.058677
posttran	.9787243	.3032597	-0.07	0.945	.5332291	1.796416
surgery	.3738278	.163204	-2.25	0.024	.1588759	.8796
year70	.8873107	.059808	-1.77	0.076	.7775022	1.012628

```
. summarize s
```

Variable	Obs	Mean	Std. Dev.	Min	Max
s	172	.629187	.2530009	.130666	.9908968

Our recentering of `age` and `year` did not affect the estimation. Also, the `s` variable we have just generated is the `s` variable we summarized above.

Here is a graph of the baseline survival curve:

```
. line s _t, sort c(J)
```

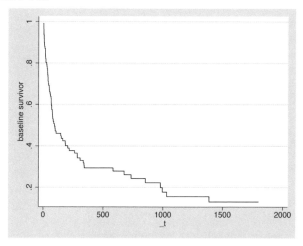

There is an easier way to graph estimated survivor, cumulative hazard, and hazard functions, both at baseline and at specified covariate values. Use `stcurve`, as we demonstrate in [ST] **stcurve**. ◁

❏ Technical Note

If you specify the `basechazard()` or `basesurv()` option, for numerical accuracy reasons, the baseline functions must correspond to something reasonable in your data. Remember, the baseline functions correspond to all covariates equal to 0 in your Cox model.

Consider, for instance, a Cox model that includes the variable calendar year among the covariates. Say that `year` varies between 1980 and 1996. The baseline functions would correspond to year 0, almost 2,000 years in the past. Say that the estimated coefficient on `year` is $-.2$, meaning that the hazard ratio for one year to the next is a reasonable 0.82.

Think carefully about the contribution to the predicted log cumulative hazard: it would be approximately $-.2 \times 2,000 = -400$. Now $e^{-400} \approx 10^{-173}$, which on a digital computer is 1. There is simply no hope that $H_0(t)e^{-400}$ will produce an accurate estimate of $H(t)$.

Even with less extreme numbers, problems arise, even in the calculation of the baseline survivor function. Baseline hazard contributions near 1 produce baseline survivor functions, with the steps differing by 10s of orders of magnitudes because the calculation of the survivor function is cumulative. Producing a meaningful graph of such a survivor function is hopeless, and adjusting the survivor function (as opposed to the hazard contribution) to other values of the covariates is too much work.

For these reasons, covariate values of 0 must be meaningful if you are going to specify the `basechazard()` or `basesurv()` option. As the baseline values move to absurdity, the first problem you will encounter is a baseline survivor function that is too hard to interpret, even though the baseline hazard contributions are estimated accurately. Further out, the procedure Stata uses to estimate the baseline hazard contributions will break down—it will produce results that are exactly 1.

This, in fact, occurs with the Stanford heart transplant data:

```
. use http://www.stata-press.com/data/r10/stan3, clear
(Heart transplant data)
. stcox age posttran surg year, basec(ch) bases(s)
 (output omitted )
. summarize ch s
```

Variable	Obs	Mean	Std. Dev.	Min	Max
ch	172	745.1134	682.8671	11.88239	2573.637
s	172	1.45e-07	9.43e-07	0	6.24e-06

The hint that there are problems is that the values of `ch` are huge and the values of `s` are close to zero. In this dataset, `age` (which ranges from 8 to 64 with a mean value of 45) and `year` (which ranges from 67 to 74) are the problems. The baseline functions correspond to a newborn at the turn of the century on the waiting list for a heart transplant!

To obtain accurate estimates of the baseline functions, type

```
. drop ch s
. generate age40 = age-40
. generate year70 = year-70
. stcox age40 posttran surg year70, basec(ch) bases(s)
 (output omitted )
. summarize ch s
```

Variable	Obs	Mean	Std. Dev.	Min	Max
ch	172	.5685743	.521076	.0090671	1.963868
s	172	.629187	.2530009	.130666	.9908968

Adjusting the variables does not affect the coefficient (and hence hazard ratio) estimates, but it changes the values at which the baseline functions are estimated to be within the range of the data. ❏

❏ Technical Note

When used with shared-frailty models, the options basehc(), basesurv(), and basechazard() produce estimates of baseline quantities that are based on the last-step penalized Cox model fit. Therefore, the term *baseline* means that not only are the covariates set to zero but ν_i also is, and thus *baseline* corresponds to $\alpha_i = 1$ (and zero covariates).

❏

Saved Results

stcox saves the following in e():

Scalars

e(N)	number of observations	e(N_g)	number of groups
e(N_sub)	number of subjects	e(g_max)	largest group size
e(N_fail)	number of failures	e(g_min)	smallest group size
e(risk)	total time at risk	e(g_avg)	average group size
e(N_clust)	number of clusters	e(ll)	log likelihood
e(df_m)	model degrees of freedom	e(ll_0)	log likelihood, constant-only model
e(r2_p)	pseudo-R-squared	e(chi2)	χ^2
e(theta)	frailty parameter	e(se_theta)	standard error of θ
e(chi2_c)	χ^2, comparison model	e(ll_c)	log likelihood, comparison model
e(p_c)	significance, comparison model		

Macros

e(cmd)	cox or stcox_fr
e(cmd2)	stcox
e(cmdline)	command as typed
e(depvar)	_t
e(t0)	_t0
e(texp)	function used for time-varying covariates
e(ties)	method used for handling ties
e(shared)	frailty grouping variable
e(offset)	offset
e(clustvar)	name of cluster variable
e(re_var)	variable containing estimated random effects
e(bases)	variable containing baseline survivor function
e(basec)	variable containing baseline cumulative hazard function
e(basehc)	variable containing baseline hazard contributions
e(mgale)	variable containing partial martingale residuals
e(vl_esr)	variables containing partial efficient score residuals
e(vl_sch)	variables containing Schoenfeld residuals
e(vl_ssc)	variables containing scaled Schoenfeld residuals
e(chi2type)	Wald or LR; type of model χ^2 test
e(vce)	*vcetype* specified in vce()
e(vcetype)	title used to label Std. Err.
e(method)	requested estimation method
e(crittype)	optimization criterion
e(properties)	b V
e(estat_cmd)	program used to implement estat
e(footnote)	program used to implement the footnote display
e(predict)	program used to implement predict

Matrices

 e(b)   coefficient vector   e(V) variance–covariance matrix of the estimators

Functions

 e(sample) marks estimation sample

Methods and Formulas

stcox is implemented as an ado-file.

The proportional hazards model with time-dependent explanatory variables was first suggested by Cox (1972). For an introductory explanation, see Hosmer and Lemeshow (1999, chap. 3, 4, and 7), Kahn and Sempos (1989, 193–198), and Selvin (2004, 412–442). For an introduction for the social scientist, see Box-Steffensmeier and Jones (2004, chap. 4). For a comprehensive review of the methods in this entry, see Klein and Moeschberger (2003). For a detailed development of these methods, see Kalbfleisch and Prentice (2002). For more Stata-specific insight, see Cleves, Gould, and Gutierrez (2004); Dupont (2002); and Vittinghoff et al. (2005).

Let $\mathbf{x}_i$ be the row vector of covariates for the time interval $(t_{0i}, t_i]$ for the ith observation in the dataset ($i = 1, \ldots, N$). stcox obtains parameter estimates $\widehat{\boldsymbol{\beta}}$ by maximizing the partial log-likelihood function

$$\ln L = \sum_{j=1}^{D} \Big[\sum_{k \in D_j} \mathbf{x}_k \boldsymbol{\beta} - d_j \ln \Big\{ \sum_{i \in R_j} \exp(\mathbf{x}_i \boldsymbol{\beta}) \Big\} \Big]$$

where j indexes the ordered failure times $t_{(j)}$ ($j = 1, \ldots, D$), D_j is the set of d_j observations that fail at $t_{(j)}$, d_j is the number of failures at $t_{(j)}$, and R_j is the set of observations k that are at risk at time $t_{(j)}$ (i.e., all k such that $t_{0k} < t_{(j)} \le t_k$). This formula for $\ln L$ is for unweighted data and handles ties by using the Peto–Breslow approximation (Peto 1972; Breslow 1974), which is the default method of handling ties in stcox.

The variance of $\widehat{\boldsymbol{\beta}}$ is estimated by the conventional inverse matrix of (negative) second derivatives of $\ln L$, unless vce(robust) is specified, in which case the method of Lin and Wei (1989) is used. If vce(cluster *clustvar*) is specified, the efficient score residuals are summed within cluster before the sandwich (robust) estimator is applied.

See [R] **maximize** for a description of the maximization algorithm and for the translation of estimated results to hazard ratios when hr is specified.

mgale() stores in each observation the observation's contribution to the martingale residual, which Stata's terminology calls the "partial" martingale residual. The derivative of $\ln L$ can be written as

$$\frac{\partial \ln L}{\partial \boldsymbol{\beta}} = \sum_{j=1}^{D} \sum_{i=1}^{N} \mathbf{x}_i \, dM_i(t_{(j)})$$

where

$$dM_i(t_{(j)}) = \delta_{ij} - I(t_{0i} < t_{(j)} \le t_i) \frac{d_j \exp(\mathbf{x}_i \boldsymbol{\beta})}{\sum_{\ell \in R_j} \exp(\mathbf{x}_\ell \boldsymbol{\beta})}$$

with $\delta_{ij} = 1$ if observation i fails at $t_{(j)}$ and 0 otherwise. $I(\cdot)$ is the indicator function. $dM_i(t_{(j)})$ is the increment of the martingale residual for the ith observation owing the failures at time $t_{(j)}$. The `mgale()` option saves the partial martingale residuals ΔM_i, which are the sum of the $dM_i(t_{(j)})$ over all failure times $t_{(j)}$, such that $t_{0i} < t_{(j)} \le t_i$. For single-record data, the partial martingale residual is the martingale residual. For multiple-record data, the martingale residual for an individual can be obtained by summing the partial martingale residuals over all observations belonging to the individual. For a discussion of martingale residuals, see Fleming and Harrington (1991, 163–197).

The increments of the efficient score residuals are

$$dF_{ij} = x_{ij}^* \, dM_i(t_{(j)})$$

where

$$x_{ij}^* = x_i - \frac{\sum_{\ell \in R_j} x_\ell \exp(x_\ell \boldsymbol{\beta})}{\sum_{\ell \in R_j} \exp(x_\ell \boldsymbol{\beta})}$$

When the `esr()` option is specified, `stcox` creates $p = \dim(x)$ new variables containing ΔF_i, which are the sum of dF_{ij} over all failure times $t_{(j)}$, such that $t_{0i} < t_{(j)} \le t_i$. The efficient score residuals for an individual can be obtained by summing ΔF_i over all observations i belonging to the individual.

The estimated baseline hazard contribution, if requested, is obtained as $h_j = 1 - \widehat{\alpha}_j$, where $\widehat{\alpha}_j$ is the solution of

$$\sum_{k \in D_j} \frac{\exp(x_k \boldsymbol{\beta})}{1 - \widehat{\alpha}_j^{\exp(x_k \boldsymbol{\beta})}} = \sum_{l \in R_j} \exp(x_l \boldsymbol{\beta})$$

(Kalbfleisch and Prentice 2002, equation (4.34), 115).

The estimated baseline survivor function, if requested, is obtained as

$$\widehat{S}_0(t_{(j)}) = \prod_{h=0}^{j-1} \widehat{\alpha}_h$$

where $\widehat{\alpha}_0 = 1$.

The estimated baseline cumulative hazard function, if requested, is related to the baseline survivor function calculation, yet the values of $\widehat{\alpha}_j$ are set at their starting values and are not iterated. Equivalently,

$$\widehat{H}_0(t_{(j)}) = \sum_{h=0}^{j-1} \frac{d_j}{\sum_{l \in R_j} \exp(x_l \boldsymbol{\beta})}$$

Tied values are handled using one of four approaches. The log likelihoods corresponding to the four approaches are given with weights (`exactp` does not allow weights) and offsets by

$$\ln L_{\text{breslow}} = \sum_{j=1}^{D} \sum_{i \in D_j} \left[w_i(\mathbf{x}_i\boldsymbol{\beta} + \text{offset}_i) - w_i \ln \left\{ \sum_{\ell \in R_j} w_\ell \exp(\mathbf{x}_\ell\boldsymbol{\beta} + \text{offset}_\ell) \right\} \right]$$

$$\ln L_{\text{efron}} = \sum_{j=1}^{D} \sum_{k=1}^{d_j} \left\{ \frac{1}{d_j} \sum_{i \in D_j} w_i(\mathbf{x}_i\boldsymbol{\beta} + \text{offset}_i) - \right.$$

$$\left. \left(\frac{1}{d_j} \sum_{i \in D_j} w_i \right) \ln \sum_{\ell \in R_j} w_\ell f_{kj\ell} \exp(\mathbf{x}_\ell\boldsymbol{\beta} + \text{offset}_\ell) \right\}$$

$$f_{kj\ell} = \begin{cases} \dfrac{d_j - k + 1}{d_j} & \text{if } \delta_{\ell j} = 1 \\ 1 & \text{otherwise} \end{cases}$$

$$\ln L_{\text{exactm}} = \sum_{j=1}^{D} \ln \int_0^\infty \prod_{\ell \in D_j} \left\{ 1 - \exp\left(-\frac{e_\ell}{s}t \right) \right\}^{w_\ell} \exp(-t)dt$$

$$e_\ell = \exp(\mathbf{x}_\ell\boldsymbol{\beta} + \text{offset}_\ell)$$

$$s = \sum_{\substack{k \in R_j \\ k \notin D_j}} w_k \exp(\mathbf{x}_k\boldsymbol{\beta} + \text{offset}_k) = \text{sum of weighted nondeath risk scores}$$

$$\ln L_{\text{exactp}} = \sum_{j=1}^{D} \left\{ \sum_{i \in R_j} \delta_{ij}(\mathbf{x}_i\boldsymbol{\beta} + \text{offset}_i) - \ln f(r_j, d_j) \right\}$$

$$f(r, d) = f(r-1, d) + f(r-1, d-1)\exp(\mathbf{x}_k\boldsymbol{\beta} + \text{offset}_k)$$

$$k = r^{\text{th}} \text{ observation in the set } R_j$$

$$r_j = \text{cardinality of the set } R_j$$

$$f(r, d) = \begin{cases} 0 & \text{if } r < d \\ 1 & \text{if } d = 0 \end{cases}$$

Calculations for the exact marginal log likelihood (and associated derivatives) are obtained with 15-point Gauss–Laguerre quadrature. The `breslow` and `efron` options both provide approximations of the exact marginal log likelihood. The `efron` approximation is a better (closer) approximation, but the `breslow` approximation is a much faster approximation. The choice of the approximation to use in a given situation should generally be driven by the proportion of ties in the data.

Weights are not allowed with the `exactp` method.

Cox–Snell residuals are calculated using

$$r_{C_i} = \delta_{i\cdot} - r_{M_i}$$

where r_{M_i} are the martingale residuals, and $\delta_{i\cdot}$ is a censoring indicator equal to 1 if the ith observation is a failure and 0 otherwise. The martingale residuals are nonnegative values following an exponential distribution with mean 1. Modified Cox–Snell residuals are defined similarly, except that the residual is augmented by some positive constant if the observation is censored. The most common modifications are to add either 1 or the Crowley–Hu adjustment of $\ln 2 \approx .693$ (which is the median of an exponential distribution with parameter 1).

Martingale residuals are calculated using

$$r_{M_i} = \delta_{i.} - \sum_{j=1}^{D} I(t_{0i} < t_{(j)} \leq t_i) \frac{d_j \exp(\mathbf{x}_i\boldsymbol{\beta} + \text{offset}_i)}{\sum_{\ell \in R_j} \exp(\mathbf{x}_\ell\boldsymbol{\beta} + \text{offset}_\ell)}$$

These residuals are in $(-\infty, 1)$.

Using the Breslow–Peto approach, we have

$$r_{M_i} = 1 - \exp(\mathbf{x}_i\boldsymbol{\beta} + \text{offset}_i) \sum_{k:t_k \leq t_i} \frac{w_k \delta_{k.}}{\sum_{\ell \in R_i} w_\ell \exp(\mathbf{x}_\ell\boldsymbol{\beta} + \text{offset}_\ell)}$$

Using the Efron approach, we have

$$r_{M_i} = \left\{ w_i - \frac{1}{d_i} \left(\sum_{j=1}^{d_i} w_j \right) \frac{\exp(\mathbf{x}_i\boldsymbol{\beta} + \text{offset}_i)}{\sum_{\ell \in R_i} w_\ell f_{ij\ell} \exp(\mathbf{x}_\ell\boldsymbol{\beta} + \text{offset}_\ell)} \right\} \bigg/ w_i$$

Deviance residuals are calculated using

$$r_{D_i} = \text{sign}(r_{M_i}) \left[-2 \left\{ r_{M_i} + \delta_{i.} \log(\delta_{i.} - r_{M_i}) \right\} \right]^{1/2}$$

These residuals are expected to be symmetric about zero but do not necessarily sum to zero.

Schoenfeld residuals are calculated using the Breslow–Peto approach as

$$r_{uS_i} = \sum_{j=1}^{D} \delta_{ij} \left\{ x_{ui} - \frac{\sum_{\ell \in R_j} w_\ell x_{u\ell} \exp(\mathbf{x}_\ell\boldsymbol{\beta} + \text{offset}_\ell)}{\sum_{\ell \in R_j} w_\ell \exp(\mathbf{x}_\ell\boldsymbol{\beta} + \text{offset}_\ell)} \right\}$$

Using the Efron approach, we have

$$r_{uS_i} = \sum_{j=1}^{D} \delta_{ij} \left\{ x_{ui} - \frac{\sum_{\ell \in R_j} w_\ell x_{u\ell} f_{ij\ell} \exp(\mathbf{x}_\ell\boldsymbol{\beta} + \text{offset}_\ell)}{\sum_{\ell \in R_j} w_\ell f_{ij\ell} \exp(\mathbf{x}_\ell\boldsymbol{\beta} + \text{offset}_\ell)} \right\}$$

These are for each of the covariates, $u = 1, \ldots, p$.

David Roxbee Cox (1924–) was born in Birmingham, England. He earned Ph.D. degrees in mathematics and statistics from the universities of Cambridge and Leeds and worked at the Royal Aircraft Establishment, the Wool Industries Research Association, and the universities of Cambridge, London (Birkbeck and Imperial Colleges), and Oxford. He was knighted in 1985. Sir David has worked on a wide range of theoretical and applied statistical problems, with outstanding contributions in areas such as experimental design, stochastic processes, binary data, survival analysis, asymptotic techniques, and multivariate dependencies.

Acknowledgment

We thank Peter Sasieni of Cancer Research UK for his statistical advice and guidance in implementing the robust variance estimator for this command.

References

Box-Steffensmeier, J. M., and B. S. Jones. 2004. *Event History Modeling: A Guide for Social Scientists.* Cambridge: Cambridge University Press.

Breslow, N. E. 1974. Covariance analysis of censored survival data. *Biometrics* 30: 89–99.

Cleves, M. A. 1999. ssa13: Analysis of multiple failure-time data with Stata. *Stata Technical Bulletin* 49: 30–39. Reprinted in *Stata Technical Bulletin Reprints*, vol. 9, pp. 338–349.

Cleves, M. A., W. W. Gould, and R. G. Gutierrez. 2004. *An Introduction to Survival Analysis Using Stata.* Rev. ed. College Station, TX: Stata Press.

Cox, D. R. 1972. Regression models and life-tables (with discussion). *Journal of the Royal Statistical Society, Series B* 34: 187–220.

——. 1975. Partial likelihood. *Biometrika* 62: 269–276.

Cox, D. R., and D. Oakes. 1984. *Analysis of Survival Data.* London: Chapman & Hall/CRC.

Cox, D. R., and E. J. Snell. 1968. A general definition of residuals (with discussion). *Journal of the Royal Statistical Society, Series B* 30: 248–275.

Crowley, J., and M. Hu. 1977. Covariance analysis of heart transplant survival data. *Journal of the American Statistical Association* 72: 27–36.

Cui, J. 2005. Buckley–James method for analyzing censored data, with an application to a cardiovascular disease and an HIV/AIDS study. *Stata Journal* 5: 517–526.

Dupont, W. D. 2002. *Statistical Modeling for Biomedical Researchers: A Simple Introduction to the Analysis of Complex Data.* Cambridge: Cambridge University Press.

Fleming, T. R., and D. P. Harrington. 1991. *Counting Processes and Survival Analysis.* New York: Wiley.

Gutierrez, R. G. 2002. Parametric frailty and shared frailty survival models. *Stata Journal* 2: 22–44.

Gutierrez, R. G., S. L. Carter, and D. M. Drukker. 2001. On boundary-value likelihood ratio tests. *Stata Technical Bulletin* 60: 15–18. Reprinted in *Stata Technical Bulletin Reprints*, vol. 10, pp. 269–273.

Hills, M., and B. L. De Stavola. 2006. *A Short Introduction to Stata for Biostatistics.* London: Timberlake.

Hosmer, D. W., Jr., and S. Lemeshow. 1999. *Applied Survival Analysis: Regression Modeling of Time to Event Data.* New York: Wiley.

Jenkins, S. P. 1997. sbe17: Discrete time proportional hazards regression. *Stata Technical Bulletin* 39: 22–32. Reprinted in *Stata Technical Bulletin Reprints*, vol. 7, pp. 109–121.

Kahn, H. A., and C. T. Sempos. 1989. *Statistical Methods in Epidemiology.* New York: Oxford University Press.

Kalbfleisch, J. D., and R. L. Prentice. 2002. *The Statistical Analysis of Failure Time Data.* 2nd ed. New York: Wiley.

Klein, J. P., and M. L. Moeschberger. 2003. *Survival Analysis: Techniques for Censored and Truncated Data.* 2nd ed. New York: Springer.

Lin, D. Y., and L. J. Wei. 1989. The robust inference for the Cox proportional hazards model. *Journal of the American Statistical Association* 84: 1074–1078.

McGilchrist, C. A., and C. W. Aisbett. 1991. Regression with frailty in survival analysis. *Biometrics* 47: 461–466.

Newman, S. C. 2001. *Biostatistical Methods in Epidemiology.* New York: Wiley.

Peto, R. 1972. Contribution to the discussion of paper by D. R. Cox. *Journal of the Royal Statistical Society, Series B* 34: 205–207.

Reid, N. 1994. A conversation with Sir David Cox. *Statistical Science* 9: 439–455.

Royston, J. P. 2001. Flexible parametric alternatives to the Cox model, and more. *Stata Journal* 1: 1–28.

——. 2006. Explained variation for survival models. *Stata Journal* 6: 83–96.

Schoenfeld, D. 1982. Partial residuals for the proportional hazards regression model. *Biometrika* 69: 239–241.

Selvin, S. 2004. *Statistical Analysis of Epidemiologic Data.* 3rd ed. New York: Oxford University Press.

Sterne, J. A. C., and K. Tilling. 2002. G-estimation of causal effects, allowing for time-varying confounding. *Stata Journal* 2: 164–182.

Therneau, T. M., and P. M. Grambsch. 2000. *Modeling Survival Data: Extending the Cox Model.* New York: Springer.

Vittinghoff, E., D. V. Glidden, S. C. Shiboski, and C. E. McCulloch. 2005. *Regression Methods in Biostatistics: Linear, Logistic, Survival, and Repeated Measures Models.* New York: Springer.

Also See

[ST] **stcox postestimation** — Postestimation tools for stcox

[ST] **stcurve** — Plot survivor, hazard, or cumulative hazard function

[ST] **stcox diagnostics** — stcox diagnostic plots

[ST] **sts** — Generate, graph, list, and test the survivor and cumulative hazard functions

[ST] **stset** — Declare data to be survival-time data

[ST] **streg** — Fit parametric survival models

[SVY] **svy estimation** — Estimation commands for survey data

[U] **20 Estimation and postestimation commands**

Title

stcox diagnostics — stcox diagnostic plots

Syntax

Check proportional-hazards assumption:

Log-log plot of survival

stphplot [*if*] , {by(*varname*) | strata(*varname*)} [*stphplot_options*]

Kaplan–Meier and predicted survival plot

stcoxkm [*if*] , by(*varname*) [*stcoxkm_options*]

stphplot_options	description
Main	
* by(*varname*)	fit separate Cox models; the default
* strata(*varname*)	fit stratified Cox model
adjust(*varlist*)	adjust to average values of *varlist*
zero	adjust to zero values of *varlist*; use with adjust()
Options	
nonegative	plot $\ln\{-\ln(\text{survival})\}$
nolntime	plot curves against analysis time
noshow	do not show st setting information
Plot	
plot#opts(*cline_options*)	affect rendition of the #th connected line
Add plots	
addplot(*plot*)	add other plots to the generated graph
Y axis, X axis, Titles, Legend, Overall	
twoway_options	any options other than by() documented in [G] *twoway_options*

* Either by(*varname*) or strata(*varname*) is required with stphplot.

(*Continued on next page*)

stcoxkm_options	description
Main	
*by(*varname*)	report the nominal or ordinal covariate
<u>ties</u>(<u>b</u>reslow)	use Breslow method to handle tied failures
<u>ties</u>(<u>ef</u>ron)	use Efron method to handle tied failures
<u>ties</u>(exactm)	use exact marginal-likelihood method to handle tied failures
<u>ties</u>(exactp)	use exact partial-likelihood method to handle tied failures
<u>separate</u>	draw separate plot for predicted and observed curves
<u>nosho</u>w	do not show st setting information
Observed plot	
<u>obsopts</u>(*connect_options*)	affect rendition of the observed curve
obs#opts(*connect_options*)	affect rendition of the #th observed curve; not allowed with <u>separate</u>
Predicted plot	
<u>predopts</u>(*connect_options*)	affect rendition of the predicted curve
pred#opts(*connect_options*)	affect rendition of the #th predicted curve; not allowed with <u>separate</u>
Add plots	
<u>addplot</u>(*plot*)	add other plots to the generated graph
Y axis, X axis, Titles, Legend, Overall	
twoway_options	any options documented in [G] ***twoway_options***
<u>byopts</u>(*byopts*)	how subgraphs are combined, labeled, etc.

* by(*varname*) is required with stcoxkm.

You must stset your data before using stphplot and stcoxkm; see [ST] **stset**.
fweights, iweights, and pweights may be specified using stset; see [ST] **stset**.

Description

stphplot plots $-\ln\{-\ln(\text{survival})\}$ curves for each category of a nominal or ordinal covariate versus ln(analysis time). These are often referred to as "log-log" plots. Optionally, these estimates can be adjusted for covariates. The proportional-hazards assumption is not violated when the curves are parallel.

stcoxkm plots Kaplan–Meier observed survival curves and compares them with the Cox predicted curves for the same variable. The closer the observed values are to the predicted, the less likely it is that the proportional-hazards assumption has been violated. Do not run stcox before running this command; stcoxkm will execute stcox itself to fit the model and obtain predicted values.

Options for stphplot

Main

by(*varname*) specifies the nominal or ordinal covariate. Either by() or strata() is required with stphplot.

strata(*varname*) is an alternative to by(). Rather than fitting separate Cox models for each value of *varname*, strata() fits one stratified Cox model. You must also specify adjust(*varlist*) with the strata(*varname*) option; see [ST] **sts graph**.

adjust(*varlist*) adjusts the estimates to that for the *average* values of the *varlist* specified. The estimates can also be adjusted to *zero* values of *varlist* by specifying the zero option. adjust(*varlist*) can be specified with by(); it is required with strata(*varname*).

zero is used with adjust() to specify that the estimates be adjusted to the 0 values of the *varlist* rather than to average values.

_____⌐ Options ⌐_____

nonegative specifies that $\ln\{-\ln(\text{survival})\}$ be plotted instead of $-\ln\{-\ln(\text{survival})\}$.

nolntime specifies that curves be plotted against analysis time instead of against ln(analysis time).

noshow prevents stphplot from showing the key st variables. This option is seldom used since most people type stset, show or stset, noshow to set whether they want to see these variables mentioned at the top of the output of every st command; see [ST] **stset**.

_____⌐ Plot ⌐_____

plot#opts(*cline_options*) affects the rendition of the #th connected line; see [G] *cline_options*.

_____⌐ Add plots ⌐_____

addplot(*plot*) provides a way to add other plots to the generated graph; see [G] *addplot_option*.

_____⌐ Y axis, X axis, Titles, Legend, Overall ⌐_____

twoway_options are any of the options documented in [G] *twoway_options*, excluding by(). These include options for titling the graph (see [G] *title_options*) and for saving the graph to disk (see [G] *saving_option*).

Options for stcoxkm

_____⌐ Main ⌐_____

by(*varname*) specifies the nominal or ordinal covariate. by() is required.

ties(breslow | efron | exactm | exactp) specifies one of the methods available to stcox for handling tied failures. If none is specified, ties(breslow) is assumed; see [ST] **stcox**.

separate produces separate plots of predicted and observed values for each value of the variable specified with by().

noshow prevents stcoxkm from showing the key st variables. This option is seldom used since most people type stset, show or stset, noshow to set whether they want to see these variables mentioned at the top of the output of every st command; see [ST] **stset**.

_____⌐ Observed plot ⌐_____

obsopts(*connect_options*) affects the rendition of the observed curve; see [G] *connect_options*.

obs#opts(*connect_options*) affects the rendition of the #th observed curve; see [G] *connect_options*. This option is not allowed with separate.

⌐ Predicted plot ⌐

predopts(*connect_options*) affects the rendition of the predicted curve; see [G] ***connect_options***.

pred#opts(*connect_options*) affects the rendition of the #th predicted curve; see [G] ***connect_options***. This option is not allowed with separate.

⌐ Add plots ⌐

addplot(*plot*) provides a way to add other plots to the generated graph; see [G] ***addplot_option***.

⌐ Y axis, X axis, Titles, Legend, Overall ⌐

twoway_options are any of the options documented in [G] ***twoway_options***, excluding by(). These include options for titling the graph (see [G] ***title_options***) and for saving the graph to disk (see [G] ***saving_option***).

byopts(*byopts*) affects the appearance of the combined graph when by() and separate are specified, including the overall graph title and the organization of subgraphs. See [G] ***by_option***.

Remarks

Cox proportional hazards models assume that the hazard ratio is proportional over time. Suppose that a group of cancer patients on an experimental treatment is monitored for 10 years. If the hazard of dying for the nontreated group is twice the rate as that of the treated group (HR = 2.0), the proportional-hazards assumption implies that this ratio is the same at 1 year, at 2 years, or at any point on the time scale. Because the Cox model, by definition, is constrained to follow this assumption, it is important to evaluate its validity. If the assumption fails, alternative modeling choices would be more appropriate (e.g., a stratified Cox model).

stphplot and stcoxkm provide graphical methods for assessing violations of the proportional-hazards assumption. Although using graphs to assess the validity of the assumption is subjective, it can be a helpful tool.

stphplot plots $-\ln\{-\ln(\text{survival})\}$ curves for each category of a nominal or ordinal covariate versus ln(analysis time). These are often referred to as "log–log" plots. Optionally, these estimates can be adjusted for covariates. If the plotted lines are reasonably parallel, the proportional-hazards assumption has not been violated, and it would be appropriate to base the estimate for that variable on one baseline survivor function.

Another graphical method of evaluating the proportional-hazards assumption, though less common, is to plot the Kaplan–Meier observed survival curves and compare them with the Cox predicted curves for the same variable. This plot is produced with stcoxkm. When the predicted and observed curves are close together, the proportional-hazards assumption has not been violated. See Garrett (1997) for more details.

▷ Example 1

These examples use data from a leukemia remission study (Garrett 1997). The data consist of 42 patients who are monitored over time to see how long (weeks) it takes them to go out of remission (relapse: 1 = yes, 0 = no). Half the patients receive a new experimental drug, and the other half receive a standard drug (treatment1: 1 = drug A, 0 = standard). White blood cell count, a strong indicator of the presence of leukemia, is divided into three categories (wbc3cat: 1 = normal, 2 = moderate, 3 = high).

```
. use http://www.stata-press.com/data/r10/leukemia
(Leukemia Remission Study)

. describe

Contains data from http://www.stata-press.com/data/r10/leukemia.dta
  obs:            42                          Leukemia Remission Study
  vars:            8                          23 Mar 2007 10:39
  size:          504 (99.9% of memory free)
```

variable name	storage type	display format	value label	variable label
weeks	byte	%8.0g		Weeks in Remission
relapse	byte	%8.0g	yesno	Relapse
treatment1	byte	%8.0g	trt1lbl	Treatment I
treatment2	byte	%8.0g	trt2lbl	Treatment II
wbc3cat	byte	%9.0g	wbclbl	White Blood Cell Count
wbc1	byte	%8.0g		wbc3cat==Normal
wbc2	byte	%8.0g		wbc3cat==Moderate
wbc3	byte	%8.0g		wbc3cat==High

```
Sorted by:  weeks

. stset weeks, failure(relapse) noshow

     failure event:  relapse != 0 & relapse < .
obs. time interval:  (0, weeks]
 exit on or before:  failure
```

```
      42   total obs.
       0   exclusions
```

```
      42   obs. remaining, representing
      30   failures in single record/single failure data
     541   total analysis time at risk, at risk from t =          0
                            earliest observed entry t =          0
                              last observed exit t =           35
```

In this example, we examine whether the proportional-hazards assumption holds for drug A versus the standard drug (treatment1). First, we will use stphplot, followed by stcoxkm.

```
. stphplot, by(treatment1)
```

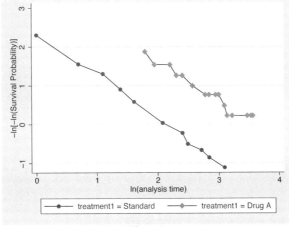

Figure 1.

```
. stcoxkm, by(treatment1)
```

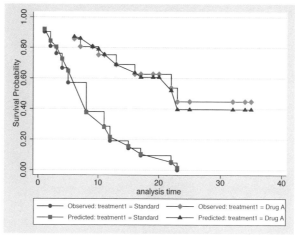

Figure 2.

Figure 1 (`stphplot`) displays lines that are parallel, implying that the proportional-hazards assumption for `treatment1` has not been violated. This is confirmed in figure 2 (`stcoxkm`), where the observed values and predicted values are close together.

The graph in figure 3 is the same as figure 1, adjusted for white blood cell count (using two dummy variables). The adjustment variables were centered temporarily by `stphplot` before the adjustment was made.

```
. stphplot, strata(treatment1) adj(wbc2 wbc3)
```

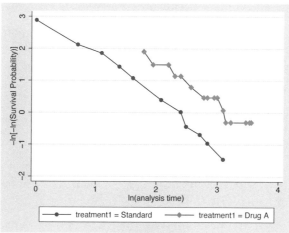

Figure 3.

The lines in figure 3 are still parallel, although they are somewhat closer together. Examining the proportional-hazards assumption on a variable without adjusting for covariates is usually adequate as a diagnostic tool before using the Cox model. However, if you know that adjustment for covariates in a final model is necessary, you may wish to reexamine whether the proportional-hazards assumption still holds.

Another variable in this dataset measures a different drug (`treatment2`: 1 = drug B, 0 = standard). We wish to examine the proportional-hazards assumption for this variable.

```
. stphplot, by(treatment2)
```

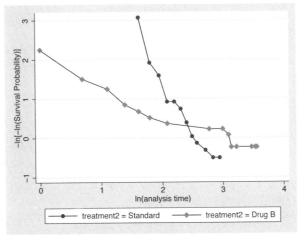

Figure 4.

```
. stcoxkm, by(treatment2) separate
```

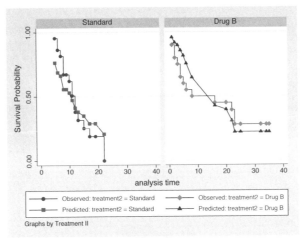

Figure 5.

This variable violates the proportional-hazards assumption. In figure 4, we see that the lines are not only nonparallel but also cross in the data region. In figure 5, we see that there are considerable differences between the observed and predicted values. We have overestimated the positive effect of drug B for the first half of the study and have underestimated it in the later weeks. One hazard ratio describing the effect of this drug would be inappropriate. We definitely would want to stratify this variable in our Cox model.

◁

Methods and Formulas

stphplot and stcoxkm are implemented as ado-files.

For one covariate, x, the Cox proportional-hazards model reduces to

$$h(t; x) = h_0(t) \exp(\mathbf{x}\boldsymbol{\beta})$$

where $h_0(t)$ is the baseline hazard function from the Cox model. Let $S_0(t)$ and $H_0(t)$ be the corresponding Cox baseline survivor and baseline cumulative hazard functions, respectively.

The proportional-hazards assumption implies that

$$H(t) = H_0(t) \exp(\mathbf{x}\boldsymbol{\beta})$$

or

$$\ln H(t) = \ln H_0(t) + \mathbf{x}\boldsymbol{\beta}$$

where $H(t)$ is the cumulative hazard function. Thus, under the proportional-hazards assumption, the logs of the cumulative hazard functions at each level of the covariate have equal slope. This is the basis for the method implemented in stphplot.

The proportional-hazards assumption also implies that

$$S(t) = S_0(t)^{\exp(\mathbf{x}\boldsymbol{\beta})}$$

Let $\widehat{S}(t)$ be the estimated survivor function based on the Cox model. This function is a step function like the Kaplan–Meier estimate and, in fact, reduces to the Kaplan–Meier estimate when $\mathbf{x} = 0$. Thus for each level of the covariate of interest, we can assess violations of the proportional-hazards assumption by comparing these survival estimates with estimates calculated independently of the model. See Kalbfleisch and Prentice (2002) or Hess (1995).

stcoxkm plots Kaplan–Meier estimated curves for each level of the covariate together with the Cox model predicted baseline survival curve. The closer the observed values are to the predicted values, the less likely it is that the proportional-hazards assumption has been violated.

Acknowledgment

The original versions of stphplot and stcoxkm were written by Joanne M. Garrett, University of North Carolina at Chapel Hill.

References

Barthel, F. M.-S., and P. Royston. 2006. Graphical representation of interactions. *Stata Journal* 6: 348–363.

Breslow, N. E. 1974. Covariance analysis of censored survival data. *Biometrics* 30: 89–99.

Cox, D. R. 1972. Regression models and life-tables (with discussion). *Journal of the Royal Statistical Society, Series B* 34: 187–220.

———. 1975. Partial likelihood. *Biometrika* 62: 269–276.

Cox, D. R., and D. Oakes. 1984. *Analysis of Survival Data*. London: Chapman & Hall/CRC.

Cox, D. R., and E. J. Snell. 1968. A general definition of residuals (with discussion). *Journal of the Royal Statistical Society, Series B* 30: 248–275.

Garrett, J. M. 1997. gr23: Graphical assessment of the Cox model proportional-hazards assumption. *Stata Technical Bulletin* 35: 9–14. Reprinted in *Stata Technical Bulletin Reprints*, vol. 6, pp. 38–44.

——. 1998. ssa12: Predicted survival curves for the Cox proportional hazards model. *Stata Technical Bulletin* 44: 37–41. Reprinted in *Stata Technical Bulletin Reprints*, vol. 8, pp. 285–290.

Hess, K. R. 1995. Graphical methods for assessing violations of the proportional-hazards assumption in Cox regression. *Statistics in Medicine* 14: 1707–1723.

Kalbfleisch, J. D., and R. L. Prentice. 2002. *The Statistical Analysis of Failure Time Data*. 2nd ed. New York: Wiley.

Rogers, W. H. 1994. ssa4: Ex post tests and diagnostics for a proportional hazards model. *Stata Technical Bulletin* 19: 23–27. Reprinted in *Stata Technical Bulletin Reprints*, vol. 4, pp. 186–191.

Also See

[ST] **stcox** — Fit Cox proportional hazards model

[ST] **sts** — Generate, graph, list, and test the survivor and cumulative hazard functions

[ST] **stset** — Declare data to be survival-time data

[U] **20 Estimation and postestimation commands**

Title

stcox postestimation — Postestimation tools for stcox

Description

The following postestimation commands are of special interest after stcox:

command	description
estat con	Harrell's C
estat phtest	tests proportional-hazards assumption on the basis of Schoenfeld residuals
stcurve	plots the survivor, hazard, and cumulative hazard functions

estat concordance and estat phtest are not appropriate after the svy prefix.

For information on estat concordance and estat phtest, see below. For information on stcurve, see [ST] **stcurve**.

The following standard postestimation commands are also available:

command	description
adjust	adjusted predictions of $\mathbf{x}\beta$ or $\exp(\mathbf{x}\beta)$
estat	AIC, BIC, VCE, and estimation sample summary
estat (svy)	postestimation statistics for survey data
estimates	cataloging estimation results
lincom	point estimates, standard errors, testing, and inference for linear combinations of coefficients
linktest	link test for model specification
lrtest[1]	likelihood-ratio test
mfx	marginal effects or elasticities
nlcom	point estimates, standard errors, testing, and inference for nonlinear combinations of coefficients
predict	predictions, residuals, influence statistics, and other diagnostic measures
predictnl	point estimates, standard errors, testing, and inference for generalized predictions
test	Wald tests for simple and composite linear hypotheses
testnl	Wald tests of nonlinear hypotheses

[1] lrtest does not work with svy estimation results.

See the corresponding entries in the *Stata Base Reference Manual* for details, but see [SVY] **estat** for details about estat (svy).

Special-interest postestimation commands

estat concordance calculates Harrell's C, which is defined as the proportion of all usable subject pairs in which the predictions and outcomes are concordant. estat concordance also reports the Somers' D rank correlation, which is obtained by calculating $2(C - 0.5)$.

estat phtest tests the proportional-hazards assumption based on Schoenfeld residuals. Using this command requires that you previously specify stcox's schoenfeld() option for the global test or stcox's scaledsch() option for the detailed test.

Syntax for predict

predict [_type_] _newvar_ [_if_] [_in_] [, _statistic_ <u>nooff</u>set]

predict [_type_] { _stub*_ | _newvarlist_ } [_if_] [_in_], <u>sc</u>ores

statistic	description
Main	
hr	predicted hazard ratio, also known as the relative hazard; the default
xb	linear prediction $\mathbf{x}_j\beta$
stdp	standard error of the linear prediction; $\mathrm{SE}(\mathbf{x}_j\beta)$
* csnell	(partial) Cox–Snell residuals
* deviance	deviance residuals
* ccsnell	cumulative Cox–Snell residuals
* cmgale	cumulative martingale residuals

Unstarred statistics are available both in and out of sample; type predict ... if e(sample) ... if wanted for only the estimation sample. Starred statistics are calculated for only the estimation sample, even when e(sample) is not specified. The (partial) martingale residuals, the efficient score residuals, the Schoenfeld residuals, and the scaled Schoenfeld residuals are available through options specified to the stcox command itself.

Options for predict

⌐ Main ⌐

hr, the default, calculates the relative hazard (hazard ratio), that is, the exponentiated linear prediction, $\exp(\mathbf{x}_j\widehat{\beta})$.

xb calculates the linear prediction from the fitted model. That is, you fit the model by estimating a set of parameters $\beta_1, \beta_2, \ldots, \beta_k$, and the linear prediction is $\widehat{y}_j = \widehat{\beta}_1 x_{1j} + \widehat{\beta}_2 x_{2j} + \cdots + \widehat{\beta}_k x_{kj}$, often written in matrix notation as $\widehat{y}_j = \mathbf{x}_j\widehat{\beta}$.

The x_{1j}, x_{2j}, ..., x_{kj} used in the calculation are obtained from the data currently in memory and do not have to correspond to the data on the independent variables used in estimating β.

stdp calculates the standard error of the prediction, that is, the standard error of $\widehat{y}_j$.

csnell calculates the (partial) Cox–Snell generalized residuals. If you have 1 observation per subject, csnell calculates the usual Cox–Snell residual; otherwise, csnell calculates the additive contribution of this observation to the subject's overall Cox–Snell residual. In such cases, see option ccsnell below.

To specify option csnell, you must have specified "stcox ..., mgale(*newvar*) ..." when you fitted the model. The name specified for the new variable does not matter, but you must have specified the mgale() option, or predict will return an error.

deviance calculates the deviance residual. For multiple-record data, only one value per subject is calculated, and it is placed on the last record for the subject.

To specify option deviance, you must have specified "stcox ..., mgale(*newvar*) ..." when you fitted the model. See the comment for option csnell above.

ccsnell calculates the cumulative Cox–Snell residual in multiple-record data by calculating the partial Cox–Snell residuals (see option csnell above) and then summing them. Only one value per subject is recorded—the overall sum—and it is placed on the last record for the subject. ccsnell is the same as csnell in single-record survival data.

To specify option ccsnell, you must have specified "stcox ..., mgale(*newvar*) ..." when you fitted the model. See the comment for option csnell above.

cmgale calculates the cumulative martingale residual in multiple-record data by summing the partial martingale residuals available from stcox. Only one value per subject is recorded—the overall sum—and it is placed on the last record for the subject. cmgale is the same as mgale in single-record survival data.

To specify option cmgale, you must have specified "stcox ..., mgale(*newvar*) ..." when you fitted the model. See the comment for option csnell above.

nooffset is relevant only if you specified offset(*varname*) for stcox. It modifies the calculations made by predict so that they ignore the offset variable; the linear prediction is treated as $x_j\widehat{\beta}$ rather than $x_j\widehat{\beta} + \text{offset}_j$.

scores calculates the partial efficient score residual for each regressor in the model. The variables generated with this option are equivalent to those generated with the esr() option of stcox during estimation.

Syntax for estat concordance

estat <u>con</u>cordance $\begin{bmatrix} if \end{bmatrix}$ $\begin{bmatrix} in \end{bmatrix}$ $\begin{bmatrix} , \ concordance\_options \end{bmatrix}$

concordance_options	description
Main	
all	compute statistic for all observations in the data
<u>nosho</u>w	do not show st setting information

Options for estat concordance

⌐ Main ⌐

all requests that the statistic be computed for all observations in the data. By default, estat concordance computes over the estimation subsample.

noshow prevents estat concordance from displaying the identities of the key st variables above its output.

Syntax for estat phtest

estat phtest [, *phtest_options*]

phtest_options	description
Main	
log	use natural logarithm time-scaling function
km	use $1 - $ KM product-limit estimate as the time-scaling function
rank	use rank of analysis time as the time-scaling function
time(*varname*)	use *varname* containing a monotone transformation of analysis time as the time-scaling function
plot(*varname*)	plot smoothed, scaled Schoenfeld residuals versus time
bwidth(#)	use bandwidth of #; default is bwidth(0.8)
detail	test proportional-hazards assumption separately for each covariate
Scatterplot	
marker_options	change look of markers (color, size, etc.)
marker_label_options	add marker labels; change look or position
Smoothed line	
lineopts(*cline_options*)	affect rendition of the smoothed line
Y axis, X axis, Titles, Legend, Overall	
twoway_options	any options other than by() documented in [G] ***twoway_options***

Options for estat phtest

⌐ Main └───

log, km, rank, and time() are used to specify the time scaling function.

By default, estat phtest performs the tests using the identity function, i.e., analysis time itself.

log specifies that the natural log of analysis time be used.

km specifies that 1 minus the Kaplan–Meier product-limit estimate be used.

rank specifies that the rank of analysis time be used.

time(*varname*) specifies a variable containing an arbitrary monotonic transformation of analysis time. You must ensure that *varname* is a monotonic transform.

plot(*varname*) specifies that a scatterplot and smoothed plot of scaled Schoenfeld residuals versus time be produced for the covariate specified by *varname*. By default, the smoothing is performed using the running-mean method implemented in lowess, mean noweight; see [R] **lowess**.

bwidth(#) specifies the bandwidth. Centered subsets of bwidth() $* N$ observations are used for calculating smoothed values for each point in the data except for endpoints, where smaller, uncentered subsets are used. The greater the bwidth(), the greater the smoothing. The default is bwidth(0.8).

detail specifies that a separate test of the proportional-hazards assumption be produced for each covariate in the Cox model. By default, estat phtest produces only the global test.

marker_options affect the rendition of markers drawn at the plotted points, including their shape, size, color, and outline; see [G] ***marker_options***.

marker_label_options specify if and how the markers are to be labeled; see [G] ***marker_label_options***.

lineopts(*cline_options*) affects the rendition of the smoothed line; see [G] ***cline_options***.

twoway_options are any of the options documented in [G] ***twoway_options***, excluding by(). These include options for titling the graph (see [G] ***title_options***) and for saving the graph to disk (see [G] ***saving_option***).

Remarks

Remarks are presented under the following headings:

>   *Cox regression residuals*
>   *estat concordance*
>   *estat phtest*

Cox regression residuals

Stata can calculate score residuals, efficient score residuals (esr), martingale residuals, Schoenfeld residuals, and scaled Schoenfeld residuals with options specified to the stcox command. Cox–Snell and deviance residuals can be calculated with options to predict. For time-varying covariates and multiple observations per subject, cumulative martingale and cumulative Cox–Snell residuals can also be calculated using predict.

Although the uses of residuals vary and depend on the data and user preferences, traditional and suggested uses are the following: Cox–Snell residuals are useful in assessing overall model fit; martingale residuals are useful in determining the functional form of covariates to be included in the model and are occasionally useful in assessing lack of fit; Schoenfeld and score residuals are useful for checking and testing the proportional-hazards assumption, examining leverage points, and identifying outliers; and deviance residuals are useful in examining model accuracy and identifying outliers.

▷ Example 1: Cox–Snell residuals

Let us first examine the use of Cox–Snell residuals. Using the cancer data introduced in example 2 in [ST] **stcox**, we first perform a Cox regression requesting that martingale residuals be calculated. Martingale residuals must be requested because these are used by predict to calculate the Cox–Snell residuals. If we forget to request martingale residuals, predict will issue an error message reminding us.

```
. use http://www.stata-press.com/data/r10/drugtr
(Patient Survival in Drug Trial)
. stset studytime, failure(died)
(output omitted )
. stcox age drug, mgale(mg)
(output omitted )
. predict double cs, csnell
```

The first command performs the Cox regression, calculates the martingale residuals, and saves them in the variable mg. In the second command, the csnell option tells predict to output the Cox–Snell residuals to a new variable, cs. If the Cox regression model fits the data, these residuals should have a standard censored exponential distribution with hazard ratio 1. We can verify the model's fit by calculating—based, for example, on the Kaplan–Meier estimated survivor function or the Aalen–Nelson estimator—an empirical estimate of the cumulative hazard function, using the Cox–Snell residuals as the time variable and the data's original censoring variable. If the model fits the data, the plot of the cumulative hazard versus cs should be a straight line with slope 1.

To do this, we first stset the data, specifying cs as our new failure-time variable and died as the failure/censoring indicator. We then use the sts generate command to generate the variable km containing the Kaplan–Meier survivor estimates. Last, we generate the cumulative hazard H by using the relationship H = −ln(km) and plot it against cs.

```
. stset cs, failure(died)
(output omitted )
. sts generate km=s
. generate double H=-ln(km)
(1 missing value generated)
. line H cs cs, sort ytitle("") clstyle(. refline) legend(nodraw)
```

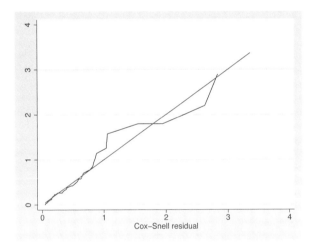

We specified cs twice in the graph command so that a reference $45°$ line is plotted. Comparing the jagged line with the reference line, we observe that the Cox model does not fit these data too badly.

◁

❏ Technical Note

The statement that "if the Cox regression model fits the data, the Cox–Snell residuals have a standard censored exponential distribution with hazard ratio 1" holds only if the true parameters β and the true cumulative baseline hazard function, $H_0(t)$, are used in calculating the residuals. Since we use estimates $\widehat{\beta}$ and $\widehat{H}_0(t)$, deviations from the $45°$ line in the above plots could be due partially to uncertainty about these estimates. This is particularly important for small sample sizes and in the right-hand tail of the distribution, where the baseline hazard is more variable because of the reduced effective sample caused by prior failures and censoring.

❏

▷ Example 2: Martingale residuals

Let us now examine the martingale residuals. Martingale residuals are useful in assessing the functional form of a covariate to be entered into a Cox model. Sometimes the covariate may need transforming so that the transformed variable will satisfy the assumptions of the proportional hazards model. To find the appropriate functional form of a variable, we fit a Cox model excluding the variable and then plot a `lowess` smooth of the martingale residuals against some transformation of the variable in question. If the transformation is appropriate, then the smooth should be approximately linear.

We apply this procedure to our cancer data to find an appropriate transformation of `age` (or to verify that `age` need not be transformed).

```
. use http://www.stata-press.com/data/r10/drugtr, clear
(Patient Survival in Drug Trial)
. stset studytime, failure(died)
(output omitted)
. stcox drug, mgale(mg)
(output omitted)
. lowess mg age, mean noweight title("") note("") m(o)
```

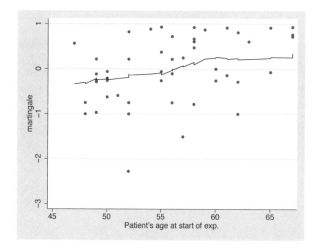

We used the `lowess` command with the options `mean` and `noweight` to obtain a plot of the running-mean smoother to ease interpretation. A lowess smoother or other smoother could also be used; see [R] **lowess**. The smooth appears nearly linear, supporting the inclusion of the untransformed version of `age` in our Cox model. Had the smooth not been linear, we would have tried smoothing the martingale residuals against various transformations of `age` until we found one that produced a near-linear smooth.

◁

Martingale residuals can also be interpreted as the difference over time of the observed number of failures minus the difference predicted by the model. Thus a plot of the martingale residuals versus the linear predictor may be used to detect outliers.

Plots of martingale residuals are sometimes difficult to interpret, however, because these residuals are skewed, taking values in $(-\infty, 1)$. For this reason, deviance residuals are preferred for examining model accuracy and identifying outliers.

▷ Example 3: Deviance residuals

Using our cancer data, we can calculate the deviance residuals with `predict`, but we first need to refit the Cox model with `age` (untransformed) included and regenerate the martingale residuals for this model. `predict, deviance` requires that martingale residuals be calculated and saved when fitting the Cox model. Deviance residuals are a rescaling of the martingale residuals so that they are symmetric about zero and thus are more like residuals obtained from linear regression. Plots of these residuals against the linear predictor, survival time, rank order of survival, or observation number can be useful in identifying aberrant observations and assessing model fit.

```
. drop mg
. stcox drug age, mgale(mg)
 (output omitted )
. predict double xb, xb
. scatter mg xb
```

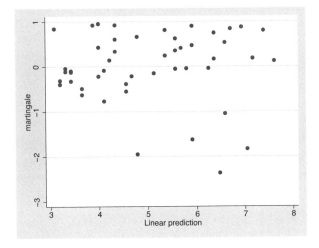

```
. predict double dev, deviance
. scatter dev xb
```

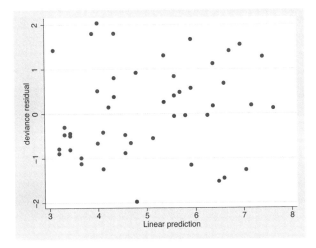

We first plotted the martingale residuals versus the linear predictor and then the deviance residuals versus the linear predictor. Given their symmetry about zero, deviance residuals are easier to interpret, although both graphs yield the same information. With uncensored data, deviance residuals should resemble white noise if the fit is adequate. Censored observations would be represented as clumps of deviance residuals near zero (Klein and Moeschberger 2003, 381). Given what we see above, there do not appear to be any outliers.

◁

In evaluating the adequacy of the fitted model, we must determine if any observation or group of observations has a disproportionate influence on the estimated parameters. This is known as influence or leverage analysis. The preferred method of performing influence or leverage analysis is to compare the estimated parameter, $\widehat{\beta}$, obtained from the full data, with estimated parameters $\widehat{\beta}_{(i)}$, obtained by fitting the model to the $n-1$ observations remaining after the ith observation is removed. If $\widehat{\beta} - \widehat{\beta}_{(i)}$ is close to zero, the ith observation has little influence on the estimate. The process is repeated for all observations included in the original model. To compute these differences for a dataset with n observations, we would have to execute stcox n additional times, which could be impractical for large datasets. In such cases, an approximation to $\widehat{\beta} - \widehat{\beta}_{(i)}$ that is based on the efficient score residuals can be calculated as

$$\Delta' \mathbf{V}(\widehat{\beta})$$

where $\mathbf{V}(\widehat{\beta})$ is the variance–covariance matrix and Δ' is the matrix of efficient score residuals. The difference $\widehat{\beta} - \widehat{\beta}_{(i)}$ is commonly referred to as dfbeta in the literature; see [R] **regress postestimation**.

▷ Example 4: Efficient score residuals

We now perform an influence analysis using the cancer data. To do this, we first obtain the efficient score residuals by typing stcox age drug, esr(esr*). This command generates two new variables, esr1 and esr2, corresponding to the two covariates in the model. The first variable, esr1, contains the efficient score residuals corresponding to the first covariate listed in the model (age), and the second variable, esr2, contains the efficient score residuals corresponding to the second covariate listed in the model (drug). We then use the mkmat command to create a matrix of the efficient score residuals, we obtain the variance–covariance matrix, and then we multiply the two matrices.

```
. use http://www.stata-press.com/data/r10/drugtr, clear
(Patient Survival in Drug Trial)
. stset studytime, fail(died)
  (output omitted)
. stcox age drug, esr(esr*)
  (output omitted)
. mkmat esr1 esr2, matrix(esr)
. mat V = e(V)
. mat Inf = esr*V
. svmat Inf, names(s)
```

The last command saves the estimates of dfbeta $= \widehat{\beta} - \widehat{\beta}_{(i)}$ in the variables s1 and s2. We can now label these new variables and plot them versus time or observation number to identify observations with disproportionate influence.

```
. label var s1 "dfbeta - Age"
. label var s2 "dfbeta - Drug"
. scatter s1 studytime, ylab(-.1(.1).2) yline(0)
```

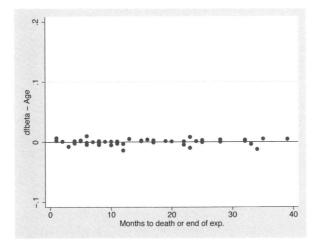

```
. scatter s2 studytime, ylab(-.1(.1).2) yline(0)
```

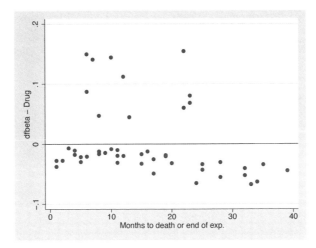

◁

estat concordance

estat concordance calculates Harrell's C, which is defined as the proportion of all usable subject pairs in which the predictions and outcomes are concordant. estat concordance also reports the Somers' D rank correlation, which is derived by calculating $2(C - 0.5)$. estat concordance may not be used after a Cox regression model with time-varying covariates and may not be applied to weighted data or to data with late entries.

▷ Example 5: Harrell's C

Using our cancer data, we wish to evaluate the predictive value of the measurement of drug and age. After fitting a Cox regression model, we use `estat concordance` to calculate Harrell's C index.

```
.use http://www.stata-press.com/data/r10/drugtr, clear
(Patient Survival in Drug Trial)
. stcox drug age
        failure _d:  died
  analysis time _t:  studytime
Iteration 0:   log likelihood = -99.911448
Iteration 1:   log likelihood = -83.551879
Iteration 2:   log likelihood = -83.324009
Iteration 3:   log likelihood = -83.323546
Refining estimates:
Iteration 0:   log likelihood = -83.323546
Cox regression -- Breslow method for ties
No. of subjects =          48                 Number of obs   =        48
No. of failures =          31
Time at risk    =         744
                                              LR chi2(2)      =     33.18
Log likelihood  =   -83.323546                Prob > chi2     =    0.0000
```

_t	Haz. Ratio	Std. Err.	z	P>|z|	[95% Conf. Interval]	
drug	.1048772	.0477017	-4.96	0.000	.0430057	.2557622
age	1.120325	.0417711	3.05	0.002	1.041375	1.20526

```
. estat concordance, noshow
  Harrell's C concordance statistic
  Number of subjects (N)                =        48
  Number of comparison pairs (P)        =       849
  Number of orderings as expected (E)   =       679
  Number of tied predictions (T)        =        15
          Harrell's C = (E + T/2) / P =    .8086
                         Somers' D =    .6172
```

The result of `stcox` shows that the drug results in a lower hazard and therefore a longer survival time, controlling for age and older patients being more likely to die. The value of Harrell's C is 0.8086, which indicates that we can correctly order survival times for pairs of patients 81% of the time on the basis of measurement of drug and age. See *Methods and Formulas* for the full definition of concordance.

◁

❑ Technical Note

`estat concordance` does not work after a Cox regression model with time-varying covariates. When the covariates are varying with time, the prognostic score, $PS = \mathbf{x}\beta$, will not capture or condense the information in given measurements. It does not make sense to calculate the rank correlation between PS and survival time any more.

❑

estat phtest

Many popular tests for proportional hazards are, in fact, tests of nonzero slope in a generalized linear regression of the scaled Schoenfeld residuals of time (see Grambsch and Therneau 1994). The estat phtest command tests, for individual covariates and globally, the null hypothesis of zero slope, which is equivalent to testing that the log hazard-ratio function is constant over time. Thus, rejection of the null hypothesis of a zero slope indicates deviation from the proportional-hazards assumption. The estat phtest command allows three common time-scaling options (log, rank and km) and allows you to specify a user-defined function of time through the time() option. When no option is specified, the tests are performed using analysis time without further transformation.

▷ Example 6: estat phtest

This example uses the same data used in example 1 of [ST] **stcox diagnostics**.

```
. use http://www.stata-press.com/data/r10/leukemia
(Leukemia Remission Study)

. describe

Contains data from http://www.stata-press.com/data/r10/leukemia.dta
  obs:            42                    Leukemia Remission Study
  vars:            8                    23 Mar 2007 10:39
  size:          504 (99.9% of memory free)
```

variable name	storage type	display format	value label	variable label
weeks	byte	%8.0g		Weeks in Remission
relapse	byte	%8.0g	yesno	Relapse
treatment1	byte	%8.0g	trt1lbl	Treatment I
treatment2	byte	%8.0g	trt2lbl	Treatment II
wbc3cat	byte	%9.0g	wbclbl	White Blood Cell Count
wbc1	byte	%8.0g		wbc3cat==Normal
wbc2	byte	%8.0g		wbc3cat==Moderate
wbc3	byte	%8.0g		wbc3cat==High

```
Sorted by:  weeks
```

In this example, we examine whether the proportional-hazards assumption holds for a model with covariates wbc2, wbc1, and treatment1. After stsetting the data, we first run stcox, saving both the scaled and the nonscaled Schoenfeld residuals. Then we use estat phtest, which requires that we request scaled Schoenfeld residuals if we want a separate test for each covariate and that we request the unscaled residuals if we want the global test. If we forget to request the residuals at estimation time, estat phtest will remind us.

```
. stset weeks, failure(relapse)

     failure event:  relapse != 0 & relapse < .
obs. time interval:  (0, weeks]
 exit on or before:  failure
```

42	total obs.		
0	exclusions		

42	obs. remaining, representing		
30	failures in single record/single failure data		
541	total analysis time at risk, at risk from t =		0
	earliest observed entry t =		0
	last observed exit t =		35

```
. stcox treatment1 wbc2 wbc3, scaledsch(sca*) schoenfeld(sch*) nolog
        failure _d:  relapse
   analysis time _t:  weeks
Cox regression -- Breslow method for ties
No. of subjects =          42                  Number of obs   =          42
No. of failures =          30
Time at risk    =         541
                                               LR chi2(3)      =       33.02
Log likelihood  =   -77.476905                 Prob > chi2     =      0.0000
```

_t	Haz. Ratio	Std. Err.	z	P>|z|	[95% Conf. Interval]	
treatment1	.2834551	.1229874	-2.91	0.004	.1211042	.6634517
wbc2	3.637825	2.201306	2.13	0.033	1.111134	11.91015
wbc3	10.92214	7.088783	3.68	0.000	3.06093	38.97284

```
. estat phtest, rank detail
     Test of proportional-hazards assumption
     Time:  Rank(t)
```

	rho	chi2	df	Prob>chi2
treatment1	-0.02802	0.02	1	0.8755
wbc2	-0.10665	0.32	1	0.5735
wbc3	-0.02238	0.02	1	0.8987
global test		0.51	3	0.9159

Because we saved both the Schoenfeld residuals and the scaled Schoenfeld residuals by specifying the `detail` option on the `estat phtest` command, both covariate-specific and global tests were produced. We can see that there is no evidence that the proportional-hazards assumption has been violated. When we saved the residuals using `stcox`, it did not matter what we named them; it just mattered that we saved them.

Another variable in this dataset measures a different drug (`treatment2`: $1 = $ drug B, $0 = $ standard). We now wish to examine the proportional-hazards assumption for the previous model by substituting `treatment2` for `treatment1`.

After dropping the previous Schoenfeld and scaled Schoenfeld residuals, we fit a new Cox model and perform the test for proportional hazards.

```
. drop sca* sch*
. stcox treatment2 wbc2 wbc3, scaledsch(sca*) schoenfeld(sch*) nolog
        failure _d:  relapse
   analysis time _t:  weeks
Cox regression -- Breslow method for ties
No. of subjects =          42                  Number of obs   =          42
No. of failures =          30
Time at risk    =         541
                                               LR chi2(3)      =       23.93
Log likelihood  =   -82.019053                 Prob > chi2     =      0.0000
```

_t	Haz. Ratio	Std. Err.	z	P>|z|	[95% Conf. Interval]	
treatment2	.8483777	.3469054	-0.40	0.688	.3806529	1.890816
wbc2	3.409628	2.050784	2.04	0.041	1.048905	11.08353
wbc3	14.0562	8.873693	4.19	0.000	4.078529	48.44314

```
. estat phtest, rank detail
    Test of proportional-hazards assumption
    Time:  Rank(t)
```

	rho	chi2	df	Prob>chi2
treatment2	-0.63673	15.47	1	0.0001
wbc2	-0.17380	0.90	1	0.3426
wbc3	-0.08294	0.21	1	0.6481
global test		15.76	3	0.0013

`treatment2` violates the proportional-hazards assumption. One hazard ratio describing the effect of this drug is inappropriate.

◁

❏ Technical Note

The test of the proportional-hazards assumption is based on the principle that the assumption restricts $\beta_j(t) = \beta$ for all t, which implies that a plot of $\beta_j(t)$ versus time will have a slope of zero. Grambsch and Therneau (1994) showed that $E(s_j^*) + \widehat{\beta} \approx \beta(t_j)$, where s_j^* is the scaled Schoenfeld residual and $\widehat{\beta}$ is the estimated coefficient from the Cox model. Thus a plot of $s_j^* + \beta$ versus some function of time provides a graphical assessment of the assumption.

❏

❏ Technical Note

The tests of the proportional-hazards assumption assume homogeneity of variance across risk sets. This allows the use of the estimated overall (pooled) variance–covariance matrix in the equations. Although these tests have been shown by Grambsch and Therneau (1994) to be fairly robust to departures from this assumption, exercise care where this assumption may not hold, particularly when performing a stratified Cox analysis. In such cases, we recommend that you check the proportional-hazards assumption separately for each stratum.

❏

Saved Results

estat concordance saves the following in r():

Scalars

r(N)	number of observations	r(n_T)	number of tied predictions
r(n_P)	number of comparison pairs	r(D)	Somers' D coefficient
r(n_E)	number of ordering as expected	r(C)	Harrell's C coefficient

estat phtest saves the following in r():

Scalars

r(df)	global test degrees of freedom	r(chi2)	global test χ^2

Methods and Formulas

All postestimation commands listed above are implemented as ado-files.

estat concordance

Harrell's C was proposed by Harrell et al. (1982) and was developed to evaluate the results of a medical test. The C index is defined as the proportion of all usable subject pairs in which the predictions and outcomes are concordant. The C index may be applied to ordinary continuous outcomes, dichotomous diagnostic outcomes, ordinal outcomes, and censored time-until-event response variables.

In predicting the time until death, C is calculated by considering all possible patient pairs for which at least one of whom has died. If the predicted survival time is larger for the patient who lived longer, the predictions for the pair are said to be concordant with the outcomes. Harrell's C is defined as $(E + T/2)/D$, where D is the total number of pairs usable for comparison, E is the number of pairs for which the predictions are concordant with the outcomes and the predictions are not identical, and T is the number of usable pairs for which the predictions are identical.

For a Cox proportional hazards model, the probability that the patient survives past the time t is given by $S_0(t)$ raised to the $\exp(\mathbf{x}\boldsymbol{\beta})$ power, where $S_0(t)$ is the baseline survivor function, $\mathbf{x}$ denotes a set of measurements for the patient, and $\boldsymbol{\beta}$ is the vector of coefficients. A Cox regression model is fitted by the `stcox` command. The hazard ratio, $\exp(\mathbf{x}\boldsymbol{\beta})$, is obtained by `predict` after `stcox`. Since the predicted survivor time and the predicted survivor function are one-to-one functions of each other, the predicted survivor function can be used to calculate C instead of the predicted survival time. The predicted survivor function decreases when predicted hazard ratio increases; therefore, Harrell's C can be calculated by computing E, T, and D, based on the observed outcomes and the predicted hazard ratios.

C takes a value between 0 and 1. A value of 0.5 indicates no predictive discrimination, and values of 0 or 1.0 indicate perfect separation of subjects with different outcomes. See Harrell, Lee, and Mark (1996) for more detail. Somers' D rank correlation is calculated by $2C - 1$, see Newson (2002) for a discussion of Somers' D.

estat phtest

Grambsch and Therneau (1994) presented a scaled adjustment for the Schoenfeld residuals that permits the interpretation of the smoothed residuals as a nonparametric estimate of the log hazard-ratio function. These are defined at each death event as

$$r_{uS_i^*} = \widehat{\beta}_u + \Delta(\mathbf{S}\widehat{\mathbf{V}}^{-1})_{ui}$$

where $\Delta = \sum_{i=1}^{N} \delta_i$ is the total number of deaths, $\mathbf{S}$ is the matrix of Schoenfeld residuals, and $\widehat{\mathbf{V}}$ is the variance matrix estimate. These residuals are centered at $\widehat{\beta}_u$ for each covariate and should have slope zero when plotted against functions of time. The `estat phtest` command uses these residuals, tests the null hypothesis that the slope is equal to zero for each covariate in the model, and performs the global test proposed by Grambsch and Therneau (1994). The test of zero slope is equivalent to testing that the log hazard-ratio function is constant over time.

For a specified function of time, $g(t)$, the statistic for testing individual covariates is (for $\overline{g}(t) = \Delta^{-1} \sum_{i=1}^{N} \delta_i g(t_i)$)

$$\frac{\left[\sum_{i=1}^{N}\{\delta_{i.}g(t_i) - \overline{g}(t)\}r_{uS_i^*}\right]^2}{\Delta\widehat{\mathbf{V}}_{uu}\sum_{i=1}^{N}\{\delta_{i.}g(t_i) - \overline{g}(t)\}^2}$$

which is asymptotically distributed as a χ^2 random variate with 1 degree of freedom.

The statistic for the global tests is calculated as

$$\left[\sum_{i=1}^{N}\{\delta_{i.}g(t_i) - \overline{g}(t)\}\mathbf{r}_i\right]'\left[\frac{\Delta\widehat{\mathbf{V}}}{\sum_{i=1}^{N}\left\{\delta_{i.}g(t_i) - \overline{g}(t)\right\}^2}\right]\left[\sum_{i=1}^{N}\{\delta_{i.}g(t_i) - \overline{g}(t)\}\mathbf{r}_i\right]$$

for $\mathbf{r}_i$, a vector of the p (unscaled) Schoenfeld residuals for the ith observation. The global test statistic is asymptotically distributed as a χ^2 random variate with p degrees of freedom.

The equations for the scaled Schoenfeld residuals and the two test statistics just described assume homogeneity of variance across risk sets. Although these tests are fairly robust to deviations from this assumption, care must be exercised, particularly when dealing with a stratified Cox model.

For shared-frailty models, the data are organized into G groups with the ith group consisting of n_i observations, $i = 1, \ldots, G$. For Therneau and Grambsch (2000, 253–255), estimation of θ takes place via maximum profile log likelihood. For fixed θ, estimates of $\boldsymbol{\beta}$ and $\nu_1, \ldots, \nu_G$ are obtained by maximizing

$$\ln L(\theta) = \ln L_{\mathrm{Cox}}(\boldsymbol{\beta}, \nu_1, \ldots, \nu_G) + \sum_{i=1}^{G}\left[\frac{1}{\theta}\{\nu_i - \exp(\nu_i)\} + \right.$$

$$\left.\left(\frac{1}{\theta} + D_i\right)\left\{1 - \ln\left(\frac{1}{\theta} + D_i\right)\right\} - \frac{\ln\theta}{\theta} + \ln\Gamma\left(\frac{1}{\theta} + D_i\right) - \ln\Gamma\left(\frac{1}{\theta}\right)\right]$$

where D_i is the number of death events in group i, and $\ln L_{\mathrm{Cox}}(\boldsymbol{\beta}, \nu_1, \ldots, \nu_G)$ is the standard Cox partial log likelihood, with the ν_i treated as the coefficients of indicator variables identifying the groups. That is, the jth observation in the ith group has log relative hazard $\mathbf{x}_{ij}\boldsymbol{\beta} + \nu_i$. The estimate of the frailty parameter, $\widehat{\theta}$, is chosen as that which maximizes $\ln L(\theta)$. The final estimates of $\boldsymbol{\beta}$ are obtained by maximizing $\ln L(\widehat{\theta})$ in $\boldsymbol{\beta}$ and the ν_i; the ν_i are not reported in the coefficient table but are available optionally. The estimated variance–covariance matrix of $\widehat{\boldsymbol{\beta}}$ is obtained as the appropriate submatrix of the variance matrix of $(\widehat{\boldsymbol{\beta}}, \widehat{\nu}_1, \ldots, \widehat{\nu}_G)$, and that matrix is obtained as the inverse of the negative Hessian of $\ln L(\widehat{\theta})$. Therefore, standard errors and inference based on $\widehat{\boldsymbol{\beta}}$ should be treated as conditional on $\theta = \widehat{\theta}$.

The likelihood-ratio test statistic for testing H_0: $\theta = 0$ is calculated as minus twice the difference between the log-likelihood for a Cox model without shared frailty and $\ln L(\widehat{\theta})$ evaluated at the final $(\widehat{\boldsymbol{\beta}}, \widehat{\nu}_1, \ldots, \widehat{\nu}_G)$. All residuals and predictions are calculated treating the estimated ν_i as fixed offsets to the linear predictor. Estimated baseline functions are interpreted as those for which $\mathbf{x}$ *and* ν equal zero.

Acknowledgment

We thank Joanne M. Garrett, University of North Carolina at Chapel Hill, for her contributions to the `estat phtest` command.

References

Grambsch, P. M., and T. M. Therneau. 1994. Proportional hazards tests and diagnostics based on weighted residuals. *Biometrika* 81: 515–526.

Harrell, F. E., R. M. Califf, D. B. Pryor, K. L. Lee, and R. A. Rosati. 1982. Evaluating the yield of medical tests. *Journal of the American Medical Association* 247: 2543–2546.

Harrell, F. E., K. L. Lee, and D. B. Mark. 1996. Multivariable prognostic models: Issues in developing models, evaluating assumptions and adequacy, and measuring and reducing errors. *Statistics in Medicine* 15: 361–387.

Klein, J. P., and M. L. Moeschberger. 2003. *Survival Analysis: Techniques for Censored and Truncated Data*. 2nd ed. New York: Springer.

Newson, R. 2002. Parameters behind "nonparametric" statistics: Kendall's tau, Somers' D and median differences. *Stata Journal* 2: 45–64.

———. 2006. Confidence intervals for rank statistics: Somers' D and extensions. *Stata Journal* 6: 309–334.

Rogers, W. H. 1994. ssa4: Ex post tests and diagnostics for a proportional hazards model. *Stata Technical Bulletin* 19: 23–27. Reprinted in *Stata Technical Bulletin Reprints*, vol. 4, pp. 186–191.

Schoenfeld, D. 1982. Partial residuals for the proportional hazards regression model. *Biometrika* 69: 239–241.

Therneau, T. M., and P. M. Grambsch. 2000. *Modeling Survival Data: Extending the Cox Model*. New York: Springer.

Also See

[ST] **stcox** — Fit Cox proportional hazards model

[ST] **stcurve** — Plot survivor, hazard, or cumulative hazard function

[U] **20 Estimation and postestimation commands**

Title

> **stcurve** — Plot survivor, hazard, or cumulative hazard function

Syntax

stcurve [, *stcurve_options*]

stcurve_options	description
Main	
* <u>surv</u>ival	plot survivor function
* <u>haz</u>ard	plot hazard function
* <u>cumh</u>az	plot cumulative hazard function
at(*varname*=# [*varname*=#...])	value of the specified covariates and mean of
[at1(*varname*=# [*varname*=#...])	unspecified covariates
[at2(*varname*=# [*varname*=#...])	
[...]]]	
Options	
<u>alpha1</u>	conditional frailty model
<u>uncond</u>itional	unconditional frailty model
<u>ran</u>ge(# #)	range of analysis time
<u>outf</u>ile(*filename* [, <u>replace</u>])	save values used to plot the curves
width(#)	override "optimal" width; use with hazard
<u>k</u>ernel(*kernel*)	kernel function; use with hazard
<u>nob</u>oundary	no boundary correction; use with hazard
Plot	
connect_options	affect rendition of plotted survivor, hazard, or cumulative hazard function
Add plots	
addplot(*plot*)	add other plots to the generated graph
Y axis, X axis, Titles, Legend, Overall	
twoway_options	any options other than by() documented in [G] *twoway_options*

*One of survival, hazard, or cumhaz must be specified.

Description

stcurve plots the survivor, hazard, or cumulative hazard function after stcox or streg.

Options

```
        Main
```

survival requests that the survivor function be plotted.

hazard requests that the hazard function be plotted.

cumhaz requests that the cumulative hazard function be plotted.

at(*varname=#*...) requests that the covariates specified by *varname* be set to *#*. By default, stcurve evaluates the function by setting each covariate to its mean value. This option causes the function to be evaluated at the value of the covariates listed in at() and at the mean of all unlisted covariates.

at1(*varname=#*...), at2(*varname=#*...), ..., at10(*varname=#*...) specify that multiple curves (up to 10) be plotted on the same graph. at1(), at2(), ..., at10() work like the at() option. They request that the function be evaluated at the value of the covariates specified and at the mean of all unlisted covariates. at1() specifies the values of the covariates for the first curve, at2() specifies the values of the covariates for the second curve, and so on.

```
        Options
```

alpha1, when used after fitting a frailty model, plots curves that are conditional on a frailty value of one. This is the default for shared-frailty models.

unconditional, when used after fitting a frailty model, plots curves that are unconditional on the frailty; i.e., the curve is "averaged" over the frailty distribution. This is the default for unshared-frailty models.

range(*# #*) specifies the range of the time axis to be plotted. If this option is not specified, stcurve plots the desired curve on an interval expanding from the earliest to the latest time in the data.

outfile(*filename* [,replace]) saves in *filename*.dta the values used to plot the curve(s).

width(*#*) is for use with hazard (and applies only after stcox) and is used to specify the bandwidth to be used in the kernel smooth used to plot the estimated hazard function. If left unspecified, a default bandwidth is used as described in [R] **kdensity**.

kernel(*kernel*) is for use with hazard and is for use only after stcox since, for Cox regression, an estimate of the hazard function is obtained by smoothing the estimated *hazard contributions*. kernel() specifies the kernel function for use in calculating the weighted kernel-density estimate required to produce a smoothed hazard function estimator. The default kernel is Epanechnikov, yet *kernel* may be any of the kernels supported by kdensity; see [R] **kdensity**.

noboundary is for use with hazard and applies only to the plotting of smoothed hazard functions after stcox. It specifies that no boundary-bias adjustments are to be made when calculating the smoothed hazard function estimator. By default, the smoothed hazards are adjusted near the boundaries; see [ST] **sts graph**. If the epan2, biweight, or rectangular kernel is used, the bias correction near the boundary is performed using boundary kernels. For other kernels, the plotted range of the smoothed hazard function is restricted to be inside of one bandwidth from each endpoint. For these other kernels, specifying noboundary merely removes this range restriction.

```
        Plot
```

connect_options affect the rendition of the plotted survivor, hazard, or cumulative hazard function; see [G] *connect_options*.

⌐‾‾ Add plots ⌐

addplot(*plot*) provides a way to add other plots to the generated graph; see [G] *addplot_option*.

⌐‾‾ Y axis, X axis, Titles, Legend, Overall ⌐

twoway_options are any of the options documented in [G] *twoway_options*, excluding by(). These include options for titling the graph (see [G] *title_options*) and for saving the graph to disk (see [G] *saving_option*).

Remarks

Remarks are presented under the following headings:

> *stcurve after stcox*
> *stcurve after streg*

stcurve after stcox

After fitting a Cox model, stcurve can be used to plot the estimated hazard, cumulative hazard, and survivor functions.

▷ Example 1

```
. use http://www.stata-press.com/data/r10/drugtr
(Patient Survival in Drug Trial)

. stcox age drug, basesurv(s) basehc(h)
  (output omitted )

. stcurve, survival
```

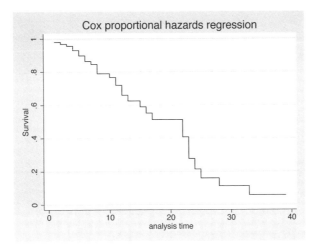

By default, the curve is evaluated at the mean values of all the predictors, but we can specify other values if we wish.

. stcurve, survival at1(drug=0) at2(drug=1)

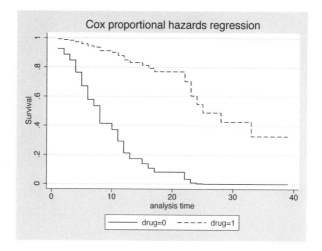

In this example, we asked for two plots, one for the placebo group and one for the treatment group. For both groups, the value of age was held at its mean value for the overall estimation sample.

◁

▷ Example 2

stcurve can also be used to plot estimated hazard functions. The hazard function is estimated by a kernel smooth of the estimated hazard contributions, which is available to us after specifying basehc(h) to stcox; see [ST] **sts graph** for details. We can thus customize the smooth as we would any other; see [R] **kdensity** for details.

. stcurve, hazard at1(drug=0) at2(drug=1) kernel(gauss) yscale(log)

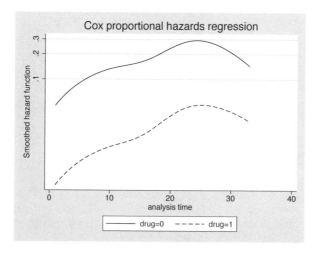

For the hazard plot, we plotted on a log scale to demonstrate the proportionality of hazards under this model; see the technical note below on smoothed hazards.

◁

When we ran stcox above, we specified the options basesurv(s) and basehc(h). When plotting the hazard, you must specify option basehc() to stcox—that is how stcurve retrieves the necessary information to estimate the hazard. When plotting the cumulative hazard, you must specify basechazard() to stcox. When plotting the survivor function, you must specify basesurv(). If you forget to specify one of these options, stcurve will complain.

❏ Technical Note

For survivor or cumulative hazard estimation, stcurve works by first estimating the baseline function and then modifying it to adhere to the specified (or by default, mean) covariate patterns. As mentioned previously, *baseline* (when all covariates are equal to zero) must correspond to something that is meaningful and preferably in the range of your data. Otherwise, stcurve could encounter numerical difficulties. We ignored our own advice above and left age unchanged. Had we encountered numerical problems, or funny-looking graphs, we would have known to try shifting age so that age==0 was in the range of our data.

For hazard estimation, stcurve works by first transforming the estimated hazard contributions (as produced by basehc()) to adhere to the necessary covariate pattern and then applying the smooth. When you plot multiple curves, each is smoothed independently, although the same bandwidth is used for each.

The smoothing takes place in the hazard scale and not in the log-hazard scale. As a result, the resulting curves will look nearly, but not exactly, parallel when plotted on a log scale. This inexactitude is a product of the smoothing and should not be interpreted as a deviation from the proportional-hazards assumption; stcurve (after stcox) assumes proportionality of hazards and will reflect this in the produced plots. If smoothing were a perfect science, the curves would be parallel when plotted on a log scale. If you encounter estimated hazards exhibiting severe disproportionality, this may signal a numerical problem as described above. Try recentering your covariates so that baseline is more reasonable.

❏

stcurve after streg

stcurve is used after streg to plot the fitted survivor, hazard, and cumulative hazard functions. By default, stcurve computes the means of the covariates and evaluates the fitted model at each time in the data, censored or uncensored. The resulting plot is therefore the survival experience of a subject with a covariate pattern equal to the average covariate pattern in the study. You can produce the plot at other values of the covariates by using the at() option or specify a time range by using the range() option.

▷ Example 3

We pick up where [ST] **streg** left off. The cancer dataset we are using has three values for variable drug: 1 corresponds to placebo, and 2 and 3 correspond to two alternative treatments. Using the cancer data with drug remapped to form an indicator of treatment, let's fit a log-logistic regression model and plot its survival curves. We can perform a log-logistic regression by issuing the following commands:

```
. use http://www.stata-press.com/data/r10/cancer, clear
(Patient Survival in Drug Trial)
. replace drug = drug==2 | drug==3        // 0, placebo : 1, nonplacebo
(48 real changes made)
```

```
. stset studytime, failure(died)
 (output omitted )

. streg age drug, d(llog) nolog

         failure _d:  died
   analysis time _t:  studytime

Log-logistic regression -- accelerated failure-time form

No. of subjects =          48                  Number of obs   =          48
No. of failures =          31
Time at risk    =         744
                                               LR chi2(2)      =       35.14
Log likelihood  =    -43.21698                 Prob > chi2     =      0.0000
```

_t	Coef.	Std. Err.	z	P>|z|	[95% Conf. Interval]
age	-.0803289	.0221598	-3.62	0.000	-.1237614 -.0368964
drug	1.420237	.2502148	5.68	0.000	.9298251 1.910649
_cons	6.446711	1.231914	5.23	0.000	4.032204 8.861218
/ln_gam	-.8456552	.1479337	-5.72	0.000	-1.1356 -.5557105
gamma	.429276	.0635044			.3212293 .5736646

Now we wish to plot the survivor and the hazard functions:

```
. stcurve, survival ylabels(0 .5 1)
```

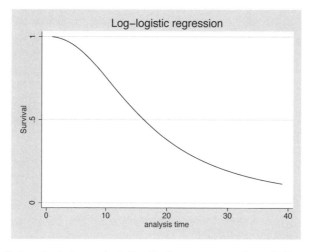

Figure 3. Log-logistic survival distribution at mean value of all covariates

```
. stcurve, hazard
```

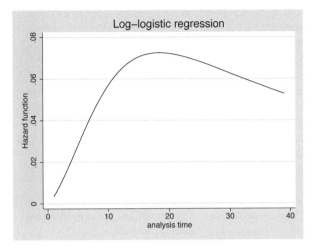

Figure 4. Log-logistic hazard distribution at mean value of all covariates

These plots show the fitted survivor and hazard functions evaluated for a cancer patient of average age receiving the average drug. Of course, the "average drug" has no meaning here since drug is an indicator variable. It makes more sense to plot the curves at a fixed value (level) of the drug. We can do this with the at option. For example, we may want to compare the average-age patient's survival curve under placebo (drug==0) and under treatment (drug==1).

We can plot both curves on the same graph:

```
. stcurve, surv at1(drug = 0) at2(drug = 1) ylabels(0 .5 1)
```

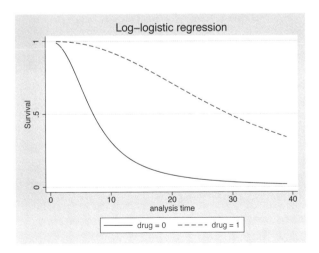

Figure 5. Log-logistic survival distribution at mean age for placebo

In the plot, we can see from the log-logistic model that the survival experience of an average-age patient receiving the placebo is worse than the survival experience of that same patient receiving treatment. We can also see the accelerated-failure-time feature of the log-logistic model. The survivor function for treatment is a time-decelerated (stretched-out) version of the survivor function for placebo.

◁

▷ Example 4

In our discussion of frailty models in [ST] **streg**, we emphasize the distinction between the individual hazard (or survivor) function and the hazard (survivor) function for the population. When significant frailty is present, the population hazard will tend to begin falling past a certain point, regardless of the shape of the individual hazard. This is due to the frailty effect—as time passes, the frailer individuals will fail, leaving a more homogeneous population comprising only the most robust individuals.

The frailty effect may be demonstrated using stcurve to plot the estimated hazard (both individual and population) after fitting a frailty model. Use option alpha1 to specify the individual hazard ($\alpha = 1$) and option unconditional to specify the population hazard. Applying this to the Weibull/inverse-Gaussian shared-frailty model on the kidney data of example 11 of [ST] **streg**,

```
. use http://www.stata-press.com/data/r10/catheter, clear
(Kidney data, McGilchrist and Aisbett, Biometrics, 1991)

. stset time infect

 (output omitted )

. qui streg age female, d(weibull) frailty(invgauss) shared(patient)

. stcurve, hazard at(female = 1) alpha1
```

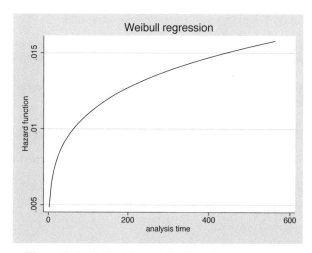

Figure 6. Individual hazard for females at mean age

Compare with

```
. stcurve, hazard at(female = 1) unconditional
```

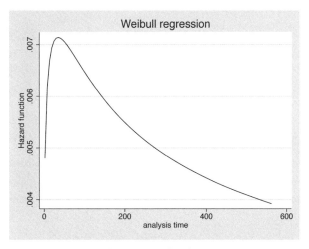

Figure 7. Population hazard for females at mean age

◁

Methods and Formulas

stcurve is implemented as an ado-file.

Reference

Cleves, M. A. 2000. stata54: Multiple curves plotted with stcurve command. *Stata Technical Bulletin* 54: 2–4. Reprinted in *Stata Technical Bulletin Reprints*, vol. 9, pp. 7–10.

Also See

[ST] **stcox** — Fit Cox proportional hazards model

[ST] **stcox postestimation** — Postestimation tools for stcox

[ST] **streg** — Fit parametric survival models

[ST] **streg postestimation** — Postestimation tools for streg

[ST] **sts** — Generate, graph, list, and test the survivor and cumulative hazard functions

[ST] **stset** — Declare data to be survival-time data

Title

stdescribe — Describe survival-time data

Syntax

stdescribe $\left[\textit{if}\right]$ $\left[\textit{in}\right]$ $\left[\text{, } \underline{\text{weight}} \underline{\text{nosh}}\text{ow}\right]$

You must stset your data before using stdescribe; see [ST] **stset**.

fweights, iweights, and pweights may be specified using stset; see [ST] **stset**.

by is allowed; see [D] **by**.

Description

stdescribe produces a summary of the st data in a computer or data-based sense rather than in an analytical or statistical sense.

stdescribe can be used with single- or multiple-record or single- or multiple-failure st data.

Options

⌐ Main ⌐

weight specifies that the summary use weighted rather than unweighted statistics. weight does nothing unless you specified a weight when you stset the data. The weight option and the ability to ignore weights are unique to stdescribe. The purpose of stdescribe is to describe the data in a computer sense—the number of records, etc.—and for that purpose, the weights are best ignored.

noshow prevents stdescribe from showing the key st variables. This option is seldom used since most people type stset, show or stset, noshow to set whether they want to see these variables mentioned at the top of the output of every st command; see [ST] **stset**.

Remarks

Here is an example of stdescribe with single-record survival data:

```
. use http://www.stata-press.com/data/r10/page2
. stdescribe
        failure _d:  dead
  analysis time _t:  time
```

		per subject			
Category	total	mean	min	median	max
no. of subjects	40				
no. of records	40	1	1	1	1
(first) entry time		0	0	0	0
(final) exit time		227.95	142	231	344
subjects with gap	0				
time on gap if gap	0				
time at risk	9118	227.95	142	231	344
failures	36	.9	0	1	1

There is one record per subject. The purpose of this summary is not analysis—it is to describe how the data are arranged. We can quickly see that there is one record per subject (the number of subjects equals the number of records, but if there is any doubt, the minimum and maximum number of records per subject is 1), that all the subjects entered at time 0, that the subjects exited between times 142 and 344 (median 231), that there are no gaps (as there could not be if there is only one record per subject), that the total time at risk is 9,118 (distributed reasonably evenly across the subjects), and that the total number of failures is 36 (with a maximum of 1 failure per subject).

Here is a description of the multiple-record Stanford heart transplant data that we introduced in [ST] **stset**:

```
. use http://www.stata-press.com/data/r10/stan3
(Heart transplant data)

. stdescribe
         failure _d:  died
   analysis time _t:  t1
                id:  id
```

Category	total	mean	min	median	max
			per subject		
no. of subjects	103				
no. of records	172	1.669903	1	2	2
(first) entry time		0	0	0	0
(final) exit time		310.0786	1	90	1799
subjects with gap	0				
time on gap if gap	0	.	.	.	.
time at risk	31938.1	310.0786	1	90	1799
failures	75	.7281553	0	1	1

Here patients have one or two records. Although this is not revealed by the output, a patient has one record if the patient never received a heart transplant and two if the patient did receive a transplant; the first reflects the patient's survival up to the time of transplantation and the second their subsequent survival:

```
. stset, noshow          /* to not show the st marker variables */
. stdescribe if !transplant
```

Category	total	mean	min	median	max
			per subject		
no. of subjects	34				
no. of records	34	1	1	1	1
(first) entry time		0	0	0	0
(final) exit time		96.61765	1	21	1400
subjects with gap	0				
time on gap if gap	0	.	.	.	.
time at risk	3285	96.61765	1	21	1400
failures	30	.8823529	0	1	1

```
. stdescribe if transplant
```

| Category | total | | per subject | | |
		mean	min	median	max
no. of subjects	69				
no. of records	138	2	2	2	2
(first) entry time		0	0	0	0
(final) exit time		415.2623	5.1	207	1799
subjects with gap	0				
time on gap if gap	0	.	.	.	.
time at risk	28653.1	415.2623	5.1	207	1799
failures	45	.6521739	0	1	1

Finally, here are the results of stdescribe from multiple-failure data:

```
. use http://www.stata-press.com/data/r10/mfail2
. stdescribe
```

| Category | total | | per subject | | |
		mean	min	median	max
no. of subjects	926				
no. of records	1734	1.87257	1	2	4
(first) entry time		0	0	0	0
(final) exit time		470.6857	1	477	960
subjects with gap	6				
time on gap if gap	411	68.5	16	57.5	133
time at risk	435444	470.2419	1	477	960
failures	808	.8725702	0	1	3

The maximum number of failures per subject observed is three, although 50% had just one failure, and that six subjects have gaps in their histories.

Saved Results

stdescribe saves the following in r():

Scalars

r(N_sub)	number of subjects	r(gap)	total gap, if gap
r(N_total)	number of records	r(gap_min)	minimum gap, if gap
r(N_min)	minimum number of records	r(gap_mean)	mean gap, if gap
r(N_mean)	mean number of records	r(gap_med)	median gap, if gap
r(N_med)	median number of records	r(gap_max)	maximum gap, if gap
r(N_max)	maximum number of records	r(tr)	total time at risk
r(t0_min)	minimum first entry time	r(tr_min)	minimum time at risk
r(t0_mean)	mean first entry time	r(tr_mean)	mean time at risk
r(t0_med)	median first entry time	r(tr_med)	median time at risk
r(t0_max)	maximum first entry time	r(tr_max)	maximum time at risk
r(t1_min)	minimum final exit time	r(N_fail)	number of failures
r(t1_mean)	mean final exit time	r(f_min)	minimum number of failures
r(t1_med)	median final exit time	r(f_mean)	mean number of failures
r(t1_max)	maximum final exit time	r(f_med)	median number of failures
r(N_gap)	number of subjects with gap	r(f_max)	maximum number of failures

Methods and Formulas

stdescribe is implemented as an ado-file.

Reference

Cleves, M. A., W. W. Gould, and R. G. Gutierrez. 2004. *An Introduction to Survival Analysis Using Stata.* Rev. ed. College Station, TX: Stata Press.

Also See

[ST] **stset** — Declare data to be survival-time data

[ST] **stsum** — Summarize survival-time data

[ST] **stvary** — Report whether variables vary over time

Title

> **stfill** — Fill in by carrying forward values of covariates

Syntax

stfill *varlist* [*if*] [*in*] , { <u>b</u>aseline | <u>f</u>orward } [*options*]

options	description
Main	
*<u>b</u>aseline	replace with values at baseline
*<u>f</u>orward	carry forward values
<u>nosh</u>ow	do not show st setting information

* Either baseline or forward is required.

You must stset your data before using stfill; see [ST] **stset**.

fweights, iweights, and pweights may be specified using stset; see [ST] **stset**.

Description

stfill is intended for use with multiple-record st data for which id() has been stset. stfill may be used with single-record data, but it does nothing. That is, stfill can be used with multiple-record or single- or multiple-failure st data.

stfill, baseline changes variables to contain the value at the earliest time each subject was observed, making the variable constant over time. stfill, baseline changes all subsequent values of the specified variables to equal the first value, whether they originally contained missing or not.

stfill, forward fills in missing values of each variable with that of the most recent time at which the variable was last observed. stfill, forward changes only missing values.

You must specify either the baseline or the forward option.

if *exp* and in *range* operate slightly differently from their usual definitions to work as you would expect. if and in restrict where changes can be made to the data, but no matter what, all stset observations are used to provide the values to be carried forward.

Options

┌─ Main ┐

baseline specifies that values be replaced with the values at baseline, the earliest time at which the subject was observed. All values of the specified variables are replaced, missing and nonmissing.

forward specifies that values be carried forward and that previously observed, nonmissing values be used to fill in later values that are missing in the specified variables.

noshow prevents stfill from showing the key st variables. This option is seldom used since most people type stset, show or stset, noshow to set whether they want to see these variables mentioned at the top of the output of every st command; see [ST] **stset**.

Remarks

stfill assists in fixing data errors and makes baseline analyses easier.

▷ Example 1

Let us begin by repairing broken data.

You have a multiple-record st dataset which, because of how it was constructed, has a problem with the gender variable:

```
. use http://www.stata-press.com/data/r10/mrecord
. stvary sex
        failure _d:  myopic
  analysis time _t:  t
               id:  id

                    subjects for whom the variable is
                                        never    always  sometimes
     variable |  constant   varying    missing   missing   missing
   -----------+-------------------------------------------------------
          sex |     131         1          22        0       110
```

For 110 subjects, sex is sometimes missing, for one more subject, the value of sex changes over time! The sex change is an error, but the missing values occurred because sometimes the subject's sex was not filled in on the revisit forms. We will assume that you have checked the changing-sex subject and determined that the baseline record is correct in that case, too.

```
. stfill sex, baseline
        failure _d:  myopic
  analysis time _t:  t
               id:  id

replace all values with value at earliest observed:
           sex:  221 real changes made
. stvary sex
        failure _d:  myopic
  analysis time _t:  t
               id:  id

                    subjects for whom the variable is
                                        never    always  sometimes
     variable |  constant   varying    missing   missing   missing
   -----------+-------------------------------------------------------
          sex |     132         0         132        0        0
```

The sex variable is now completely filled in.

In this same dataset, there is another variable—bp, blood pressure—that is not always filled in because readings were not always taken.

```
. stvary bp
        failure _d:  myopic
  analysis time _t:  t
               id:  id

                    subjects for whom the variable is
                                        never    always  sometimes
     variable |  constant   varying    missing   missing   missing
   -----------+-------------------------------------------------------
           bp |      18        114          9        0       123
```

(bp is constant for 18 patients because it was taken only once—at baseline.) Anyway, you decide that it will be good enough, when bp is missing, to use the previous value of bp:

```
. stfill bp, forward noshow
replace missing values with previously observed values:
        bp:  263 real changes made
. stvary bp, noshow
```

| | subjects for whom the variable is | | | | |
variable	constant	varying	never missing	always missing	sometimes missing
bp	18	114	132	0	0

So much for data repair and fabrication.

◁

▷ Example 2

Much later, deep in analysis, you are concerned about the bp variable and decide to compare results with a model that simply includes blood pressure at baseline. You are undecided on the issue and want to have both variables in your data:

```
. stset, noshow
. gen bp0 = bp
. stfill bp0, baseline
replace all values with value at earliest observed:
        bp0:  406 real changes made
. stvary bp bp0
```

| | subjects for whom the variable is | | | | |
variable	constant	varying	never missing	always missing	sometimes missing
bp	18	114	132	0	0
bp0	132	0	132	0	0

◁

Methods and Formulas

stfill is implemented as an ado-file.

Also See

[ST] **stbase** — Form baseline dataset

[ST] **stgen** — Generate variables reflecting entire histories

[ST] **stset** — Declare data to be survival-time data

[ST] **stvary** — Report whether variables vary over time

Title

---

stgen — Generate variables reflecting entire histories

Syntax

stgen [*type*] *newvar* = *function*

where *function* is

                    ever(*exp*)
                    never(*exp*)
                    always(*exp*)
                    min(*exp*)
                    max(*exp*)
                    when(*exp*)
                    when0(*exp*)
                    count(*exp*)
                    count0(*exp*)
                    minage(*exp*)
                    maxage(*exp*)
                    avgage(*exp*)
                    nfailures()
                    ngaps()
                    gaplen()
                    hasgap()

You must stset your data before using stgen; see [ST] **stset**.

Description

stgen provides a convenient way to generate new variables reflecting entire histories—variables you could create for yourself by using generate (and especially, generate with the by *varlist*: prefix), but that would require too much thought, and there would be too much chance of making a mistake.

These functions are intended for use with multiple-record survival data but may be used with single-record data. With single-record data, each function reduces to one generate, and generate would be a more natural way to approach the problem.

stgen can be used with multiple-record or single- or multiple-failure st data.

If you want to generate calculated values, such as the survivor function, see [ST] **sts**.

Functions

In the description of the functions below, time units refer to the same units as *timevar* from stset *timevar*, ... For instance, if *timevar* is the number of days since 01 January 1960 (a Stata date), time units are days. If *timevar* is in years—years since 1960, years since diagnosis, or whatever—time units are years.

When we say variable X records a "time", we mean a variable that records when something occurred in the same units and with the same base as *timevar*. If *timevar* is a Stata date, "time" is correspondingly a Stata date.

t units, or analysis time units, refer to a variable in the units $timevar/\texttt{scale()}$ from $\texttt{stset}$ $timevar$, $\texttt{scale(...)}$ .... If you did not specify a $\texttt{scale()}$, t units are the same as time units. Alternatively, say that $timevar$ is recorded as a Stata date and you specified $\texttt{scale(365.25)}$. Then t units are years. If you specified a nonconstant scale—$\texttt{scale(myvar)}$, where $\texttt{myvar}$ varies from subject to subject—t units are different for every subject.

"An analysis time" refers to the time something occurred, recorded in the units $(timevar-\texttt{origin()})/\texttt{scale()}$. We speak about analysis time only in terms of the beginning and end of each time-span record.

Although in *Description* above we said that $\texttt{stgen}$ creates variables reflecting entire histories, $\texttt{stgen}$ restricts itself to the $\texttt{stset}$ observations, so "entire history" means the entire history as it is currently $\texttt{stset}$. If you really want to use entire histories as recorded in the data, type $\texttt{streset}$, $\texttt{past}$ or $\texttt{streset, past future}$ before using $\texttt{stgen}$. Then type $\texttt{streset}$ to reset to the original analysis sample.

The following functions are available:

$\texttt{ever}(exp)$ creates *newvar* containing 1 (true) if the expression is ever true (nonzero) and 0 otherwise. For instance,

    . stgen everlow = ever(bp<100)

would create $\texttt{everlow}$ containing, for each subject, uniformly 1 or 0. Every record for a subject would contain $\texttt{everlow} = 1$ if, on any $\texttt{stset}$ record for the subject, $\texttt{bp} < 100$; otherwise, $\texttt{everlow}$ would be 0.

$\texttt{never}(exp)$ is the reverse of $\texttt{ever()}$; it creates *newvar* containing 1 (true) if the expression is always false (0) and 0 otherwise. For instance,

    . stgen neverlow = never(bp<100)

would create $\texttt{neverlow}$ containing, for each subject, uniformly 1 or 0. Every record for a subject would contain $\texttt{neverlow} = 1$ if, on every $\texttt{stset}$ record for the subject, $\texttt{bp} < 100$ is false.

$\texttt{always}(exp)$ creates *newvar* containing 1 (true) if the expression is always true (nonzero) and 0 otherwise. For instance,

    . stgen lowlow = always(bp<100)

would create $\texttt{lowlow}$ containing, for each subject, uniformly 1 or 0. Every record for a subject would contain $\texttt{lowlow} = 1$ if, on every $\texttt{stset}$ record for a subject, $\texttt{bp} < 100$.

$\texttt{min}(exp)$ and $\texttt{max}(exp)$ create $\texttt{newvar}$ containing the minimum or maximum nonmissing value of exp within $\texttt{id()}$. $\texttt{min()}$ and $\texttt{max()}$ are often used with variables recording a time (see definition above), such as $\texttt{min(visitdat)}$.

$\texttt{when}(exp)$ and $\texttt{when0}(exp)$ create $\texttt{newvar}$ containing the time when exp first became true within the previously $\texttt{stset id()}$. The result is in time, not t units; see the definition above.

$\texttt{when()}$ and $\texttt{when0()}$ differ about when the exp became true. Records record time spans $(time0, time1]$. $\texttt{when()}$ assumes that the expression became true at the end of the time span, $time1$. $\texttt{when0()}$ assumes that the expression became true at the beginning of the time span, $time0$.

Assume that you previously $\texttt{stset myt, failure}(eventvar = ...)$ .... $\texttt{when()}$ would be appropriate for use with $eventvar$, and presumably $\texttt{when0()}$ would be appropriate for use with the remaining variables.

count(*exp*) and count0(*exp*) create *newvar* containing the number of occurrences when *exp* is true within id().

count() and count0() differ in when they assume that *exp* occurs. count() assumes that *exp* corresponds to the end of the time-span record. Thus even if *exp* is true in this record, the count would remain unchanged until the next record.

count0() assumes that *exp* corresponds to the beginning of the time-span record. Thus if *exp* is true in this record, the count is immediately updated.

For example, assume that you previously stset myt, failure(*eventvar*=...) .... count() would be appropriate for use with *eventvar*, and presumably count0() would be appropriate for use with the remaining variables.

minage(*exp*), maxage(*exp*), and avgage(*exp*) return the elapsed time, in time units, since *exp* at the beginning, end, or middle of the record, respectively. *exp* is expected to evaluate to a time in time units. minage(), maxage(), and avgage() would be appropriate for use with the result of when(), when0(), min(), and max(), for instance.

Also see [ST] **stsplit**; stsplit will divide the time-span records into new time-span records that record specified intervals of ages.

nfailures() creates *newvar* containing the cumulative number of failures for each subject as of the entry time for the observation. nfailures() is intended for use with multiple-failure data; with single-failure data, nfailures() is always 0. In multiple-failure data,

    . stgen nfail = nfailures()

might create, for a particular subject, the following:

id	time0	time1	fail	x	nfail
93	0	20	0	1	0
93	20	30	1	1	0
93	30	40	1	2	1
93	40	60	0	1	2
93	60	70	0	2	2
93	70	80	1	1	2

The total number of failures for this subject is 3, and yet the maximum of the new variable nfail is 2. At time 70, the beginning of the last record, there had been two failures previously, and there were two failures up to but not including time 80.

ngaps() creates *newvar* containing the cumulative number of gaps for each subject as of the entry time for the record. Delayed entry (an opening gap) is not considered a gap. For example,

    . stgen ngap = ngaps()

might create, for a particular subject, the following:

id	time0	time1	fail	x	ngap
94	10	30	0	1	0
94	30	40	0	2	0
94	50	60	0	1	1
94	60	70	0	2	1
94	82	90	1	1	2

gaplen() creates *newvar* containing the time on gap, measured in analysis time units, for each subject as of the entry time for the observation. Delayed entry (an opening gap) is not considered a gap. Continuing with the previous example,

```
. stgen gl = gaplen()
```

would produce

id	time0	time1	fail	x	ngap	gl
94	10	30	0	1	0	0
94	30	40	0	2	0	0
94	50	60	0	1	1	10
94	60	70	0	2	1	0
94	82	90	1	1	2	12

hasgap() creates *newvar* containing uniformly 1 if the subject ever has a gap and 0 otherwise. Delayed entry (an opening gap) is not considered a gap.

Remarks

stgen does nothing you cannot do in other ways, but it is convenient.

Consider how you would obtain results like those created by stgen should you need something that stgen will not create for you. Say that we have an st dataset for which we have previously

```
. stset t, failure(d) id(id)
```

Assume that these are some of the data:

id	t	d	bp
27	30	0	90
27	50	0	110
27	60	1	85
28	11	0	120
28	40	1	130

If we were to type

```
. stgen everlow = ever(bp<100)
```

the new variable everlow would contain for these two subjects

id	t	d	bp	everlow
27	30	0	90	1
27	50	0	110	1
27	60	1	85	1
28	11	0	120	0
28	40	1	130	0

Variable everlow is 1 for subject 27 because, in two of the three observations, bp < 100, and everlow is 0 for subject 28 because everlow is never less than 100 in either observation.

Here is one way we could have created everlow for ourselves:

```
. generate islow = bp<100
. sort id
. by id: generate sumislow = sum(islow)
. by id: generate everlow = sumislow[_N]>0
. drop islow sumislow
```

The generic term for code like this is explicit subscripting; see [U] **13.7 Explicit subscripting**.

Anyway, that is what stgen did for us, although, internally, stgen used denser code that was equivalent to

```
. by id, sort: generate everlow=sum(bp<100)
. by id: replace everlow = everlow[_N]>0
```

Obtaining things like the time on gap is no more difficult. When we `stset` the data, `stset` created variable _t0 to record the entry time. `stgen`'s `gaplen()` function is equivalent to

```
. sort id _t
. by id: generate gaplen = _t0-_t[_n-1]
. by id: replace gaplen = 0 if _n == 1
```

Seeing this, you should realize that if all you wanted was the cumulative length of the gap before the current record, you could type

```
. sort id _t
. by id: generate curgap = sum(_t0-_t[_n-1])
```

If, instead, you wanted a variable that was 1 if there were a gap just before this record and 0 otherwise, you could type

```
. sort id _t
. by id: generate iscurgap = (_t0-_t[_n-1])>0
```

▷ Example 1

Let us use the `stgen` commands to real effect. We have a multiple-record, multiple-failure dataset.

```
. use http://www.stata-press.com/data/r10/mrmf
. st
-> stset t, id(id) failure(d) time0(t0) exit(time .) noshow

                id:  id
     failure event:  d != 0 & d < .
obs. time interval:  (t0, t]
 exit on or before:  time .

. stdescribe
```

			per subject		
Category	total	mean	min	median	max
no. of subjects	926				
no. of records	1734	1.87257	1	2	4
(first) entry time		0	0	0	0
(final) exit time		470.6857	1	477	960
subjects with gap	6				
time on gap if gap	411	68.5	16	57.5	133
time at risk	435444	470.2419	1	477	960
failures	808	.8725702	0	1	3

Also in this dataset are two covariates, x1 and x2. We wish to fit a Cox model on these data but wish to assume that the baseline hazard for first failures is different from that for second and later failures.

Our data contain six subjects with gaps. Since failures might have occurred during the gap, we begin by dropping those six subjects:

```
. stgen hg = hasgap()
. drop if hg
(14 observations deleted)
```

The six subjects had 14 records among them. We can now create variable nf containing the number of failures and, from that, create variable group, which will be 0 when subjects have experienced no previous failures and 1 thereafter:

```
. stgen nf = nfailures()
. generate byte group = nf>0
```

We can now fit our stratified model:

```
. stcox x1 x2, strata(group) vce(robust)
Iteration 0:   log pseudolikelihood = -4499.9966
Iteration 1:   log pseudolikelihood = -4444.7797
Iteration 2:   log pseudolikelihood = -4444.4596
Iteration 3:   log pseudolikelihood = -4444.4596
Refining estimates:
Iteration 0:   log pseudolikelihood = -4444.4596

Stratified Cox regr. -- Breslow method for ties

No. of subjects    =         920          Number of obs   =       1720
No. of failures    =         800
Time at risk       =      432153
                                          Wald chi2(2)    =     102.78
Log pseudolikelihood =   -4444.4596       Prob > chi2     =     0.0000

                          (Std. Err. adjusted for 920 clusters in id)
```

_t	Haz. Ratio	Robust Std. Err.	z	P>|z|	[95% Conf. Interval]	
x1	2.087903	.1961725	7.84	0.000	1.736738	2.510074
x2	.2765613	.052277	-6.80	0.000	.1909383	.4005806

Stratified by group

◁

Methods and Formulas

stgen is implemented as an ado-file.

Also See

[ST] **stci** — Confidence intervals for means and percentiles of survival time

[ST] **sts** — Generate, graph, list, and test the survivor and cumulative hazard functions

[ST] **stset** — Declare data to be survival-time data

[ST] **stvary** — Report whether variables vary over time

Title

stir — Report incidence-rate comparison

Syntax

stir *exposedvar* $\left[\textit{if}\right]$ $\left[\textit{in}\right]$ $\left[\,,\,\textit{options}\right]$

options	description
Main	
<u>stra</u>ta(*varname*)	stratify on *varname*
<u>nosh</u>ow	do not show st setting information
Options	
ird	report incidence-rate difference rather than ratio
estandard	combine external weights with within-stratum statistics
istandard	combine internal weights with within-stratum statistics
<u>stand</u>ard(*varname*)	combine user-specified weights with within-stratum statistics
<u>poo</u>l	display pooled estimate
<u>noc</u>rude	do not display crude estimate
<u>noh</u>om	do not display homogeneity test
tb	calculate test-based confidence intervals
<u>lev</u>el(#)	set confidence level; default is level(95)

Options except noshow, tb, and level(#) are relevant only if strata() is specified.

You must stset your data before using stir; see [ST] **stset**.

by is allowed; see [D] **by**.

fweights and iweights may be specified using stset; see [ST] **stset**. stir may not be used with pweighted data.

Description

stir reports point estimates and confidence intervals for the incidence-rate ratio and difference. stir is an interface to the ir command; see [ST] **epitab**.

By the logic of ir, *exposedvar* should be a 0/1 variable, 0 meaning unexposed and 1 meaning exposed. stir, however, allows any two-valued coding and even allows *exposedvar* to be a string variable.

stir may not be used with pweighted data.

stir can be used with single- or multiple-record or single- or multiple-failure st data.

Options

> **Main**

<u>stra</u>ta(*varname*) specifies that the calculation be stratified on *varname*, which may be a numeric or string variable. Within-stratum statistics are shown and then combined with Mantel–Haenszel weights.

noshow prevents stir from showing the key st variables. This option is seldom used since most people type stset, show or stset, noshow to set whether they want to see these variables mentioned at the top of the output of every st command; see [ST] **stset**.

___Options___

ird, estandard, istandard, standard(*varname*), pool, nocrude, and nohom are relevant only if strata() is specified; see [ST] **epitab**.

tb and level(#) are relevant in all cases; see [ST] **epitab**.

Remarks

stir examines the incidence rate and time at risk.

```
. use http://www.stata-press.com/data/r10/page2
. stir group, noshow
note:  Exposed <-> group==2 and Unexposed <-> group==1
```

	group Exposed	Unexposed	Total
Failure	19	17	36
Time	5023	4095	9118
Incidence Rate	.0037826	.0041514	.0039482

	Point estimate	[95% Conf. Interval]		
Inc. rate diff.	−.0003688	−.002974	.0022364	
Inc. rate ratio	.9111616	.4484366	1.866047	(exact)
Prev. frac. ex.	.0888384	−.8660469	.5515634	(exact)
Prev. frac. pop	.04894			

(midp)	Pr(k<=19) =		0.3900	(exact)
(midp)	2*Pr(k<=19) =		0.7799	(exact)

Saved Results

stir saves the following in r():

Scalars

r(p)	one-sided *p*-value	r(ub_irr)	upper bound of CI for irr
r(ird)	incidence-rate difference	r(afe)	attributable (prev.) fraction among exposed
r(lb_ird)	lower bound of CI for ird	r(lb_afe)	lower bound of CI for afe
r(ub_ird)	upper bound of CI for ird	r(ub_afe)	upper bound of CI for afe
r(irr)	incidence-rate ratio	r(afp)	attributable fraction for the population
r(lb_irr)	lower bound of CI for irr		

Methods and Formulas

stir is implemented as an ado-file.

stir simply accumulates numbers of failures and time at risk by exposed and unexposed (by strata, if necessary) and passes the calculation to ir; see [ST] **epitab**.

Reference

Dupont, W. D. 2002. *Statistical Modeling for Biomedical Researchers: A Simple Introduction to the Analysis of Complex Data.* Cambridge: Cambridge University Press.

Also See

[ST] **stset** — Declare data to be survival-time data

[ST] **stsum** — Summarize survival-time data

[ST] **epitab** — Tables for epidemiologists

Title

> **stpower** — Sample-size, power, and effect-size determination for survival analysis

Syntax

Sample-size determination

> stpower cox $\left[\ldots\right]$ $\left[,\ldots\right]$

> stpower logrank $\left[\ldots\right]$ $\left[,\ldots\right]$

> stpower exponential $\left[\ldots\right]$ $\left[,\ldots\right]$

Power determination

> stpower cox $\left[\ldots\right]$, n(*numlist*) $\left[\ldots\right]$

> stpower logrank $\left[\ldots\right]$, n(*numlist*) $\left[\ldots\right]$

> stpower exponential $\left[\ldots\right]$, n(*numlist*) $\left[\ldots\right]$

Effect-size determination

> stpower cox, n(*numlist*) { power(*numlist*) | beta(*numlist*) } $\left[\ldots\right]$

> stpower logrank $\left[\ldots\right]$, n(*numlist*) { power(*numlist*) | beta(*numlist*) } $\left[\ldots\right]$

See [ST] **stpower cox**, [ST] **stpower logrank**, and [ST] **stpower exponential**.

Description

stpower computes sample size and power for survival analysis comparing two survivor functions using the log-rank test or the *exponential test* (to be defined later), as well as for more general survival analysis investigating the effect of a single covariate in a Cox proportional hazards regression model, possibly in the presence of other covariates. It provides the estimate of the number of events required to be observed (or the expected number of events) in a study. The minimal effect size (minimal detectable difference, expressed as the hazard ratio or the log hazard ratio) may also be obtained for the log-rank test and for the Wald test on a single coefficient from the Cox model.

This entry provides an overview of the relevant terminology, theory, and a few examples. For more details, see the entries specific to each stpower subcommand.

Remarks

Remarks are presented under the following headings:

> *Theory and terminology*
> *Introduction to stpower subcommands*
> *Sample-size determination for survival studies*
> *Creating output tables*
> *Power curves*

Theory and terminology

The prominent feature of survival data is that the outcome is the time from an origin to the occurrence of a given event (failure), often referred to as the analysis time. Analyses of such data use the information from all subjects in a study, both those who experience an event by the end of the study and those who do not. However, inference about the survival experience of subjects is based on the event times and therefore depends on the number of events observed in a study. Indeed, if none of the subjects fails in a study, the survival rate cannot be estimated and survivor functions of subjects from different groups cannot be compared. Therefore, power depends on the number of events observed in a study and not directly on the number of subjects recruited to the study. As a result, to obtain the estimate of the required number of subjects, the probability that a subject experiences an event during the course of the study needs to be estimated in addition to the required number of events. This distinguishes sample-size determination for survival studies from that for other studies in which the endpoint is not measured as a time to failure.

All the above leads us to consider the following two types of survival studies. The first type (a *type I study*) is a study in which all subjects experience an event by the end of the study (no censoring), and the second type (a *type II study*) is a study that terminates after a fixed period regardless of whether all subjects experienced an event by that time. For a type II study, subjects who did not experience an event at the end of the study are known to be right-censored. For a type I study, when all subjects fail by the end of the study, the estimate of the probability of a failure in a study is one and the required number of subjects is equal to the required number of failures. For a type II study, the probability of a failure needs to be estimated and therefore various aspects that affect this probability (and usually do not come into play at the analysis stage) must be taken into account for the computation of the sample size.

Under the assumption of random censoring (Lachin 2000, 355; Lawless 2003, 52; Chow and Liu 2004, 388), the type of censoring pattern is irrelevant to the analysis of survival data in which the goal is to make inferences about the survival distribution of subjects. It becomes important, however, for sample-size determination since the probability that a subject experiences an event in a study depends on the censoring distribution. We consider the following two types of random censoring: administrative censoring and loss to follow-up.

Under administrative censoring, a subject is known to have experienced either of the two outcomes at the end of a study: survival or failure. The probability of a subject failing in a study depends on the duration of the study. Often in practice, subjects may withdraw from a study, say, because of severe side effects from a treatment or may be lost to follow-up because of moving to a different location. Here the information about the outcome that subject would have experienced at the end of the study had he completed the course of the study is unavailable, and the probability of experiencing an event by the end of the study is affected by the process governing withdrawal of subjects from the study. In the literature, this type of censoring is often referred to as subject loss to follow-up, subject withdrawal, or sometimes subject dropout (Freedman 1982, Machin and Campbell 2005). Generally, great care must be taken when using this terminology since it may have slightly different meanings in different contexts. `stpower logrank` and `stpower cox` apply a conservative adjustment to the estimate of the sample size for withdrawal. `stpower exponential` assumes that losses to follow-up are exponentially distributed.

Another important component of sample-size and power determination that affects the estimate of the probability of a failure is the pattern of accrual of subjects into the study. The duration of a study is often divided into two phases: an accrual phase, during which subjects are recruited to the study, and a follow-up phase, during which subjects are followed up until the end of the study and no new subjects enter the study. For a fixed-duration study, fast accrual increases the average analysis time (average follow-up time) and increases the chance of a subject failing in a study, whereas slow accrual decreases the average analysis time and consequently decreases this probability. `stpower logrank` and `stpower exponential` provide facilities to take into account uniform accrual, and for `stpower exponential` only, truncated exponential accrual.

All sample-size formulas used by `stpower` rely on the proportional-hazards assumption, that is, the assumption that the hazard ratio does not depend on time. See the documentation entry of each subcommand for the additional assumptions imposed by the methods it uses. In the case when the proportional-hazards assumption is suspect, or in the presence of other complexities associated with the nature of the trial (for example, lagged effect of a treatment, more than two treatment groups, clustered data) and with the behavior of participants (for example, noncompliance of subjects with the assigned treatment, competing risks), one may consider obtaining required sample size or power by simulation. Feiveson (2002) demonstrates an example of such simulation for clustered survival data. Barthel et al. (2006); Barthel, Royston, and Babiker (2005); and Royston and Babiker (2002) present sample-size and power computation for multiarm trials under more flexible design conditions.

Introduction to stpower subcommands

`stpower cox` provides estimates of sample size, power, or the minimal detectable value of the coefficient when an effect of a single covariate on subject survival is to be explored using Cox proportional hazards regression. It is assumed that the effect is to be tested using the partial likelihood from the Cox model (for example, score or Wald test) on the coefficient of the covariate of interest.

`stpower logrank` reports estimates of sample size, power, or minimal detectable value of the hazard ratio in the case when the two survivor functions are to be compared using the log-rank test. The only requirement about the distribution of the survivor functions is that the two survivor functions must satisfy the proportional-hazards assumption.

`stpower exponential` reports estimates of sample size or power when the disparity in the two exponential survivor functions is to be tested using the *exponential test*, the parametric test comparing the two exponential hazard rates. In particular, we refer to (exponential) *hazard-difference test* as the exponential test for the difference between hazards and (exponential) *log hazard-ratio test* as the exponential test for the log of the hazard ratio or, equivalently, for the difference between log hazards.

All subcommands share a common syntax. Sample-size determination with a power of 80% or, equivalently, a probability of a *type II error*, a failure to reject the null hypothesis when the alternative hypothesis is true, of 20% is the default. Other values of power or type II error probability may be supplied via options `power()` or `beta()`, respectively. If power determination is desired, sample size `n()` must be specified. If the minimal detectable difference is of interest, both sample size `n()` and `power()` (or type II error probability `beta()`) must be specified.

For sample-size and power computations, the default effect size corresponds to a value of the hazard ratio of 0.5 and may be changed by specifying option `hratio()`. The hazard ratio is defined as a ratio of hazards of the experimental group to the control group (or the less favorable of the two groups). Other ways of specifying the effect size are available, and these are particular to each subcommand.

The default probability of a *type I error*, a rejection of the null hypothesis when the null hypothesis is true, of a test is 0.05 but may changed by using option `alpha()`. Results for one-sided tests may be requested by using option `onesided`. To change the default setting of equal-sized groups in `stpower logrank` and `stpower exponential`, one of options `p1()` or `nratio()` must be specified.

By default, all subcommands assume a type I study, that is, perform computations for uncensored survival data. The censoring information may be taken into account by specifying the appropriate arguments or options. See [ST] **stpower cox**, [ST] **stpower logrank**, and [ST] **stpower exponential** for details.

All subcommands can report results in a table. Results may be tabulated for various values of input parameters. See *Creating output tables* for examples. An example of how to produce a power curve is given in *Power curves.*

Sample-size determination for survival studies

Here we demonstrate using stpower to obtain an estimate of the sample size for three different survival studies.

▷ Example 1: Sample size for the test of the effect of a covariate in the Cox model

Consider a hypothetical study for which the goal is to investigate the effect of the expression of one gene on subject survival with the Cox proportional hazards regression model. Suppose that the Wald test is to be used to test the coefficient on the gene after fitting the Cox model. Gene expression values measure the level of activity of the gene. Consider the scenario described in Simon, Radmacher, and Dobbin (2002) in which the hazard ratio of 3 associated with a one-unit change in the $\log_2$-intensity of a gene (or, respectively, with a twofold change in gene expression level) is desired to be detected with 95% power using a two-sided 0.001 level test. The estimate of the standard deviation of the $\log_2$-intensity level of the gene over the entire set of samples is assumed to be 0.75.

```
. stpower cox, hratio(3) sd(0.75) power(0.95) alpha(0.001)

Estimated sample size for Cox PH regression
Wald test, log-hazard metric
Ho: [b1, b2, ..., bp] = [0, b2, ..., bp]

Input parameters:

        alpha =    0.0010  (two sided)
           b1 =    1.0986
           sd =    0.7500
        power =    0.9500

Estimated number of events and sample size:

            E =         36
            N =         36
```

◁

Provided that all subjects experience an event in this study, a total of 36 events is required to be observed in the study to ensure the specified power.

See [ST] **stpower cox** for more details.

▷ Example 2: Sample size for the log-rank test

Consider an example from Machin and Campbell (2005) of a study comparing two forms of surgical resection for patients with gastric cancer. From a prestudy survey, the baseline 5-year survival rate was expected to be 20% and an anticipated increase in survival in the experimental group expressed as a hazard ratio of 0.6667 (corresponding to approximately a 5-year survival rate of 34%) was desired to be detected with 90% power using a two-sided 0.05 level log-rank test under 1:1 randomization. To obtain the estimate of the sample size for this study, we use stpower logrank with survival proportion in the control group 0.2 supplied as an argument, option hratio(0.6667) to request a hazard ratio of 0.6667, and option power(0.9) to request 90% power.

```
. stpower logrank 0.2, hratio(0.6667) power(0.9)

Estimated sample sizes for two-sample comparison of survivor functions
Log-rank test, Freedman method
Ho: S1(t) = S2(t)

Input parameters:
        alpha =    0.0500  (two sided)
           s1 =    0.2000
           s2 =    0.3420
       hratio =    0.6667
        power =    0.9000
           p1 =    0.5000

Estimated number of events and sample sizes:
            E =       264
            N =       362
           N1 =       181
           N2 =       181
```

From the output, 264 events (failures) are required to be observed in this study to ensure 90% power to detect a hazard ratio of 0.6667 using the log-rank test. The respective estimate of the total number of subjects required to observe 264 events in a 5-year study is 362 with 181 subjects per surgical group. Our estimate, 181, of each group's sample size is close to the manually computed estimate of 180 from Machin and Cambell (2005). This study is an example of a type II study as previously described, since 20% of subjects were expected to survive (be censored) by the end of the study.

◁

See [ST] **stpower logrank** for more detailed examples and other available methods of sample-size computation for this type of analysis.

▷ Example 3: Sample size for two-sample test of exponential survivor functions

Consider an example from Lachin (2000, 412) of a study comparing two therapies, the combination of a new therapy with the standard one versus the standard alone, in the treatment of lupus nephritis patients. From previous studies, the survivor function of the control group treated with the standard therapy was log linear with a constant yearly hazard rate of 0.3. The number of events (failures) required to ensure 90% power to detect a 50% risk reduction, $\Delta = 0.5$, (or, respectively, the log hazard ratio of $\ln(0.5) = -0.6931$) with a one-sided test at a 0.05 significance level was obtained to be 72 under equal-group allocation. In the absence of censoring, Lachin (2000) determined that a total of 72 subjects (36 per group) would have to be recruited to the study. To obtain this same estimate with `stpower exponential`, we supply the control hazard rate 0.3 as an argument and specify options `power(0.9)`, `onesided`, and `loghazard` to request 90% power, a one-sided test, and sample-size determination for the exponential log hazard-ratio test (or, test for the log-hazard difference), respectively.

```
. stpower exponential 0.3, power(0.9) onesided loghazard
Note: input parameters are hazard rates.
```

```
Estimated sample sizes for two-sample comparison of survivor functions
Exponential test, log-hazard difference, conditional
Ho: ln(h2/h1) = 0
```

```
Input parameters:
        alpha =    0.0500  (one sided)
           h1 =    0.3000
           h2 =    0.1500
    ln(h2/h1) =   -0.6931
        power =    0.9000
           p1 =    0.5000
```

```
Estimated sample sizes:
            N =        72
           N1 =        36
           N2 =        36
```

Further, the study was planned to continue for 6 years with a recruitment period of 4 years. Subjects who did not experience an event by the end of 6 years were censored. For this fixed-duration study with uniform entry (recruitment), the estimate of the sample size increases from 72 to 128. We specify the length of the accrual and the follow-up periods in options aperiod() and fperiod(), respectively. We also request to display the expected number of events by using option detail.

```
. stpower exponential 0.3, power(0.9) onesided loghazard aperiod(4) fperiod(2) detail
Note: input parameters are hazard rates.
```

```
Estimated sample sizes for two-sample comparison of survivor functions
Exponential test, log-hazard difference, conditional
Ho: ln(h2/h1) = 0
```

```
Input parameters:
        alpha =    0.0500  (one sided)
           h1 =    0.3000
           h2 =    0.1500
    ln(h2/h1) =   -0.6931
        power =    0.9000
           p1 =    0.5000
```

```
Accrual and follow-up information:
     duration =    6.0000
    follow-up =    2.0000
       accrual =    4.0000  (uniform)
```

```
Estimated sample sizes:
            N =       128
           N1 =        64
           N2 =        64
```

```
Estimated expected number of events:
        E|Ha =        72      E|Ho =        74
       E1|Ha =        44     E1|Ho =        37
       E2|Ha =        28     E2|Ho =        37
```

◁

Under the alternative hypothesis of H_a: $\ln(\Delta) = -0.6931$, we expect to observe 44 events in the control group and 28 events in the experimental group. A total of 128 subjects (64 per group) is required to be enrolled into the study to observe an expected total of 72 events under the alternative.

See [ST] **stpower exponential** for more examples.

Creating output tables

stpower subcommands offer options table and columns() to display results in a table. All tables in the examples below are produced for a default screen width of 79 characters. You may need to resize your Results window if you wish to clearly reproduce these tables.

▷ Example 4: Displaying results in a table with default columns

Continuing example 1, we display results in a table with the default columns.

```
. stpower cox, hratio(3) sd(0.75) power(0.95) alpha(0.001) table
Estimated sample size for Cox PH regression
Wald test, log-hazard metric
Ho: [b1, b2, ..., bp] = [0, b2, ..., bp]
```

Power	N	E	B1	SD	Alpha*
.95	36	36	1.09861	.75	.001

```
* two sided
```

Suppose that we would now like to take into account that only 90% of subjects survived until the end of the study by using option failprob(0.9).

```
. stpower cox, hratio(3) sd(0.75) power(0.95) alpha(0.001) failprob(0.9) table
Estimated sample size for Cox PH regression
Wald test, log-hazard metric
Ho: [b1, b2, ..., bp] = [0, b2, ..., bp]
```

Power	N	E	B1	SD	Alpha*	Pr(E)
.95	40	36	1.09861	.75	.001	.9

```
* two sided
```

The specified options determine what table columns are displayed by default. See the documentation entry of each command for the details on the default columns.

◁

▷ Example 5: Producing tables when options contain multiple values

Recall example 2. Suppose that we would like to tabulate values of power for sample-size values of 200, 250, and 300 and for three different values of the survival probability in the experimental group, 0.34, 0.5, and 0.65. To fit the table on a screen of width 79, we specify option colwidth(7), requesting a width of 7 for all table columns.

```
. stpower logrank 0.2 (0.34 0.5 0.65), n(200 250 300) colwidth(7)
```

Estimated power for two-sample comparison of survivor functions
Log-rank test, Freedman method
Ho: S1(t) = S2(t)

Power	N	N1	N2	E	S1	S2	HR	Alpha*
.6646	200	100	100	146	.2	.34	.6703	.05
.7601	250	125	125	183	.2	.34	.6703	.05
.8318	300	150	150	219	.2	.34	.6703	.05
.995	200	100	100	130	.2	.5	.4307	.05
.9991	250	125	125	163	.2	.5	.4307	.05
.9998	300	150	150	195	.2	.5	.4307	.05
1	200	100	100	115	.2	.65	.2677	.05
1	250	125	125	144	.2	.65	.2677	.05
1	300	150	150	173	.2	.65	.2677	.05

* two sided

Optionally, the width of each column may be changed by specifying respective column widths in colwidth(), as we demonstrate in example 6. Using colwidth(7) is equivalent to colwidth(7 7 7 7 7 7 7 7 7) in the above.

By default, the results are displayed for all possible combinations of values of n() and the second argument list. If a table is desired instead with results for sequential pairs of values (0.34, 200), (0.5, 250), and (0.65, 300), one can specify option parallel.

```
. stpower logrank 0.2 (0.34 0.5 0.65), n(200 250 300) colwidth(7) parallel
```

Estimated power for two-sample comparison of survivor functions
Log-rank test, Freedman method
Ho: S1(t) = S2(t)

Power	N	N1	N2	E	S1	S2	HR	Alpha*
.6646	200	100	100	146	.2	.34	.6703	.05
.9991	250	125	125	163	.2	.5	.4307	.05
1	300	150	150	173	.2	.65	.2677	.05

* two sided

If option parallel is specified, options with multiple values must each contain the same number of values.

◁

▷ Example 6: Customized tables

In the previous examples, we used table to display the default columns. One can construct a customized table by specifying *colnames* within columns(). The columns will be displayed in the same order as they are specified in columns(). Continuing example 3, we display the total and per group expected number of events under the null and under the alternative hypotheses for two values of the hazard ratio, 0.5 and 0.6 (Lachin 2000, 413). To obtain this table, we also specify options hratio(0.5 0.6) and columns(power ea ea1 ea2 eo eo1 eo2 hr alpha) and omit option detail in the earlier syntax. We request that the columns widths of the first six columns be as specified in colwidth(7 6 7 7 6 7). Remaining columns will be displayed with the width of 7 (the last specified columns width). If the widths of the remaining columns are desired to be unchanged, a missing (.), denoting the default column width of 9, may be specified as the last column width.

```
. stpower exponential 0.3, power(0.9) hratio(0.5 0.6) onesided loghazard
> aperiod(4) fperiod(2) columns(power ea ea1 ea2 eo eo1 eo2 hr alpha)
> colwidth(7 6 7 7 6 7)
Note: input parameters are hazard rates.

Estimated sample sizes for two-sample comparison of survivor functions
Exponential test, log-hazard difference, conditional
Ho: ln(h2/h1) = 0
```

Power	E|Ha	E1|Ha	E2|Ha	E|Ho	E1|Ho	E2|Ho	HR	Alpha*
.9	72	44	28	74	37	37	.5	.05
.9	132	76	56	134	67	67	.6	.05

```
* one sided
```

◁

The displayed table values may be saved to a Stata data file by using option saving(). Also, table and columns() in conjunction with noheader and continue may be used to produce tables for various values in options that do not allow specifying a number list. This task may be done by issuing a stpower subcommand repeatedly within a forvalues loop. See example 5 in [ST] **stpower exponential**.

Power curves

Here we demonstrate how to produce a graph of a power curve as a function of sample size.

▷ Example 7: Plotting a simple power curve

Continuing example 2, we plot power for sample-size values in a range from 200 to 400 for this study. We supply the integers in this range with a step size of 1 to option n() and use option saving() to save table values in a Stata dataset named mypower.dta.

```
. quietly stpower logrank 0.2, hratio(0.6667) n(200(1)400) saving(mypower)
```

We specify quietly to avoid displaying the resulting table. The values of columns of the table are saved in mypower.dta. We generate the power graph by plotting the values of power and sample size saved in variables power and n:

```
. use mypower

. line power n,
> title("Power vs sample size for the log-rank test")
> ytitle("Power") xtitle("Number of subjects")
> yline(.9, lpattern("-.")) xline(362, lpattern("-."))
> xlabel(200(20)400, grid) text(.915 345 "(.9, 362)")
> ylabel(.65(.05).95, grid)
> note("S1(5) = .2, S2(5) = .342, HR = .6667, alpha = .05 (two sided)")
```

◁

Power curves may also be plotted for combinations of values of different options. For an example of plotting two power curves, see example 7 in [ST] **stpower logrank**.

Methods and Formulas

`stpower` is implemented as an ado-file.

`stpower cox` adopts the method of Hsieh and Lavori (2000) to compute sample size and power for the test of a covariate obtained after the Cox model fit.

`stpower logrank` uses the approach of Freedman (1982) and Schoenfeld (1981) for sample-size and power computation. The approach of Schoenfeld (1983) is used to obtain the estimates in the presence of uniform accrual.

`stpower exponential` implements methods of Lachin (1981); Lachin and Foulkes (1986); George and Desu (1974); and Rubinstein, Gail, and Santner (1981) for the two-sample test of exponential survivor functions. The explicit sample-size formula for the last method was given in Lakatos and Lan (1992).

See *Methods and Formulas* in [ST] **stpower cox**, [ST] **stpower logrank**, and [ST] **stpower exponential** for more details.

References

Barthel, F. M.-S., P. Royston, and A. Babiker. 2005. A menu-driven facility for complex sample size calculation in randomized controlled trials with a survival or a binary outcome: update. *Stata Journal* 5: 123–129.

Barthel, F. M.-S., A. Babiker, P. Royston, and M. K. B. Parmar. 2006. Evaluation of sample size and power for multi-arm survival trials allowing for non-uniform accrual, non-proportional hazards, and loss to follow-up and cross-over. *Statistics in Medicine* 25: 2521–2542.

Chow, S.-C., and J.-P. Liu. 2004. *Design and Analysis of Clinical Trials: Concepts and Methodologies*. 2nd ed. Hoboken, NJ: Wiley.

Chow, S.-C., J. Shao, and H. Wang. 2003. *Sample Size Calculations in Clinical Research*. New York: Marcel Dekker.

Collett, D. 2003. *Modelling Survival Data in Medical Research*. 2nd ed. London: Chapman & Hall/CRC.

Cox, D. R. 1972. Regression models and life-tables (with discussion). *Journal of the Royal Statistical Society, Series B* 34: 187–220.

Cox, D. R., and D. Oakes. 1984. *Analysis of Survival Data*. London: Chapman & Hall/CRC.

Feiveson, A. H. 2002. Power by simulation. *Stata Journal* 2: 107–124.

Freedman, L. S. 1982. Tables of the number of patients required in clinical trials using the logrank test. *Statistics in medicine* 1: 121–129.

George, S. L., and M. M. Desu. 1974. Planning the size and duration of a clinical trial studying the time to some critical event. *Journal of Chronic Diseases* 27: 15–24.

Hosmer, D. W., Jr., and S. Lemeshow. 1999. *Applied Survival Analysis: Regression Modeling of Time to Event Data*. New York: Wiley.

Hsieh, F. Y. 1999. Comparing sample size formulae for trials with unbalanced allocation using the logrank test. *Statistics in medicine* 11: 1091–1098.

Hsieh, F. Y., and P. W. Lavori. 2000. Sample size calculations for the Cox proportional hazards regression models with nonbinary covariates. *Controlled Clinical Trials* 21: 552–560.

Klein, J. P., and M. L. Moeschberger. 2003. *Survival Analysis: Techniques for Censored and Truncated Data*. 2nd ed. New York: Springer.

Lachin, J. M. 1981. Introduction to sample size determination and power analysis for clinical trials. *Controlled Clinical Trials* 2: 93–113.

——. 2000. *Biostatistical Methods: The Assessment of Relative Risks*. New York: Wiley.

Lachin, J. M., and M. A. Foulkes. 1986. Evaluation of sample size and power for analysis of survival with allowance for nonuniform patient entry, losses to follow-up, noncompliance, and stratification. *Biometrics* 42: 507–519.

Lakatos, E., and K. K. G. Lan. 1992. A comparison of sample size methods for the logrank statistic. *Statistics in medicine* 11: 179–191.

Lawless, J. F. 2003. *Statistical Models and Methods for Lifetime Data*. 2nd ed. Hoboken, NJ: Wiley.

Machin, D. 2004. On the evolution of statistical methods as applied to clinical trials. *Journal of internal medicine* 255: 521–528.

Machin, D., and M. Campbell. 2005. *Design of Studies for Medical Research*. Chichester, UK: Wiley.

Machin, D., M. Campbell, P. Fayers, and A. Pinol. 1997. *Sample Size Tables for Clinical Studies*. 2nd ed. Oxford: Blackwell Science.

Marubini, E., and M. G. Valsecchi. 1997. *Analysing Survival Data from Clinical Trials and Observational Studies*. Chichester, UK: Wiley.

Royston, P., and A. Babiker. 2002. A menu-driven facility for complex sample size calculation in randomized controlled trials with a survival or a binary outcome. *Stata Journal* 2: 151–163.

Rubinstein, L. V., M. H. Gail, and T. J. Santner. 1981. Planning the duration of a comparative clinical trial with loss to follow-up and a period of continued observation. *Journal of Chronic Diseases* 34: 469–479.

Schoenfeld, D. 1981. The asymptotic properties of nonparametric tests for comparing survival distributions. *Biometrika* 68: 316–319.

——. 1983. Sample-size formula for the proportional-hazards regression model. *Biometrics* 39: 499–503.

Schoenfeld, D. A., and J. R. Richter. 1982. Nomograms for calculating the number of patients needed for a clinical trial with survival as an endpoint. *Biometrics* 38: 163–170.

Simon, R., R. D. Radmacher, and K. Dobbin. 2002. Design of studies using DNA microarrays. *Genetic Epidemiology* 23: 21–36.

Væth M., and E. Skovlund. 2004. A simple approach to power and sample size calculations in logistic regression and Cox regression models. *Statistics in Medicine* 23: 1781–1792.

Wittes, J. 2002. Sample size calculations for randomized control trials. *Epidemiologic Reviews* 24: 39–53.

Also See

[ST] **stpower cox** — Sample size, power, and effect size for the Cox proportional hazards model

[ST] **stpower exponential** — Sample size and power for the exponential test

[ST] **stpower logrank** — Sample size, power, and effect size for the log-rank test

[R] **sampsi** — Sample size and power determination

[ST] **glossary** — Glossary of terms

Title

stpower cox — Sample size, power, and effect size for the Cox proportional hazards model

Syntax

Sample-size determination

> stpower cox [*coef*] [, *options*]

Power determination

> stpower cox [*coef*] , n(*numlist*) [*options*]

Effect-size determination

> stpower cox , n(*numlist*) { power(*numlist*) | beta(*numlist*) } [*options*]

where *coef* is the regression coefficient (effect size) of a covariate of interest, in a Cox proportional hazards model, desired to be detected by a test with a prespecified power. *coef* may be specified either as one number or as a list of values (see [U] **11.1.8 numlist**) enclosed in parentheses.

options	description
Main	
* alpha(*numlist*)	significance level; default is alpha(0.05)
* power(*numlist*)	power; default is power(0.8)
* beta(*numlist*)	probability of type II error; default is beta(0.2)
* n(*numlist*)	sample size; required to compute power or effect size
* hratio(*numlist*)	hazard ratio (effect size) associated with a one-unit increase in covariate of interest; default is hratio(0.5)
onesided	one-sided test; default is two sided
sd(#)	standard deviation of covariate of interest; default is sd(0.5)
r2(#)	squared coefficient of multiple correlation with other covariates; default is r2(0)
failprob(#)	probability of an event (failure) of interest; default is failprob(1) meaning no censoring
wdprob(#)	the proportion of subjects anticipated to withdraw from the study; default is wdprob(0)
parallel	treat number lists in starred options as parallel (do not enumerate all possible combinations of values) when multiple values per option are specified

Reporting

hr	report hazard ratio, not coefficient
table	display results in a table with default columns
columns(*colnames*)	display results in a table with specified *colnames* columns
notitle	suppress table title
nolegend	suppress table legend
colwidth(# [# ...])	column widths; default is colwidth(9)
separator(#)	draw a horizontal separator line every # lines; default is separator(0) meaning no separator lines
saving(*filename* [, replace])	save the table data to *filename*; use replace to overwrite existing *filename*
†noheader	suppress table header; seldom used
†continue	draw a continuation border in the table output; seldom used

Starred options may be specified either as one number or as a list of values (see [U] **11.1.8 numlist**).

†noheader and continue are not shown in the dialog box.

colnames	description
alpha	significance level
power	power
beta	type II error probability
n	total number of subjects
e	total number of events (failures)
hr	hazard ratio
coef	coefficient (log hazard ratio)
sd	standard deviation
r2	squared multiple correlation coefficient
pr	overall probability of an event (failure)
w	proportion of withdrawals

By default, the following *colnames* are displayed:

   power, n, e, sd, and alpha are always displayed;

   coef is displayed, unless the hr option is specified, in which case, hr is displayed;

   pr if overall probability of an event (failprob());

   r2 if squared multiple correlation coefficient (r2()) is specified; and

   w if withdrawal proportion (wdprob()) is specified.

Description

stpower cox estimates required sample size, power, and effect size for survival analyses that use Cox proportional hazards (PH) models. It also reports the number of events (failures) required to be observed in a study. The estimates of sample size or power are obtained for the test of the effect of one covariate x_1 (binary or continuous) on time to failure adjusted for other predictors $x_2, \ldots, x_p$ in a PH model. The command provides options to account for possible correlation between a covariate of interest and other predictors and for withdrawal of subjects from the study. Optionally, the minimal effect size (minimal detectable difference in a regression coefficient, β_1, or hazard ratio) may be obtained for given sample size and power.

You can use `stpower cox` to

1. calculate required number of events and sample size when you know power and effect size expressed as a hazard ratio or a coefficient (log hazard ratio),

2. calculate power when you know sample size (number of events) and effect size expressed as a hazard ratio or a coefficient (log hazard ratio), and

3. calculate effect size and display it as a coefficient (log hazard ratio) or a hazard ratio when you know sample size (number of events) and power.

`stpower cox`'s input parameter *coef* is the value, β_{1a}, of the regression coefficient β_1 of a covariate of interest x_1 from a Cox PH model, which is desired to be detected by a test with prespecified power.

Options

> **Main**

alpha(*numlist*) sets the significance level of the test. The default is `alpha(0.05)`.

power(*numlist*) sets the power of the test. The default is `power(0.8)`. If `beta()` is specified this value is set to be $1 - beta()$. Only one of `power()` or `beta()` may be specified.

beta(*numlist*) sets the probability of a type II error of the test. The default is `beta(0.2)`. If `power()` is specified, this value is set to be $1 - power()$. Only one of `beta()` or `power()` may be specified.

n(*numlist*) specifies the number of subjects in the study to be used to compute the power of the test or the minimal effect size (minimal detectable value of the regression coefficient, β_1, or hazard ratio) if `power()` or `beta()` is also specified.

hratio(*numlist*) specifies the hazard ratio associated with a one-unit increase in the covariate of interest, x_1, when other covariates are held constant. The default is `hratio(0.5)`. This value defines the minimal clinically significant effect of a covariate on the response to be detected by a test with a certain power, specified in `power()`, in a Cox PH model. If *coef* is specified, `hratio()` is not allowed and the hazard ratio is instead computed as $\exp(coef)$.

onesided indicates a one-sided test. The default is two sided.

sd(*#*) specifies the standard deviation of the covariate of interest, x_1. The default is `sd(0.5)`.

r2(*#*) specifies the squared multiple correlation coefficient between x_1 and other predictors $x_2, \ldots, x_p$ in a Cox PH model. The default is `r2(0)`, meaning that x_1 is independent of other covariates. This option defines the proportion of variance explained by the regression of x_1 on $x_2, \ldots, x_p$ (see [R] **regress**).

failprob(*#*) specifies the overall probability of a subject failing (or experiencing an event of interest, or not being censored) in the study. The default is `failprob(1)`, meaning that all subjects experience an event (or fail) in the study; that is, no censoring of subjects occurs.

wdprob(*#*) specifies the proportion of subjects anticipated to withdraw from a study. The default is `wdprob(0)`. `wdprob()` may not be combined with `n()`.

parallel reports results sequentially (in parallel) over the list of numbers supplied to options allowing *numlist*. By default, results are computed over all combinations of the number lists in the following order of nesting: `alpha()`, `hratio()` or list of coefficients *coef*, `power()` or `beta()`, and `n()`. This option requires that options with multiple values each contain the same number of elements.

Reporting

`hr` specifies that the hazard ratio be displayed rather than the regression coefficient. This option affects how results are displayed and not how they are estimated.

`table` displays results in a tabular format and is implied if any number list contains more than one element. This option is useful if you are producing results one case at a time and wish to construct your own custom table by using a `forvalues` loop.

`columns(`*colnames*`)` specifies results in a table with specified *colnames* columns. The order of columns in the output table is the same as the order of *colnames* specified in `columns()`. Column names in `columns()` must be space separated.

`notitle` prevents the table title from displaying.

`nolegend` prevents the table legend from displaying and column headers from being marked.

`colwidth(`# $\left[\ \#\ \ldots\right]$`)` specifies column widths. The default is 9 for all columns. The number of specified values may not exceed the number of columns in the table. A missing value (.) may be specified for any column to indicate the default width (9). If fewer widths are specified than the number of columns in the table, the last width specified is used for the remaining columns.

`separator(`#`)` specifies how often separator lines should be drawn between rows of the table. The default is `separator(0)`, meaning that no separator lines should be displayed.

`saving(`*filename* $\left[\ \right.$, `replace` $\left]\right.$`)` creates a Stata data file (`.dta` file) containing the table values with variable names corresponding to the displayed *colnames*. `replace` indicates that *filename* be overwritten, if it exists. `saving()` is appropriate only with tabular output.

The following options are available with `stpower cox` but are not shown in the dialog box:

`noheader` prevents the table header from displaying. This option is useful when the command is issued repeatedly, such as within a loop. `noheader` implies `notitle`.

`continue` draws a continuation border at the bottom of the table. This option is useful when the command is issued repeatedly within a loop.

Remarks

Remarks are presented under the following headings:

> *Introduction*
> *Computing sample size in the absence of censoring*
> *Computing sample size in the presence of censoring*
> *Link to the sample-size and power computation for the log-rank test*
> *Power and effect-size determination*
> *Performing the analysis with the Cox PH model*

Introduction

Consider a survival study for which the goal is to investigate the effect of a covariate of interest, x_1, on time to failure, possibly adjusted for other predictors, $x_2, \ldots, x_p$, using the Cox proportional hazards model (Cox 1972). For continuous x_1, the effect is measured as a hazard ratio, Δ, or a log hazard ratio, $\ln(\Delta)$, associated with a one-unit increase in x_1 when the other covariates $x_2, \ldots, x_p$ are held constant. For a binary predictor, the effect is a ratio of hazards or log hazards corresponding to the two categories of x_1 when other covariates are held constant. In both cases, to measure the effect of a covariate, a test of a hazard or a log hazard ratio is performed.

In a Cox PH model, the hazard function is assumed to be

$$h(t) = h_0(t) \exp(\beta_1 x_1 + \ldots + \beta_p x_p)$$

where no distributional assumption is made about the baseline hazard $h_0(t)$. Under this assumption, the regression coefficient β_1 is the log hazard ratio, $\ln(\Delta)$, associated with a one-unit increase in x_1 when the other predictors are held constant, and the exponentiated regression coefficient $\exp(\beta_1)$ is the hazard ratio Δ. Therefore, the effect of x_1 on time to failure can be investigated by performing an appropriate test based on the partial likelihood (Hosmer and Lemeshow 1999, Klein and Moeschberger 2003) for the regression coefficient β_1 from a Cox model. Negative values of β_1 correspond to the reduction in hazard for a one-unit increase in x_1 and, conversely, positive values correspond to the increase in hazard for a one-unit increase in x_1.

stpower cox provides the estimates of sample size or power for a test of the regression coefficient β_1 with the null hypothesis $H_o: (\beta_1, \beta_2, \ldots, \beta_p) = (0, \beta_2, \ldots, \beta_p)$ against the alternative $H_a: (\beta_1, \beta_2, \ldots, \beta_p) = (\beta_{1a}, \beta_2, \ldots, \beta_p)$. The methods used are derived for the score test of H_o versus H_a. In practice, however, the obtained results may be used in the context of the Wald test as well since the two tests usually lead to the same conclusions about the significance of the regression coefficient. Refer to section *The conditional versus unconditional approaches* in [ST] **stpower exponential** for more details about the results based on conditional and unconditional tests. From now on, we will refer to H_a as $H_a: \beta_1 = \beta_{1a}$ for simplicity.

stpower cox implements the method of Hsieh and Lavori (2000) for the sample-size and power computation, which reduces to the method of Schoenfeld (1983) for a binary covariate. The sample size is related to the power of a test through the number of events observed in the study; that is, for a fixed number of events the power of a test is independent of the sample size. As a result, the sample size is estimated as the number of events divided by the overall probability of a subject failing in the study.

The argument *coef* or `hratio()` may be used to specify the effect size desired to be detected by a test. If argument *coef* is omitted, the value of the log of the hazard ratio specified in option `hratio()` or the log of the default hazard-ratio value of 0.5 is used to compute β_{1a}. If argument *coef* is specified, `hratio()` is not allowed and the hazard ratio is computed as $\exp(coef)$.

If power determination is desired, sample size `n()` must be specified. Otherwise, sample-size determination is assumed with `power(0.8)` (or, equivalently, `beta(0.2)`). The default setting for power or, alternatively, the probability of a *type II error*, a failure to reject the null hypothesis when the alternative hypothesis is true, may be changed by using `power()` or `beta()`, respectively. If both `n()` and `power()` (or `beta()`) are specified, the value of the regression coefficient, β_{1a} (or hazard ratio if option `hr` is specified), which can be detected by a test with requested `power()` for fixed sample size `n()`, is computed.

The default probability of a *type I error*, a rejection of the null hypothesis when the null hypothesis is true, of a test is 0.05 but may be changed by using option `alpha()`. One-sided tests may be requested by using `onesided`. By default, no censoring, no correlation between x_1 and other predictors, and no withdrawal of subjects from the study are assumed. This may be changed by specifying `failprob()`, `r2()`, and `wdprob()`, respectively.

Optionally, the results may be displayed in a table by using `table` or `columns()`, as demonstrated in [ST] **stpower**. Refer to [ST] **stpower** and example 7 in section *Power and effect-size determination* in [ST] **stpower logrank** to see how to obtain a graph of a power curve.

Computing sample size in the absence of censoring

First, consider a *type I study* in which all subjects fail by the end of the study (no censoring). Then the required sample size is the same as the number of events required to be observed in a study.

▷ Example 1: Sample size for a model with a binary covariate of interest

Consider a survival study for which the goal is to investigate the effect of a treatment on survival times of subjects. The covariate of interest is binary with levels defining whether a subject receives the treatment (the experimental group) or a placebo (the control or placebo group). Prior to conducting the study, investigators need an estimate of the sample size that ensures that a ratio of hazards of the experimental group to the control group of 0.5 ($\beta_{1a} = \ln(0.5) = -0.6931$) can be detected with a power of 80% with a two-sided 0.05 level test. Under 1:1 randomization, a subject has a 50% chance of receiving the treatment. The corresponding binary covariate follows a Bernoulli distribution with the probability of a subject receiving a treatment, p, equal to 0.5. As such, the standard deviation of the covariate is $\{p(1-p)\}^{1/2} = 0.5$. Since these study parameters correspond to default values of stpower cox, to obtain the sample size for the above study we simply type

```
. stpower cox
Estimated sample size for Cox PH regression
Wald test, log-hazard metric
Ho: [b1, b2, ..., bp] = [0, b2, ..., bp]

Input parameters:
           alpha =    0.0500  (two sided)
              b1 =   -0.6931
              sd =    0.5000
           power =    0.8000

Estimated number of events and sample size:
               E =         66
               N =         66
```

Recall that if argument *coef* is omitted, a default value of $\ln(0.5) = -0.6931$ is assumed. From the output, we see that 66 events (failures) are required to be observed in the study to ensure a power of 80% to detect an alternative $H_a: \beta_1 = -0.6931$ using a two-sided test with a 0.05 significance level. Because we have no censoring, a total of 66 subjects is needed in the study to observe 66 events.

One can also request that the results be displayed in the hazard metric by specifying option hr.

```
. stpower cox, hr
Estimated sample size for Cox PH regression
Wald test, hazard metric
Ho: [b1, b2, ..., bp] = [0, b2, ..., bp]

Input parameters:
           alpha =    0.0500  (two sided)
          hratio =    0.5000
              sd =    0.5000
           power =    0.8000

Estimated number of events and sample size:
               E =         66
               N =         66
```

◁

Suppose now that the covariate of interest x_1 is continuous. Hsieh and Lavori (2000) extend the formula of Schoenfeld (1983) for the number of events to the case when a covariate is continuous. They also relax the assumption of Schoenfeld (1983) about the independence of x_1 of other covariates and provide an adjustment to the estimate of the number of events for possible correlation.

▷ Example 2: Sample size for a model with a continuous covariate of interest

Consider an example from Hsieh and Lavori (2000) of a study of multiple-myeloma patients treated with alkylating agents (Krall, Uthoff, and Harley 1975). Although in the original study of multiple-myeloma patients, 17 of a total of 65 patients are censored; here we assume that all patients die by the end of the study (a type I study, no censoring). Suppose that the covariate of interest x_1 is the log of the amount of blood urea nitrogen (BUN) measured in a patient. The sample size for a one-sided 0.05 level test to detect a coefficient (log hazard ratio) of 1 for a unit increase in x_1 with a power of 80% is required. The standard deviation of x_1 is 0.3126. To obtain an estimate of the sample size, we supply coefficient, 1, as an argument, option sd(0.3126), and option onesided for a one-sided test.

```
. stpower cox 1, sd(0.3126) onesided
Estimated sample size for Cox PH regression
Wald test, log-hazard metric
Ho: [b1, b2, ..., bp] = [0, b2, ..., bp]

Input parameters:
         alpha =    0.0500  (one sided)
            b1 =    1.0000
            sd =    0.3126
         power =    0.8000

Estimated number of events and sample size:
             E =         64
             N =         64
```

The estimate of the required number of events and the sample size is 64.

◁

Based on the derivation in Schoenfeld (1983) and Hsieh and Lavori (2000), sample-size estimates in the above examples may be used if other covariates are also present in the model as long as these covariates are independent of the covariate of interest. The independence assumption holds for randomized studies but it is not true for nonrandomized studies, often encountered in practice. Also, in many studies the main covariate of interest will often be correlated with other covariates. For example, age and gender will often be confounded with the covariate of interest such as smoking. Below we investigate the effect of the confounding factor on the estimate of the required number of events.

▷ Example 3: Sample size when covariates are not independent

Continuing example 2, the effect of a covariate BUN is desired to be adjusted for eight other covariates in the model. Hsieh and Lavori (2000) report the coefficient of determination of $R^2 = 0.1837$ from regression of the log of BUN, x_1, on the eight other covariates.

```
. stpower cox 1, sd(0.3126) onesided r2(0.1837)
Estimated sample size for Cox PH regression
Wald test, log-hazard metric
Ho: [b1, b2, ..., bp] = [0, b2, ..., bp]

Input parameters:
         alpha =    0.0500  (one sided)
            b1 =    1.0000
            sd =    0.3126
         power =    0.8000
            R2 =    0.1837

Estimated number of events and sample size:
             E =         78
             N =         78
```

The number of events required to be observed in a study and, respectively, the number of subjects increase from 64 to 78 after adjusting for the inflation of the variance of the estimate of β_1 because of the correlation with other covariates. The variance of x_1 decreases by the factor $1 - R^2$, so the estimate of the number of events must also be adjusted by a variance inflation factor $\text{VIF} = 1/(1 - R^2)$.

◁

Computing sample size in the presence of censoring

In the previous section we assumed that all subjects fail by the end of the study. In practice, the study often terminates after a fixed time T. As a result, some subjects may not experience an event by the end of study (a *type II study*). These subjects are censored. To obtain an estimate of the sample size in the presence of censoring, an estimate of the overall probability of a subject not being censored is required. The investigator may already have such an estimate from previous studies, or this probability may be computed as suggested in the literature (Schoenfeld 1983, Lachin and Foulkes 1986, Barthel et al. 2006, Barthel, Royston, and Babiker 2005; also see [ST] **stpower logrank** and [ST] **stpower exponential**).

▷ Example 4: Sample size in the presence of censoring

Consider the study from example 2. In reality, as mentioned earlier, 17 of a total of 65 patients survived until the end of the study. The overall death rate is estimated as $1 - 17/65 = 0.738$.

```
. stpower cox 1, sd(0.3126) onesided failprob(0.738)

Estimated sample size for Cox PH regression
Wald test, log-hazard metric
Ho: [b1, b2, ..., bp] = [0, b2, ..., bp]

Input parameters:

          alpha =    0.0500  (one sided)
             b1 =    1.0000
             sd =    0.3126
          power =    0.8000
      Pr(event) =    0.7380

Estimated number of events and sample size:

              E =          64
              N =          86
```

In the presence of censoring, the number of subjects required in the study increases from 64 to 86. The number of events remains the same (64) since the only change in the study is the presence of censoring, and censoring is assumed to be independent of failure (event) times.

If we also adjust for the correlation between the log of BUN and other covariates, we obtain the estimate of the sample size to be 106:

```
. stpower cox, hratio(2.7182) sd(0.3126) onesided r2(0.1837) failprob(0.738)

Estimated sample size for Cox PH regression
Wald test, log-hazard metric
Ho: [b1, b2, ..., bp] = [0, b2, ..., bp]

Input parameters:

          alpha =    0.0500  (one sided)
             b1 =    1.0000
             sd =    0.3126
          power =    0.8000
      Pr(event) =    0.7380
             R2 =    0.1837

Estimated number of events and sample size:

              E =          78
              N =         106
```

In the above example, we also demonstrate the alternative syntax. Rather than supplying the coefficient (log hazard ratio) of 1, we use option `hratio()` to specify the size of the effect expressed as the hazard ratio $\exp(1) = 2.7182$.

◁

❑ Technical Note

Supplying the coefficient (log hazard ratio) of 1 or -1 (or, respectively, a hazard ratio of $\exp(1) = 2.7182$ or $\exp(-1) = 1/2.7182 = .36788$) is irrelevant for sample-size and power determination since it results in the same estimates of sample size and power. However, the sign of the coefficient (or the value of the hazard ratio being larger or smaller than one) is important at the analysis stage since it determines the direction of the effect associated with a one-unit increase of a covariate value.

❑

Often in practice, subjects may withdraw from a study before it terminates. As a result, the information about the subjects' response is lost. The proportion of subjects anticipated to withdraw from a study may be specified by using `wdprob()`. Refer to [ST] **stpower** and *Withdrawal of subjects from the study* in [ST] **stpower logrank** for a more detailed description and an example.

Link to the sample-size and power computation for the log-rank test

When there are no other covariates in a Cox regression model, the score test of the regression coefficient of a binary covariate is the same as the log-rank test (in the absence of tied observations). Powers of the two tests are the same and therefore so are the formulas for the number of events. The formula for the total number of events for a test of a binary covariate in the context of a PH model in the presence of other covariates is derived in Schoenfeld (1983) under the assumption that the covariate of interest is independent of the other covariates. This formula is also the same as the formula for the number of events when the log-rank test is used to compare survivor functions of two groups without covariates (Schoenfeld 1981). Indeed, using `stpower logrank` for the study described in example 1

```
. stpower logrank, schoenfeld

Estimated sample sizes for two-sample comparison of survivor functions
Log-rank test, Schoenfeld method
Ho: S1(t) = S2(t)

Input parameters:
        alpha =    0.0500   (two sided)
    ln(hratio) =   -0.6931
        power =    0.8000
           p1 =    0.5000

Estimated number of events and sample sizes:
            E =         66
            N =         66
           N1 =         33
           N2 =         33
```

yields the same estimates of 66 for both the required number of events and the required sample size.

Schoenfeld (1983) notes that although the formulas for the number of events are the same for the two approaches (based on the log-rank test and based on the score test of a regression coefficient from a Cox regression model adjusting for other covariates), the powers are different. Suppose that the two groups defined by a binary covariate follow the PH model. Then, if covariates are ignored, the ratio of hazards will be nonproportional at every time t and the power of the log-rank test will be smaller than the power of the test based on a Cox PH model.

If a covariate of interest is binary, either `stpower cox` or `stpower logrank` with option `schoenfeld` can be used to obtain the estimate of the sample size or power regardless of the presence of other covariates. However, if covariates are present, it is important to use the appropriate test that adjusts for other covariates when analyzing the data.

Væth and Skovlund (2004) demonstrate that for a continuous covariate the sample-size formula for the log-rank test (assuming the equal-group allocation) may be used to obtain the sample size or power with the value of the hazard ratio equal to $\exp(2\beta_{1a}\sigma)$. By typing this expression into the sample-size formula for the log-rank test, one obtains the formula derived in Hsieh and Lavori (2000).

For example, we obtain the same estimate of the total number of events as computed in example 2 using `stpower logrank` with option `schoenfeld` and with the value of the hazard ratio equal to $\exp(2\beta_{1a}\sigma) = \exp(2 \times 1 \times 0.3126) = 1.8686$.

```
. stpower log, hratio(1.8686) onesided schoenfeld

Estimated sample sizes for two-sample comparison of survivor functions
Log-rank test, Schoenfeld method
Ho: S1(t) = S2(t)

Input parameters:

        alpha =    0.0500  (one sided)
    ln(hratio) =    0.6252
        power =    0.8000
           p1 =    0.5000

Estimated number of events and sample sizes:

            E =         64
            N =         64
           N1 =         32
           N2 =         32
```

Power and effect-size determination

Suppose that for some reason the number of subjects required to ensure a certain power of a test to detect a specified effect size is not achieved by the end of the recruitment phase of a study. Investigators may want to know by how much the power of a test is decreased for the obtained sample size. If the decrease is significant, then what is the minimal effect size that can be detected with an acceptable level of power for this sample size?

▷ Example 5: Power determination

Consider the data of Krall, Uthoff, and Harley (1975) from the study described in example 2. Suppose that we want to test the effect of the log of BUN on patients' survival times adjusted for eight other covariates. In example 4, the required number of patients is estimated to be 106 to ensure a power of 80% of a 0.05 one-sided test to detect a value of 1 in the regression coefficient. This study, however, had only 65 patients. How does this reduction in sample size affect the power of the test to detect the alternative H_a: $\beta_1 = 1$?

```
. stpower cox 1, sd(0.3126) onesided r2(0.1837) failprob(0.738) n(65)

Estimated power for Cox PH regression
Wald test, log-hazard metric
Ho: [b1, b2, ..., bp] = [0, b2, ..., bp]

Input parameters:
              alpha =     0.0500   (one sided)
                 b1 =     1.0000
                 sd =     0.3126
                  N =        65
          Pr(event) =     0.7380
                 R2 =     0.1837

Estimated number of events and power:
                  E =        48
              power =     0.6222
```

When the sample size decreases from 106 to 65, power decreases from 80% to 62%.

◁

▷ Example 6: Effect-size determination

Continuing the above example: if a power of 62% is unacceptable to investigators, they may want to find out what is the smallest value of the regression coefficient that can be detected with a preserved power of 80%. To obtain this estimate, we specify both options n() and power().

```
. stpower cox, sd(0.3126) onesided r2(0.1837) failprob(0.738) n(65) power(0.8)

Estimated coefficient for Cox PH regression
Wald test, log-hazard metric
Ho: [b1, b2, ..., bp] = [0, b2, ..., bp]

Input parameters:
              alpha =     0.0500   (one sided)
                 sd =     0.3126
                  N =        65
              power =     0.8000
          Pr(event) =     0.7380
                 R2 =     0.1837

Estimated number of events and coefficient:
                  E =        48
                 b1 =    -1.2711
```

Stata reports the estimate of the regression coefficient of -1.2711. We can disregard the sign since, as mentioned earlier, it is irrelevant in the context of sample-size or power determination. Refer to *Methods and Formulas* for details.

With only 65 subjects, the smallest change in log hazards for a one-unit increase in the log of BUN which can be detected with a preserved 80% power is roughly 1.27, corresponding to a 27% increase in the log hazard ratio of 1 desired to be detected originally in example 4.

◁

Performing the analysis with the Cox PH model

After the data are collected, one can use stcox and test to fit the Cox PH model and perform a Wald test as we demonstrate below.

▷ Example 7: Performing a Wald test

We demonstrate how to perform a Wald test for the regression coefficient of the log of BUN from a Cox model using the data from Krall, Uthoff, and Harley (1975) described in example 2. The dataset myeloma.dta consists of 11 variables described below.

```
. use http://www.stata-press.com/data/r10/myeloma
(Multiple myeloma patients)

. describe
Contains data from http://www.stata-press.com/data/r10/myeloma.dta
  obs:          65                          Multiple myeloma patients
  vars:         11                          11 Feb 2007 19:26
  size:      1,950 (99.9% of memory free)
```

variable name	storage type	display format	value label	variable label
time	float	%9.0g		Survival time from diagnosis to nearest month + 1
died	byte	%9.0g		0 - Alive, 1 - Dead
lnbun	float	%9.0g		log BUN at diagnosis
hemo	float	%9.0g		Hemoglobin at diagnosis
platelet	byte	%9.0g	normal	Platelets at diagnosis
age	byte	%9.0g		Age (complete years)
lnwbc	float	%9.0g		Log WBC at diagnosis
fracture	byte	%9.0g	present	Fractures at diagnosis
lnbm	float	%9.0g		log % of plasma cells in bone marrow
protein	byte	%9.0g		Proteinuria at diagnosis
scalcium	byte	%9.0g		Serum calcium (mgm%)

```
Sorted by:
```

Prior to using stcox to fit a Cox model, we need to set up the data by using stset (see [ST] **stset**). The analysis time variable is time and the failure variable is died.

```
. stset time, failure(died)
     failure event:  died != 0 & died < .
obs. time interval:  (0, time]
 exit on or before:  failure

       65  total obs.
        0  exclusions

       65  obs. remaining, representing
       48  failures in single record/single failure data
   1560.5  total analysis time at risk, at risk from t =          0
                              earliest observed entry t =          0
                               last observed exit t =           92
```

We include all nine covariates in the model and perform a fit by using stcox. Then we perform a Wald test of H_o: $\beta_1 = 1$ for the coefficient of lnbun using test.

```
. stcox lnbun hemo platelet age lnwbc fracture lnbm protein scalcium, nohr

        failure _d:  died
  analysis time _t:  time
Iteration 0:   log likelihood = -154.85799
Iteration 1:   log likelihood = -146.68114
Iteration 2:   log likelihood = -146.29446
Iteration 3:   log likelihood = -146.29404
Refining estimates:
Iteration 0:   log likelihood = -146.29404

Cox regression -- Breslow method for ties

No. of subjects =          65                    Number of obs   =         65
No. of failures =          48
Time at risk    =      1560.5
                                                 LR chi2(9)      =      17.13
Log likelihood  =   -146.29404                   Prob > chi2     =     0.0468
```

_t	Coef.	Std. Err.	z	P>|z|	[95% Conf. Interval]	
lnbun	1.798354	.6483293	2.77	0.006	.5276519	3.069056
hemo	-.1263119	.0718333	-1.76	0.079	-.2671026	.0144789
platelet	-.2505915	.5074656	-0.49	0.621	-1.245206	.7440228
age	-.0127949	.019475	-0.66	0.511	-.0509653	.0253755
lnwbc	.3537259	.7131935	0.50	0.620	-1.044108	1.75156
fracture	.3378767	.4072774	0.83	0.407	-.4603722	1.136126
lnbm	.3589346	.4860298	0.74	0.460	-.5936663	1.311535
protein	.0130672	.0261696	0.50	0.618	-.0382243	.0643587
scalcium	.1259479	.1034015	1.22	0.223	-.0767153	.3286112

```
. test lnbun = 1

 ( 1)  lnbun = 1

         chi2(  1) =     1.52
       Prob > chi2 =    0.2182
```

By default, stcox reports estimates of hazard ratios and the two-sided tests of the equality of a coefficient to zero. We use option nohr to request estimates of coefficients. From the output table, a one-sided test of H_o: $\beta_1 = 0$ versus H_a: $\beta_1 > 0$ is rejected at a 0.05 level (one-sided p-value is $0.006/2 = 0.003 < 0.05$). The estimate of the log-hazard difference associated with a one-unit increase of lnbun is $\widehat{\beta}_1 = 1.8$. From the test output, we cannot reject the hypothesis of H_o: $\beta_1 = 1$.

For these data, the observed effect size (coefficient) of 1.8 is large enough for the sample size of 65 to be sufficient to reject the null hypothesis of no effect of the BUN on the survival of subjects (H_o: $\beta_1 = 0$). However, if the goal of the study were to ensure that the test detects the effect size corresponding to the coefficient of at least 1 with 80% power, a sample of approximately 106 subjects would have been required.

◁

Saved Results

stpower cox saves the following in r():

Scalars

r(N)	total number of subjects
r(E)	total number of events (failures)
r(power)	power of test
r(alpha)	significance level of test
r(hratio)	hazard ratio
r(onesided)	1 if one-sided test, 0 otherwise
r(sd)	standard deviation
r(Pr_E)	probability of an event (failure) (if specified)
r(r2)	squared multiple correlation (if specified)
r(w)	proportion of withdrawals (if specified)

Macros

r(metric)	displayed metric (log-hazard or hazard)

Methods and Formulas

stpower cox is implemented as an ado-file.

Let β_1 denote the regression coefficient of the covariate of interest x_1 from a Cox PH model, possibly in the presence of other covariates $x_2, \ldots, x_p$; and let Δ denote the hazard ratio associated with a one-unit increase of x_1 when other covariates are held constant. Under the PH model, $\beta_1 = \ln(\Delta)$, where $\ln(\Delta)$ is the change in log hazards associated with a one-unit increase in x_1 when other covariates are held constant.

Define E and N to be the total number of events (failures) and the total number of subjects required in the study; σ to be the standard deviation of x_1; p_{E} to be the overall probability of an event (failure); R^2 to be the proportion of variance explained by the regression of x_1 on $x_2, \ldots, x_p$ (or squared multiple correlation coefficient); w to be the proportion of subjects withdrawn from a study (lost to follow-up); α to be the significance level; β to be the probability of a type II error; $z_{(1-\alpha/k)}$ and $z_{(1-\beta)}$ to be the $(1 - \alpha/k)$th and the $(1 - \beta)$th quantiles of the standard normal distribution, with $k = 1$ for the one-sided test and $k = 2$ for the two-sided test.

The total number of events required to be observed in a study to ensure a power of $1 - \beta$ of a test to detect the regression coefficient β_1 with a significance level α, according to Hsieh and Lavori (2000) is

$$E = \frac{(z_{1-\alpha/k} + z_{1-\beta})^2}{\sigma^2 \beta_1^2 (1 - R^2)}$$

For the case of randomized study and a binary covariate x_1, this formula was derived in Schoenfeld (1983). The formula is an approximation and relies on a set of assumptions such as distinct failure times, all subjects completing the course of the study (no withdrawal), and a local alternative under which $\ln(\Delta)$ is assumed to be of order $O(N^{-1/2})$. The formula is derived for the score test but may be applied to other tests (Wald, for example) that are based on the partial likelihood of a Cox model since all these tests are asymptotically equivalent (Schoenfeld 1983, Hosmer and Lemeshow 1999, Klein and Moeschberger 2003).

The total sample size required to observe the total number of events E is given by

$$N = \frac{E}{p_{\mathrm{E}}}$$

The estimate of the sample size is rounded up to the nearest integer.

To account for a proportion of subjects, w, withdrawn from a study, a conservative adjustment to the total sample size suggested in the literature (Freedman 1982, Machin and Campbell 2005) is applied as follows:

$$N_w = \frac{N}{1 - w}$$

Withdrawal is assumed to be independent of administrative censoring and failure (event) times.

Power is estimated using the formula

$$1 - \beta = \Phi\left[|\beta_1| \sigma \{ N p_{\mathrm{E}} (1 - R^2) \}^{1/2} - z_{1-\alpha/k} \right]$$

where $\Phi(\cdot)$ is the standard normal cumulative distribution function.

The estimate of the regression coefficient for a fixed power $1 - \beta$ and a sample size N is computed as

$$\beta_1^2 = \frac{(z_{1-\alpha/k} + z_{1-\beta})^2}{\sigma^2 N p_{\mathrm{E}} (1 - R^2)}$$

Either of the two values $|\beta_1|$ and $-|\beta_1|$ satisfy the above equation. `stpower cox` reports the negative of the two values that corresponds to the reduction in a hazard of a failure for a one-unit increase in x_1. Similarly, if option `hr` is used, the corresponding value of the hazard ratio less than 1 is reported to reflect the reduction in hazard for a one-unit increase in x_1.

References

Barthel, F. M.-S., P. Royston, and A. Babiker. 2005. A menu-driven facility for complex sample size calculation in randomized controlled trials with a survival or a binary outcome: update. *Stata Journal* 5: 123–129.

Barthel, F. M.-S., A. Babiker, P. Royston, and M. K. B. Parmar. 2006. Evaluation of sample size and power for multi-arm survival trials allowing for non-uniform accrual, non-proportional hazards, and loss to follow-up and cross-over. *Statistics in Medicine* 25: 2521–2542.

Cox, D. R. 1972. Regression models and life-tables (with discussion). *Journal of the Royal Statistical Society, Series B* 34: 187–220.

Freedman, L. S. 1982. Tables of the number of patients required in clinical trials using the logrank test. *Statistics in Medicine* 1: 121–129.

Hosmer, D. W., Jr., and S. Lemeshow. 1999. *Applied Survival Analysis: Regression Modeling of Time to Event Data.* New York: Wiley.

Hsieh, F. Y., and P. W. Lavori. 2000. Sample size calculations for the Cox proportional hazards regression models with nonbinary covariates. *Controlled Clinical Trials* 21: 552–560.

Klein, J. P., and M. L. Moeschberger. 2003. *Survival Analysis: Techniques for Censored and Truncated Data.* 2nd ed. New York: Springer.

Krall, J. M., V. A. Uthoff, and J. B. Harley. 1975. A step-up procedure for selecting variables associated with survival. *Biometrics* 31: 49–57.

Lachin, J. M., and M. A. Foulkes. 1986. Evaluation of sample size and power for analysis of survival with allowance for nonuniform patient entry, losses to follow-up, noncompliance, and stratification. *Biometrics* 42: 507–519.

Machin, D., and M. Campbell. 2005. *Design of Studies for Medical Research*. Chichester: Wiley.

Schoenfeld, D. 1981. The asymptotic properties of nonparametric tests for comparing survival distributions. *Biometrika* 68: 316–319.

——. 1983. Sample-size formula for the proportional-hazards regression model. *Biometrics* 39: 499–503.

Væth M., and E. Skovlund. 2004. A simple approach to power and sample size calculations in logistic regression and Cox regression models. *Statistics in Medicine* 23: 1781–1792.

Also see [ST] **stpower**.

Also See

[ST] **stpower** — Sample-size, power, and effect-size determination for survival analysis

[ST] **stpower logrank** — Sample size, power, and effect size for the log-rank test

[ST] **stpower exponential** — Sample size and power for the exponential test

[R] **sampsi** — Sample size and power determination

[ST] **stcox** — Fit Cox proportional hazards model

[R] **test** — Test linear hypotheses after estimation

[ST] **sts test** — Test equality of survivor functions

[ST] **glossary** — Glossary of terms

Title

> **stpower exponential** — Sample size and power for the exponential test

Syntax

Sample-size determination

Specifying hazard rates

stpower exponential $\left[\, h_1 \,\left[\, h_2 \,\right]\,\right]$ $\left[\,$, *options* $\,\right]$

Specifying survival probabilities

stpower exponential s_1 $\left[\, s_2 \,\right]$, t(*#*) $\left[\, options \,\right]$

Power determination

Specifying hazard rates

stpower exponential $\left[\, h_1 \,\left[\, h_2 \,\right]\,\right]$, n(*numlist*) $\left[\, options \,\right]$

Specifying survival probabilities

stpower exponential s_1 $\left[\, s_2 \,\right]$, t(*#*) n(*numlist*) $\left[\, options \,\right]$

where

h_1 is the hazard rate in the control group;

h_2 is the hazard rate in the experimental group;

s_1 is the survival probability in the control group at reference (base) time t; and

s_2 is the survival probability in the experimental group at reference (base) time t. h_1, h_2 and s_1, s_2 may each be specified either as one number or as a list of values (see [U] **11.1.8 numlist**) enclosed in parentheses.

options	description
Main	
t(#)	reference time t for survival probabilities s_1 and s_2
*alpha(*numlist*)	significance level; default is alpha(0.05)
*power(*numlist*)	power; default is power(0.8)
*beta(*numlist*)	probability of type II error; default is beta(0.2)
*n(*numlist*)	sample size; required to compute power
*hratio(*numlist*)	hazard ratio of the experimental group to the control group, h_2/h_1 or $\ln(s_2)/\ln(s_1)$; default is hratio(0.5)
onesided	one-sided test; default is two sided
*p1(*numlist*)	the proportion of subjects in the control group; default is p1(0.5) meaning equal group sizes
*nratio(*numlist*)	ratio of sample sizes, N_2/N_1; default is nratio(1) meaning equal group sizes
loghazard	power or sample-size computation for the test of the difference between log hazards; default is the test of the difference between hazards
unconditional	power or sample-size computation using the unconditional approach
parallel	treat number lists in starred options as parallel (do not enumerate all possible combinations of values) when multiple values per option are specified
Accrual/Follow-up	
fperiod(#)	length of the follow-up period; if not specified the study is assumed to continue until all subjects experience an event (fail)
aperiod(#)	length of the accrual period; default is aperiod(0) meaning no accrual
aprob(#)	proportion of subjects accrued by time t^* under truncated exponential accrual; default is aprob(0.5)
aptime(#)	proportion of the accrual period, $t^*/$aperiod(), by which proportion of subjects in aprob() is accrued; default is aptime(0.5)
atime(#)	reference accrual time t^* by which the proportion of subjects in aprob() is accrued; default value is $0.5 \times$ aperiod()
ashape(#)	shape of the truncated exponential accrual distribution; default is ashape(0) meaning uniform accrual
lossprob(# #)	proportion of subjects lost to follow-up by time losstime() in the control and the experimental groups; default is lossprob(0 0) meaning no losses to follow-up
losstime(#)	(reference) time by which the proportion of subjects specified in lossprob() is lost to follow-up; default is losstime(1)
losshaz(# #)	loss hazard rates in the control and the experimental groups; default is losshaz(0 0) meaning no losses to follow-up

Reporting

detail	more detailed output
table	display results in a table with default columns
columns(*colnames*)	display results in a table with specified *colnames* columns
notitle	suppress table title
nolegend	suppress table legend
colwidth(# [# ...])	column widths; default is colwidth(9)
separator(#)	draw a horizontal separator line every # lines; default is separator(0) meaning no separator lines
saving(*filename* [, replace])	save the table data to *filename*; use replace to overwrite existing *filename*
†noheader	suppress table header; seldom used
†continue	draw a continuation border in the table output; seldom used

Starred options may be specified either as one number or as a list of values (see [U] **11.1.8 numlist**).

†noheader and continue are not shown in the dialog box.

colnames	description
alpha	significance level
power	power
beta	type II error probability
n	total number of subjects
n1	number of subjects in the control group
n2	number of subjects in the experimental group
hr	hazard ratio
loghr	log of the hazard ratio (difference between log hazards)
diff	difference between hazards
h1	hazard rate in the control group
h2	hazard rate in the experimental group
s1	survival probability in the control group
s2	survival probability in the experimental group
t	reference survival time
p1	proportion of subjects in the control group
nratio	ratio of sample sizes, experimental to control
fperiod	follow-up period
aperiod	accrual period
aprob	% of subjects accrued by time atime (or by aptime % of accrual period)
aptime	% of an accrual period by which aprob % of subjects are accrued
atime	reference accrual time
ashape	shape of the accrual distribution
lpr1	proportion of subjects lost to follow-up in the control group
lpr2	proportion of subjects lost to follow-up in the experimental group
losstime	reference loss to follow-up time

lh1	loss hazard rate in the control group
lh2	loss hazard rate in the experimental group
eo	total expected number of events (failures) under the null
eo1	number of events in the control group under the null
eo2	number of events in the experimental group under the null
ea	total expected number of events (failures) under the alternative
ea1	number of events in the control group under the alternative
ea2	number of events in the experimental group under the alternative
lo	total expected number of losses to follow-up under the null
lo1	number of losses in the control group under the null
lo2	number of losses in the experimental group under the null
la	total expected number of losses to follow-up under the alternative
la1	number of losses in the control group under the alternative
la2	number of losses in the experimental group under the alternative

By default, the following *colnames* are displayed:

power, n, n1, n2, and alpha are always displayed;

h1 and h2 are displayed if hazard rates are specified, or s1 and s2 if survival probabilities are specified;

diff if hazard difference test is specified, or loghr if log-hazard difference test is specified;

aperiod if accrual period (aperiod()) is specified;

fperiod if follow-up period (fperiod()) is specified; and

lh1 and lh2 if losshaz() or lpr1 and lpr2 if lossprob() is specified.

Description

stpower exponential estimates required sample size and power for survival analysis comparing two exponential survivor functions by using parametric tests for the difference between hazards or, optionally, for the difference between log hazards. It accommodates unequal allocation between the two groups, flexible accrual of subjects into the study and group-specific losses to follow-up. The accrual distribution may be chosen to be uniform over the fixed accrual period R or truncated exponential over the period $[0, R]$. Losses to follow-up are assumed to be exponentially distributed. Also, the computations may be carried out using the conditional or the unconditional approach.

You can use stpower exponential to

1. calculate expected number of events and required sample size when you know power and effect size (supplied as hazard rates, survival probabilities, or hazard ratio) for studies with or without follow-up and accrual periods allowing for different accrual patterns and in the presence of losses to follow-up and

2. calculate power when you know sample size and effect size (supplied as hazard rates, survival probabilities, or hazard ratio) for studies with or without follow-up and accrual periods allowing for different accrual patterns and in the presence of losses to follow-up.

If option t() is specified, the command's input parameters are the values of survival probabilities in the control (or the less favorable of the two groups) group, $S_1(t)$, and in the experimental group, $S_2(t)$, at a fixed time t (reference survival time) specified in t(), given as s_1 and s_2, respectively. Otherwise, the input parameters are assumed to be the values of the hazard rates in the control group, λ_1, and in the experimental group, λ_2, given as h1 and h2, respectively. If survival probabilities are specified, they are converted to hazard rates by using the formula for the exponential survivor function and the value of time t in t().

Options

t(*#*) specifies a fixed time t (reference survival time) such that the proportions of subjects in the control and experimental groups still alive past this time point are as specified in s_1 and s_2. If this option is specified, the input parameters, s_1 and s_2, are the survival probabilities $S_1(t)$ and $S_2(t)$. Otherwise, the input parameters are assumed to be hazard rates, λ_1 and λ_2, given as h_1 and h_2, respectively.

alpha(*numlist*) sets the significance level of the test. The default is alpha(0.05).

power(*numlist*) sets the power of the test. The default is power(0.8). If beta() is specified, this value is set to be 1−beta(). Only one of power() or beta() may be specified.

beta(*numlist*) sets the probability of a type II error of the test. The default is beta(0.2). If power() is specified, this value is set to be 1−power(). Only one of beta() or power() may be specified.

n(*numlist*) specifies the number of subjects in the study to be used to compute the power of the test. By default, the sample-size calculation is assumed. This option may not be combined with beta() or power().

hratio(*numlist*) specifies the hazard ratio of the experimental group to the control group. The default is hratio(0.5). This value defines the clinically significant improvement of the experimental procedure over the control desired to be detected by a test, with a certain power specified in power(). If h_1 and h_2 (or s_1 and s_2) are given, hratio() is not allowed and the hazard ratio is computed as h_2/h_1 (or $\ln(s_2)/\ln(s_1)$).

onesided indicates a one-sided test. The default is two sided.

p1(*numlist*) specifies the proportion of subjects in the control group. The default is p1(0.5), meaning equal allocation of subjects to the control and the experimental groups. Only one of p1() or nratio() may be specified.

nratio(*numlist*) specifies the sample-size ratio of the experimental group relative to the control group, N_2/N_1. The default is nratio(1), meaning equal allocation between the two groups. Only one of nratio() or p1() may be specified.

loghazard requests sample-size or power computation for the test of the difference between log hazards (or the test of the log of the hazard ratio). This option implies uniform accrual. By default, the test of the difference between hazards is assumed.

unconditional requests that the unconditional approach be used for sample-size or power computation; see *The conditional versus unconditional approaches* and *Methods and Formulas* for details.

parallel reports results sequentially (in parallel) over the list of numbers supplied to options allowing *numlist*. By default, results are computed over all combinations of the number lists in the following order of nesting: alpha(), p1() or nratio(), list of hazard rates h_1 and h_2 or survival probabilities s_1 and s_2, hratio(), power() or beta(), and n(). This option requires that options with multiple values each contain the same number of elements.

fperiod(*#*) specifies the follow-up period of the study, f. By default, it is assumed that subjects are followed up until the last subject experiences an event (fails). The (minimal) follow-up period is defined as the length of the period after the recruitment of the last subject to the study until the end of the study. If T is the duration of a study and R is the length of an accrual period, then the follow-up period is $f = T - R$.

aperiod(#) specifies the accrual period, R, during which subjects are to be recruited into the study. The default is aperiod(0) meaning no accrual.

aprob(#) specifies the proportion of subjects expected to be accrued by time t^* according to the truncated exponential distribution. The default is aprob(0.5). This option is useful when the shape parameter is unknown but the proportion of accrued subjects at a certain time is known. aprob() is often used in conjunction with aptime() or atime(). This option may not be specified with ashape() or loghazard and requires specifying a nonzero accrual period in aperiod().

aptime(#) specifies the proportion of the accrual period, t^*/R, by which the proportion of subjects specified in aprob() is expected to be accrued according to the truncated exponential distribution. The default is aptime(0.5). This option may not be combined with atime(), ashape(), or loghazard and requires specifying a nonzero accrual period in aperiod().

atime(#) specifies the time point t^*, reference accrual time, by which the proportion of subjects specified in aprob() is expected to be accrued according to the truncated exponential distribution. The default value is $0.5 \times R$. This option may not be combined with aptime(), ashape(), or loghazard and requires specifying a nonzero accrual period in aperiod(). The value in atime() may not exceed the value in aperiod().

ashape(#) specifies the shape, γ, of the truncated exponential accrual distribution. The default is ashape(0), meaning uniform accrual. This option is not allowed in conjunction with loghazard and requires specifying a nonzero accrual period in aperiod().

lossprob(# #) specifies the proportion of subjects lost to follow-up by time losstime() in the control and the experimental groups, respectively. The default is lossprob(0 0) meaning no losses to follow-up. This option requires specifying aperiod() or fperiod() and may not be combined with losshaz().

losstime(#) specifies the time at which the proportion of subjects specified in lossprob() is lost to follow-up, also referred to as the reference loss to follow-up time. The default is losstime(1). This option requires specifying lossprob().

losshaz(# #) specifies exponential hazard rates of losses to follow-up, η_1 and η_2, in the control and the experimental groups, respectively. The default is losshaz(0 0) meaning no losses to follow-up. This option requires specifying aperiod() or fperiod() and may not be combined with lossprob().

    ⌐ Reporting ⌐

detail displays more detailed output; the expected number of events (failures) and losses to follow-up under the null and alternative hypotheses are displayed. This option is not appropriate with tabular output.

table displays results in a tabular format and is implied if any number list contains more than one element. This option is useful if you are producing results one case at a time and wish to construct your own custom table by using a forvalues loop.

columns(colnames) specifies results in a table with specified colnames columns. The order of the columns in the output table is the same as the order of colnames specified in columns(). Column names in columns() must be space separated.

notitle prevents the table title from displaying.

nolegend prevents the table legend from displaying and column headers from being marked.

colwidth(# $\big[$ # ... $\big]$) specifies column widths. The default is 9 for all columns. The number of specified values may not exceed the number of columns in the table. A missing value (.) may be specified for any column to indicate the default width (9). If fewer widths are specified than the number of columns in the table, the last width specified is used for the remaining columns.

separator(#) specifies how often separator lines should be drawn between rows of the table. The default is separator(0), meaning that no separator lines should be displayed.

saving(*filename*[, replace]) creates a Stata data file (.dta file) containing the table values with variable names corresponding to the displayed *colnames*. replace indicates that *filename* be overwritten, if it exists. saving() is only appropriate with tabular output.

The following options are available with stpower exponential but are not shown in the dialog box:

noheader prevents the table header from displaying. This option is useful when the command is issued repeatedly, such as within a loop. noheader implies notitle.

continue draws a continuation border at the bottom of the table. This option is useful when the command is issued repeatedly within a loop.

Remarks

Remarks are presented under the following headings:

Introduction
Other ways of specifying the effect size
Sample-size determination by using different approximations
Sample-size determination in the presence of censoring
Nonuniform accrual and exponential losses to follow-up
The conditional versus unconditional approaches
Link to the sample-size and power computation for the log-rank test
Power determination

Introduction

Let $S_1(t)$ and $S_2(t)$ be the exponential survivor functions with hazard rates λ_1 and λ_2 in the control and experimental groups, respectively. Define ψ to be the treatment effect that can be expressed as a difference, $\delta = \lambda_2 - \lambda_1$, between hazard rates or as the log of the hazard ratio (a difference between log-hazard rates), $\ln(\Delta) = \ln(\lambda_2/\lambda_1) = \ln(\lambda_2) - \ln(\lambda_1)$. Negative values of the treatment effect ψ imply the superiority of the experimental treatment over the standard (control) treatment. Denote R and T to be the length of the accrual period and the total duration of the study, respectively. Then, the follow-up period f is $f = T - R$.

Consider a study designed to compare the exponential survivor functions, $S_1(t) = e^{-\lambda_1 t}$ and $S_2(t) = e^{-\lambda_2 t}$, of the two treatment groups. The disparity in survivor functions may be tested using the hazards λ_1 and λ_2 for the exponential model. Depending on the definition of the treatment effect ψ, two test statistics based on the difference and on the log ratio of the hazards may be used to conduct tests of the difference between survivor functions using respective null hypotheses, H_o: $\delta = 0$ and H_o: $\ln(\Delta) = 0$.

The basic formula for the sample-size and power calculations for the test of H_o: $\delta = 0$ is proposed by Lachin (1981). He also derives the equation relating the sample size and power allowing for uniform accrual of subjects into the study over the period from 0 to R. Lachin and Foulkes (1986) extend this formula to truncated exponential accrual over the interval 0 to R and exponential losses to follow-up over the interval 0 to T.

The simplest method for the sample-size and power calculations for the test of H_o: $\ln(\Delta) = 0$ is presented by George and Desu (1974). Rubinstein, Gail, and Santner (1981) extend their method to account for uniform accrual and exponential losses to follow-up and apply it to planning the duration of a survival study. The formula that relates the sample size and power for this test and takes into account the uniform accrual and exponential losses to follow-up is formulated by Lakatos and Lan (1992), based on the derivations of Rubinstein, Gail, and Santner (1981).

By default, `stpower exponential` computes the sample size required to achieve a specified power to detect a difference between hazard rates $\delta_a = \lambda_{2a} - \lambda_{1a}$ using the method of Lachin (1981). If `loghazard` is specified, the sample size required to detect a log of the hazard ratio $\ln(\Delta_a) = \ln(\lambda_{2a}/\lambda_{1a})$ with specified power is reported using the formula derived by George and Desu (1974). In the presence of an accrual period, the methods of Lachin and Foulkes (1986) or, for uniform accrual only, Rubinstein, Gail, and Santner (1981) (if `loghazard` and `unconditional` are specified), are used.

If power determination is desired, sample size `n()` must be specified. Otherwise, sample-size determination is assumed with `power(0.8)` (or, equivalently, `beta(0.2)`). The default setting for power or, the probability of a *type II error*, a failure to reject the null hypothesis when the alternative hypothesis is true, may be changed by using `power()` or `beta()`, respectively.

The default probability of a *type I error*, a rejection of the null hypothesis when the null hypothesis is true, of a test is 0.05 but may be changed by using option `alpha()`. One-sided tests may be requested by using option `onesided`. The default equal-group allocation may be changed by specifying either `p1()` or `nratio()`.

By default, the estimates of sample sizes or power for the test of the difference between hazards are reported. This may be changed to the test versus the difference between log hazards by using option `loghazard`. The default conditional approach may be replaced with the unconditional approach by using `unconditional`; see *The conditional versus unconditional approaches*.

If neither the length of a follow-up period, f, nor the length of an accrual period, R, is specified in `fperiod()` or `aperiod()`, respectively, the study is assumed to continue until all subjects experience an event (failure), regardless of how much time is required. If either of the two options is supplied, a study of length $T = R + f$ is assumed.

If an accrual period of length R is specified in option `aperiod()`, uniform accrual over the period $[0, R]$ is assumed. The accrual distribution may be changed to truncated exponential when the shape parameter is specified in `ashape()`. The combination of options `aprob()` and `aptime()` (or `atime()`) may be used in place of option `ashape()` to request the desired shape of the truncated exponential accrual. To take into account exponential losses to follow-up, options `losshaz()` or `lossprob()` and `losstime()` may be used. For examples, see *Nonuniform accrual and exponential losses to follow-up*.

Optionally, results may be displayed in a table by using `table` or `columns()` as demonstrated in *Sample-size determination in the presence of censoring* below and in *Creating output tables* of [ST] **stpower**. Refer to example 7 in *Power and effect-size determination* in [ST] **stpower logrank** and [ST] **stpower** to see how to obtain a graph of a power curve.

Other ways of specifying the effect size

Here we demonstrate how to provide the information about the disparity in the two exponential survivor functions, also known as the effect size, to `stpower exponential`. We separately consider the two tests, based on the hazard difference and based on the log of the hazard ratio (or on the log-hazard difference).

▷ Example 1: Effect size for the test on the difference between hazards

Consider a fictional study for which the goal is to compare the two exponential survivor functions of the control and the experimental groups, using the test based on the difference between hazard rates. The yearly hazard rate in the control group is known to be 0.4, corresponding to roughly 45% survival by 2 years. The effect size, expressed as the hazard ratio, of 0.5 corresponding to the reduction in hazard of the experimental group from 0.4 to 0.2 (or increase in survival to 67% by 2 years), is of interest. The investigators need an estimate of the required sample size to detect this effect size with 80% power with a two-sided 0.05-level test, the default settings of stpower exponential. For simplicity, we also assume that there are enough resources to monitor the subjects until all of them fail (a type I study as defined in the next section).

The hazard rate in the control group and the effect size are required in the computation. The value of the hazard rate in the control group may be supplied directly as argument h_1 (the first syntax) or computed using the supplied value of the survival probability s_1 at reference time specified in option t() (the second syntax). The effect size may be supplied by using option hratio(), or by directly supplying the hazard rate in the experimental group as argument h_2 or, if option t() is specified, by supplying the survival probability in the experimental group as argument s_2 at reference time t().

We demonstrate all the above by using our fictional example. To obtain the required sample size, we supply the hazard rate in the control group, 0.4, as argument h_1 and the hazard ratio of 0.5 in hratio().

```
. stpower exponential 0.4, hratio(0.5)
Note: input parameters are hazard rates.

Estimated sample sizes for two-sample comparison of survivor functions
Exponential test, hazard difference, conditional
Ho: h2-h1 = 0

Input parameters:
          alpha =    0.0500   (two sided)
             h1 =    0.4000
             h2 =    0.2000
          h2-h1 =   -0.2000
          power =    0.8000
             p1 =    0.5000

Estimated sample sizes:
              N =         74
             N1 =         37
             N2 =         37
```

Instead of the hazard rate, we specify the survival probability of 0.45 in the control group as argument s_2 and a reference survival time 2 in option t().

```
. stpower exponential 0.45, t(2) hratio(0.5)
Note: input parameters are survival probabilities.

Estimated sample sizes for two-sample comparison of survivor functions
Exponential test, hazard difference, conditional
Ho: h2-h1 = 0

Input parameters:
        alpha =    0.0500   (two sided)
           s1 =    0.4500
           s2 =    0.6708
            t =    2.0000
        h2-h1 =   -0.1996
        power =    0.8000
           p1 =    0.5000
Estimated sample sizes:
            N =        74
           N1 =        37
           N2 =        37
```

Since the hazard ratio of 0.5 is the default of `hratio()`, we could have omitted this option from the above syntaxes.

Now rather than specifying the effect size by using option `hratio(0.5)` above, we supply the hazard rate in the experimental group 0.2 as argument h_2,

> `. stpower exponential 0.4 0.2`
>
> *(output omitted)*

or the survival probability in the experimental group 0.67 as argument s_2 and the reference survival time of 2 years in `t()`,

> `. stpower exponential 0.45 0.67, t(2)`
>
> *(output omitted)*

and obtain the same estimates, 74 of the total sample and 37 of the group sample sizes, as in the above output.

◁

▷ Example 2: Effect size for the test on the log of the hazard ratio

Continuing with the above example, suppose that the two survivor functions are to be compared using the test based on the difference between the log hazards (or test based on the log of the hazard ratio). To request this test, option `loghazard` must be specified.

Unlike the hazard-difference test, the log hazard-ratio test does not require the hazard rate in the control group for the computation when the study is continued until all subjects fail. The only required information is the size of the effect desired to be detected by this test.

To obtain the estimate of the sample size for the test based on the log of the hazard ratio, we specify option `loghazard` and use the default value of the hazard ratio of 0.5:

(Continued on next page)

```
. stpower exponential, loghazard

Estimated sample sizes for two-sample comparison of survivor functions
Exponential test, log-hazard difference, conditional
Ho: ln(h2/h1) = 0

Input parameters:
          alpha =    0.0500   (two sided)
      ln(h2/h1) =   -0.6931
          power =    0.8000
             p1 =    0.5000

Estimated sample sizes:
              N =        66
             N1 =        33
             N2 =        33
```

Similar to the examples for the hazard-difference test, the effect size may also be supplied via hazard rates,

```
. stpower exponential 0.4 0.2, loghazard
```
   (*output omitted*)

or survival probabilities and reference survival time,

```
. stpower exponential 0.45 0.67, t(2) loghazard
```
   (*output omitted*)

For a fixed-duration study, when either `fperiod()` or `aperiod()` is specified (see *Sample-size determination in the presence of censoring*), the sample-size computations for the log hazard-ratio test does require the value of the hazard rate in the control group.

◁

Sample-size determination by using different approximations

Consider the following two types of survival studies. The first type, a *type I study*, is when investigators have enough resources to monitor the subjects until all of them experience an event (failure) and the second type, a *type II study*, is when the study terminates after a fixed period of time, regardless of whether all subjects experienced an event by that time.

Here we explore sample-size estimates using different approximations for a type I study. Examples of sample-size determination for a type II study are presented in the next section.

In survival studies, the requirement for the sample size is based on the requirement to observe a certain number of events (failures) to ensure a prespecified power of a test to detect a difference in survivor functions. For a type I study, the number of subjects required for the study is the same as the number of events required to be observed in the study since all subjects experience an event by the end of the study.

▷ Example 3: Sample size using the Lachin method

Consider an example from Lachin (1981, 107). A clinical trial is to be conducted to compare the survivor functions in the control and the experimental groups with a one-sided exponential test, based on the difference between hazards, of the superiority of a new treatment ($H_a: \delta < 0$) for a disease with moderate levels of mortality. Subjects in the control group get a standard treatment and subjects in the experimental group receive a new treatment. From previous studies the yearly hazard rate for the standard treatment was found to be $\lambda_1 = 0.3$, corresponding to 50% survival after 2.3 years. The investigators would like to know how many subjects are required to detect a reduction in hazard to $\lambda_2 = 0.2$ (H_a: $\delta = -0.1$), which corresponds to an increase in survival to 63% at 2.3 years, with 90% power, equal-sized groups, and a significance level, α, of 0.05.

To obtain the estimate of the sample size for the above study, we supply hazard rates 0.3 and 0.2 as arguments and specify options `power(0.9)` for 90% power and `onesided` for a one-sided test.

```
. stpower exponential 0.3 0.2, power(0.9) onesided
Note: input parameters are hazard rates.

Estimated sample sizes for two-sample comparison of survivor functions
Exponential test, hazard difference, conditional
Ho: h2-h1 = 0

Input parameters:

        alpha =     0.0500   (one sided)
           h1 =     0.3000
           h2 =     0.2000
        h2-h1 =    -0.1000
        power =     0.9000
           p1 =     0.5000

Estimated sample sizes:

            N =        218
           N1 =        109
           N2 =        109
```

From the output, a total of 218 events (subjects) must be observed (recruited) in a study to ensure a power of 90% of a one-sided exponential test to detect a 13% increase in survival probability of subjects in the experimental group with $\alpha = 0.05$. Our estimate of 218 of the total number of subjects (109 per group) required for the study is the same as the one reported in Lachin (1981, 107).

◁

▷ Example 4: Sample size using the George–Desu method

The syntax above reports the sample size obtained using the approximation of Lachin (1981) for the test based on the hazard difference. To obtain the sample size using the approximation of George and Desu (1974), for the equivalent alternative H_a: $\ln(\Delta) = -0.4055$ (a test based on the log of the hazard ratio), we need to specify option `loghazard`.

```
. stpower exponential 0.3 0.2, power(0.9) onesided loghazard
Note: input parameters are hazard rates.

Estimated sample sizes for two-sample comparison of survivor functions
Exponential test, log-hazard difference, conditional
Ho: ln(h2/h1) = 0

Input parameters:

        alpha =     0.0500   (one sided)
           h1 =     0.3000
           h2 =     0.2000
    ln(h2/h1) =    -0.4055
        power =     0.9000
           p1 =     0.5000

Estimated sample sizes:

            N =        210
           N1 =        105
           N2 =        105
```

The George–Desu method yields a slightly smaller estimate, 210, of the total number of events (subjects). George and Desu (1974) studied the accuracy of the two approximations based on δ and $\ln(\Delta)$ and concluded that the former is slightly conservative; that is, it gives slightly larger sample-size estimates. The latter was found to be accurate to one or two units of the exact solution for equal-sized groups.

We could have also obtained the same results by using option `hratio()` to specify the hazard ratio $0.2/0.3 = 0.66667$ instead of suppling arguments 0.3 and 0.2:

```
. stpower exponential, hratio(0.66667) power(0.9) onesided loghazard
(output omitted)
```

◁

❏ Technical Note

The above approach may also be used to obtain an approximation to the sample size or power for the exact F test of equality of two exponential mean analysis (life) times (using the relation between a mean and a hazard rate of the exponential distribution, $\mu = 1/\lambda$).

For example, the sample size of 210 obtained above may be used as an approximation to the number of subjects required in a study of which the goal is to detect an increase in a mean analysis (life) time of the experimental group from $3.33 = 1/0.3$ to $5 = 1/0.2$ by using the exact one-sided 0.05 level F test with 90% power.

The test statistic of the F test is a ratio of two sample means from two exponential distributions that has an exact F distribution. The George–Desu method is based on the normal approximation of the distribution of the log of this test statistic. George and Desu (1974) studied this approximation for equal-sized groups and some common values of significance levels, powers, and hazard ratios and found it to be accurate to one or two units of the exact solution.

❏

❏ Technical Note

We can obtain the same results from `stpower exponential` as in the examples above by using the respective survival probabilities 0.5 and 0.63 at $t = 2.3$ as arguments in place of hazard rates 0.3 and 0.2. For example,

```
. stpower exponential 0.5 0.63, t(2.3) power(0.9) onesided
Note: input parameters are survival probabilities.
(output omitted)
```

Other alternative syntaxes, using option `hratio()`, are

```
. stpower exponential 0.3, hratio(0.66667) power(0.9) onesided
Note: input parameters are hazard rates.
(output omitted)
```

where 0.3 is interpreted as a hazard rate since `t()` is not specified, and

```
. stpower exponential 0.5, t(2.3) hratio(0.6667) power(0.9) onesided
Note: input parameters are survival probabilities.
(output omitted)
```

❏

Sample-size determination in the presence of censoring

Often in practice, investigators may not have enough resources to continue a study until all subjects experience an event and therefore plan to terminate the study after a fixed period, T. Some subjects may not experience an event by the end of the study in which case the (administrative) censoring of subjects occurs. In the presence of censoring, the number of subjects required in a study will be larger than the number of events required to be observed in the study.

We investigate how terminating the study after some fixed period, T, before all subjects experience an event, affects the requirements for the sample size. The duration of a study is divided into two phases: an accrual phase of a length R, during which subjects are recruited to the study, and a follow-up phase of a length f, during which subjects are followed up until the end of the study and no new subjects enter the study. The duration of a study, T, is the sum of the lengths of two phases.

Consider the following study designs. In the first study design, A, each subject is followed up for a length of time T. Here the minimum follow-up time f is equal to T, and, consequently, $R = 0$. In practice, however, subjects will often enter the study at random times and will be followed up until the end of a study at time T, in which case the subjects who come under observation later in time will have a shorter follow-up than subjects who entered the study at the beginning. Therefore, the minimum follow-up time f will be less than T and R will be equal to $T - f$. Here the length of the accrual period R must be taken into account in the computations. In the presence of an accrual period, subjects may be recruited continuously during a period of length T ($R = T$, $f = 0$), the second study design, B, or subjects may be recruited for a fixed period R and then followed up for a period of time f, during which no new subjects enter the trial, so that the total duration of study is $T = R + f$, the third design, C.

▷ Example 5: Sample size in the presence of accrual and follow-up periods

Continuing example 3, assume that the investigators have resources to continue the study for only 5 years, $T = 5$. We tabulate sample-size values for different combinations of an accrual period R and a minimum follow-up period f such that $T = f + R = 5$. Since options aperiod() and fperiod() allow specifying only one number, we can obtain the table by issuing stpower exponential repeatedly within a forvalues loop.

```
. local cont continue
. local columns columns(power n aperiod fperiod h1 h2 alpha)
. local T = 5
. forvalues R = 0/'T' {
  2.          if 'R' == 'T' {
  3.                  local cont
  4.          }
  5.          local f = 'T' - 'R'
  6.          stpower exponential 0.3 0.2, power(0.9) onesided \\\
  >                  aperiod('R') fperiod('f') 'header' 'cont' 'columns'
  7.          local header noheader
  8. }
Note: input parameters are hazard rates.
```

(Continued on next page)

```
Estimated sample sizes for two-sample comparison of survivor functions
Exponential test, hazard difference, conditional
Ho: h2-h1 = 0
```

Power	N	AP+	FP	H1	H2	Alpha*
.9	304	0	5	.3	.2	.05
.9	322	1	4	.3	.2	.05
.9	344	2	3	.3	.2	.05
.9	378	3	2	.3	.2	.05
.9	426	4	1	.3	.2	.05
.9	502	5	0	.3	.2	.05

```
* one sided
+ uniform accrual; 50.00% accrued by 50.00% of AP
```

For each iteration of the loop, the value of a follow-up period f, stored in macro f (see [P] **macro**), is computed using the current value of an accrual period R and the fixed-time study T, defined by macros R and T, respectively. The values 'R' and 'f' are then passed to options aperiod() and fperiod(), respectively. We use option columns() to obtain a customized table with columns power, n, aperiod, fperiod, h1, h2, and alpha. We store this option in local columns simply to avoid specifying a long expression in stpower exponential. We specify noheader in the syntax of stpower exponential each time it is called in the loop except for the first time, and we specify continue each time except for the final one.

The first and the last entries of the above table correspond to the extreme cases of no accrual (design A) and no follow-up (design B), respectively.

For a design A, the estimate of the sample size 304 is larger than the earlier estimate of 218 from example 3. That is, if the study in example 3 terminates after 5 years, the requirement for the sample size increases by 39% to ensure that the same number of 218 events is observed.

By trying different values of the follow-up period, we may find that a 30-year follow-up is required if the investigators can recruit no more than 218 subjects: 30 years is required to observe all subjects to fail in this study.

```
. stpower exponential 0.3 0.2, power(0.9) onesided fperiod(30)
Note: input parameters are hazard rates.

Estimated sample sizes for two-sample comparison of survivor functions
Exponential test, hazard difference, conditional
Ho: h2-h1 = 0

Input parameters:
         alpha =    0.0500  (one sided)
            h1 =    0.3000
            h2 =    0.2000
         h2-h1 =   -0.1000
         power =    0.9000
            p1 =    0.5000

Accrual and follow-up information:
      duration =   30.0000
     follow-up =   30.0000

Estimated sample sizes:
             N =       218
            N1 =       109
            N2 =       109
```

For design B, instead of being monitored for 5 years, subjects are being continuously recruited during all of those 5 years; the total sample size increases from 304 to 502. The reason for such an increase is that the average analysis time (the time when a subject is at risk of a failure) decreases from 5 to 2.5 and therefore reduces the probability of a subject failing by the end of the study.

In general, the estimates of the total sample size steadily increase as the length of the follow-up decreases. That is, the presence of a follow-up period reduces the requirement for the number of subjects in the study. For example, a clinical trial with a 3-year uniform accrual and a 2-year follow-up needs a total of 378 subjects (189 per group) compared with the total of 502 subjects required for a study with no follow-up and a 5-year accrual.

Nonuniform accrual and exponential losses to follow-up

In the presence of an accrual period, `stpower exponential` performs computations assuming uniform accrual over the period of time R, specified in `aperiod()`. The assumption of uniform accrual may be relaxed by requesting a truncated exponential accrual over the interval 0 to R with shape γ as specified in `ashape(#)`. If the estimate of the shape parameter γ is unavailable, an alternative is to specify the proportion of subjects, $G(t^*)$, expected to be recruited by a fixed time t^* (or by a proportion of the accrual period R, t^*/R) in options `aprob()` and `atime()` (or `aptime()`), respectively. This information is used to find the corresponding γ using

$$G(t^*) = \{1 - \exp(-\gamma t^*)\}/\{1 - \exp(-\gamma R)\}$$

Also see *Methods and Formulas*.

▷ Example 6: Truncated exponential entry distribution

Continuing example 5, we investigate the influence of nonuniform accrual on the estimate of the sample size for a study with a 3-year accrual and a 2-year follow-up. Suppose that the recruitment of subjects to the study is slow for most of the accrual period and increases rapidly toward the end of the recruitment. Consider an extreme case of such an accrual corresponding to a shape parameter -6. The graph of uniform and truncated exponential with shape -6 entry distributions over $[0, 3]$ is given below.

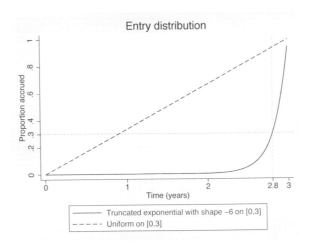

From the above graph, the accrual of subjects is extremely slow during most of the recruitment period, with 70% of subjects being recruited within the last few months of a 3-year accrual period. More precisely, according to the graph, 30% of subjects are expected to be recruited after 2.8 years.

To obtain the estimate of the sample size for this study, we type

```
. stpower exponential 0.3 0.2, power(0.9) onesided aperiod(3) fperiod(2) ashape(-6)
Note: input parameters are hazard rates.

Estimated sample sizes for two-sample comparison of survivor functions
Exponential test, hazard difference, conditional
Ho: h2-h1 = 0

Input parameters:
        alpha =    0.0500  (one sided)
           h1 =    0.3000
           h2 =    0.2000
        h2-h1 =   -0.1000
        power =    0.9000
           p1 =    0.5000

Accrual and follow-up information:
     duration =    5.0000
    follow-up =    2.0000
      accrual =    3.0000  (exponential)
   accrued(%) =      50.00 (by time t*)
           t* =    2.8845  (96.15% of accrual)

Estimated sample sizes:
            N =       516
           N1 =       258
           N2 =       258
```

and conclude that 516 subjects have to be recruited to this study. This sample size ensures 90% power of a one-sided 0.05 level test to detect a reduction in hazard from 0.3 to 0.2 when the accrual of subjects follows the considered truncated exponential distribution. For this extreme case of a negative truncated exponential entry distribution (the concave entry distribution), the estimate of the sample 516 increases significantly compared with an estimate of 378 for a uniform entry distribution. On the other hand, a truncated exponential distribution with positive values of the shape parameter (convex entry distribution) will reduce the requirement for the sample size when compared with uniform accrual.

Suppose that we do not know (or do not wish to guess) the value of the shape parameter. The only information available to us from the above graph is that 30% of subjects are expected to be recruited after 2.8 years (or, equivalently, 50% of subjects are expected to be recruited by 96.15% of the accrual period from the previous output). We submit this information in options aprob() and atime() or aprob() and aptime() as shown below and obtain the same estimate of the sample size 516.

```
. stpower exponential 0.3 0.2, power(0.9) onesided aperiod(3) fperiod(2) aprob(0.3)
> atime(2.8)
Note: input parameters are hazard rates.

Estimated sample sizes for two-sample comparison of survivor functions
Exponential test, hazard difference, conditional
Ho: h2-h1 = 0

Input parameters:
           alpha =      0.0500   (one sided)
              h1 =      0.3000
              h2 =      0.2000
           h2-h1 =     -0.1000
           power =      0.9000
              p1 =      0.5000

 Accrual and follow-up information:
        duration =      5.0000
       follow-up =      2.0000
         accrual =      3.0000   (exponential)
      accrued(%) =        30.00  (by time t*)
              t* =      2.8000   (93.33% of accrual)

 Estimated sample sizes:
               N =         516
              N1 =         258
              N2 =         258
```

or, equivalently,

```
. stpower exponential 0.3 0.2, power(0.9) onesided aperiod(3) fperiod(2) aptime(0.9615)
```
  (*output omitted*)

Since 50% is the default value of `aprob()`, we omit this option in the above.

◁

Apart from administrative censoring, subjects may not experience an event by the end of the study because of being lost to follow-up for various reasons. See *Theory and terminology* in [ST] **stpower** and [ST] **glossary** for a more detailed description. Rubinstein, Gail, and Santner (1981) and Lachin and Foulkes (1986) extend sample-size and power computations to take into account exponentially distributed losses to follow-up. In addition to being exponentially distributed, losses to follow-up are assumed to be independent of the survival times.

▷ Example 7: Exponential losses to follow-up

Suppose that in example 5, in the study with a 3-year uniform accrual and a 2-year follow-up, yearly loss hazards in the control and the experimental groups are 0.2. Groups may have different loss hazards, which can be specified in `losshaz()`.

(*Continued on next page*)

```
. stpower exponential 0.3 0.2, power(0.9) onesided aperiod(3) fperiod(2)
> losshaz(0.2 0.2) detail
Note: input parameters are hazard rates.

Estimated sample sizes for two-sample comparison of survivor functions
Exponential test, hazard difference, conditional
Ho: h2-h1 = 0

Input parameters:
          alpha =    0.0500  (one sided)
             h1 =    0.3000
             h2 =    0.2000
          h2-h1 =   -0.1000
          power =    0.9000
             p1 =    0.5000

Accrual and follow-up information:
       duration =    5.0000
      follow-up =    2.0000
        accrual =    3.0000  (uniform)
            lh1 =    0.2000
            lh2 =    0.2000

Estimated sample sizes:
              N =       500
             N1 =       250
             N2 =       250

Estimated expected number of events:
         E|Ha =       213      E|Ho =       216
        E1|Ha =       121     E1|Ho =       108
        E2|Ha =        92     E2|Ho =       108

Estimated expected number of losses to follow-up:
         L|Ha =       173      L|Ho =       172
        L1|Ha =        81     L1|Ho =        86
        L2|Ha =        92     L2|Ho =        86
```

The sample size required for a one-sided 0.05-level test to detect a reduction in hazard from 0.3 to 0.2 with 90% power increases from 378 (see example 5) to 500. We observe that for the extreme case of losses to follow-up, sample size increases significantly. A conservative adjustment commonly applied in practice is $N(1 + p_L)$, where p_L is the expected proportion of losses to follow-up in both groups combined. For this example, p_L may be computed as $0.5(0.369+0.324) \approx 0.35$ from table 2 of Lachin and Foulkes (1986). Then the conservative estimate of the sample size is $378(1+0.35) = 510$, which is slightly greater than 500, the actual required sample size.

We also requested that additional information about the expected number of events and losses to follow-up under the null and under the alternative hypothesis be displayed by using option detail. From the above output, a total of 173 subjects (81 from the control and 92 from the experimental groups) are expected to be lost in the study with exponentially distributed losses with yearly rates 0.2 in each group under the alternative hypothesis.

If the proportion of subjects lost to follow-up by a fixed period in each group is available rather than loss to follow-up rates, it can also be supplied by using options lossprob() and losstime(). For example, in the above study approximately 33%, $1 - \exp(-0.2 \times 2) \approx 0.33$, of subjects in each group are lost at time 2 (years). We can obtain the same estimates of sample sizes with

```
. stpower exponential 0.3 0.2, power(0.9) onesided aperiod(3) fperiod(2)
> lossprob(0.33 0.33) losstime(2)
```

  (*output omitted*)

◁

The conditional versus unconditional approaches

Denote ψ to be the effect size, and $\widehat{\lambda}_1$ and $\widehat{\lambda}_2$ to be the maximum likelihood estimates of the respective hazard-rate parameters. Consider the two effect-size estimators based on the difference between the hazard rates, $\widehat{\lambda}_2 - \widehat{\lambda}_1$, and based on the log of the hazard ratio, $\ln(\widehat{\lambda}_2/\widehat{\lambda}_1)$. Both estimators are asymptotically normal under the null and under the alternative hypothesis.

We adopt Chow, Shao, and Wang (2003, 171) terminology when referring to the conditional and unconditional tests. The *conditional test* is the test that uses the constraint $\lambda_2 = \lambda_1$ (conditional on H_o) when computing the variance of the effect-size estimator under the null. The *unconditional test* is the test that does not use the above constraint when computing the variance of the effect-size estimator under the null. The score and the Wald tests are each one of the examples of conditional and unconditional tests, respectively. Chow, Shao, and Wang (2003) note that neither of the two tests (conditional or unconditional) is always more powerful than the other under the alternative hypothesis. Therefore, there is no definite recommendation of which one is preferable to be used in practice.

The *conditional approach* relies on the following relationship between sample size and power (given in Lachin 1981) to compute estimates of required sample size or power,

$$|\psi| = z_{1-\alpha}\left\{\mathrm{Var}(\psi, H_o)\right\}^{1/2} + z_{1-\beta}\left\{\mathrm{Var}(\psi, H_a)\right\}^{1/2}$$

where $z_{1-\alpha}$ and $z_{1-\beta}$ are the $(1-\alpha)$th and the $(1-\beta)$th quantiles of the standard normal distribution, and $\mathrm{Var}(\psi, H_o)$ and $\mathrm{Var}(\psi, H_a)$ are the asymptotic variances under the null and under the alternative, respectively, of the effect-size estimator, $\widehat{\psi}$. This approach uses the variance of the estimator conditional on the hypothesis type.

The *unconditional approach* replace $\mathrm{Var}(\psi, H_o)$ with $\mathrm{Var}(\psi, H_a)$ in the above and uses the variance under the alternative to compute the estimates of sample size and power:

$$|\psi| = (z_{1-\alpha} + z_{1-\beta})\left\{\mathrm{Var}(\psi, H_a)\right\}^{1/2}$$

Therefore, the resulting formulas based on the two approaches are different.

Lakatos and Lan (1992) formulate the sample-size formula for the test of the log of the hazard ratio based on the method of Rubinstein, Gail, and Santner (1981). This formula is based on the unconditional approach. Lachin and Foulkes (1986) provide the sample-size formula for the test of the log of the hazard ratio that uses the conditional approach. They also present both conditional and unconditional versions of formulas for the test based on the difference between hazards. As noted by Lachin and Foulkes (1986), sample sizes estimated based on the unconditional approach will be larger than the estimates based on the conditional approach for equal-sized groups.

Both approaches are available with `stpower exponential`; the conditional is the default and the unconditional may be requested by specifying option `unconditional`. Refer to *Methods and Formulas* for the formulas underlying these approaches.

◁

▷ Example 6: Sample size using the Rubinstein–Gail–Santner method

Consider the following scenario in Lakatos and Lan (1992, table I). A 10-year survival study with a 1-year accrual period and a 9-year follow-up is conducted to compare the survivor functions of the two groups by using a two-sided 0.05 exponential test based on the log of the hazard ratio. The probability of surviving to the end of a study for subjects in the control group is 0.8 ($S_1(t) = 0.8$, $t = 10$).

Subjects are recruited uniformly over the interval $[0, 1]$. Lakatos and Lan (1992) report an estimate of 664 for the sample size required to detect a change in the hazard of the experimental group corresponding to the hazard ratio $\Delta = 0.5$ with 90% power by using the Rubinstein–Gail–Santner method. To obtain the estimates according to this method, we need to specify both loghazard and unconditional.

```
. stpower exponential 0.8, t(10) power(0.9) aperiod(1) fperiod(9) loghazard
> unconditional
Note: input parameters are survival probabilities.

Estimated sample sizes for two-sample comparison of survivor functions
Exponential test, log-hazard difference, unconditional
Ho: ln(h2/h1) = 0

Input parameters:
            alpha =     0.0500   (two sided)
               s1 =     0.8000
               s2 =     0.8944
                t =    10.0000
        ln(h2/h1) =    -0.6931
            power =     0.9000
               p1 =     0.5000

Accrual and follow-up information:
         duration =    10.0000
        follow-up =     9.0000
           accrual =     1.0000   (uniform)

Estimated sample sizes:
                N =        664
               N1 =        332
               N2 =        332
```

◁

Since the default value of the hazard ratio is 0.5, we omit option hratio(0.5) in the above. From the output, we obtain the same estimate of 664 of the sample size as reported in Lakatos and Lan (1992).

❏ Technical Note

In the absence of censoring, the estimates of the sample size or power based on the test of log of the hazard ratio are the same for the conditional and the unconditional approaches. For example, both

```
. stpower exponential 0.8, t(10) power(0.9) loghazard
  (output omitted )
```

and

```
. stpower exponential 0.8, t(10) power(0.9) loghazard unconditional
  (output omitted )
```

produce the same estimate of the sample size (88). The asymptotic variance of maximum likelihood estimates of the log of the hazard ratio does not depend on hazard rates when there is no censoring and therefore does not depend on the type of hypothesis, $\mathrm{Var}(\widehat{\psi}, H_o) = \mathrm{Var}(\widehat{\psi}, H_a) = 2/N$.

❏

Although all the above examples demonstrated sample-size computation for equal-sized groups, unequal allocation may be taken into account by using option p1() or nratio().

Link to the sample-size and power computation for the log-rank test

▷ Example 7: Sample size using the Freedman and the Schoenfeld methods

Continuing examples 3 and 4, Lachin (1981, 106) gives another approximation to obtain the estimate of the sample size under the equal-group allocation. This approximation coincides with the formula derived by Freedman (1982) for the number of events in the context of the log-rank test. We can obtain such an estimate by using `stpower logrank` and by specifying the hazard ratio computed earlier of 0.66667:

```
. stpower logrank, hratio(0.66667) power(0.9) onesided

Estimated sample sizes for two-sample comparison of survivor functions
Log-rank test, Freedman method
Ho: S1(t) = S2(t)

Input parameters:
        alpha =    0.0500  (one sided)
        hratio =    0.6667
        power =    0.9000
            p1 =    0.5000
Estimated number of events and sample sizes:
            E =         216
            N =         216
           N1 =         108
           N2 =         108
```

The estimate, 216, of the sample size is the same as given in Lachin (1981, 107) and is slightly smaller than the estimate, 218, obtained in example 3, and larger than 210, obtained using the George–Desu method in example 4.

The approximation due to George and Desu (1974) is the same as the approximation to the number of events derived by Schoenfeld (1981) in application to the log-rank test. We can confirm that by using

```
. stpower logrank, hratio(0.66667) power(0.9) onesided schoenfeld
  (output omitted)
```

and obtain the same estimate of 210 as using `stpower exponential` with option `loghazard` in example 4.

◁

Power determination

Power determination may be requested by specifying option `n()`. We verify the power computation for the study from example 6. We expect the power estimate to be close to 0.9.

▷ Example 8: Power determination

The only thing we change in the syntax of `stpower exponential` from example 6 is replacing option `power(0.9)` with option `n(664)`:

```
. stpower exponential 0.8, t(10) n(664) aperiod(1) fperiod(9) loghazard unconditional
Note: input parameters are survival probabilities.

Estimated power for two-sample comparison of survivor functions
Exponential test, log-hazard difference, unconditional
Ho: ln(h2/h1) = 0

Input parameters:
            alpha =    0.0500   (two sided)
               s1 =    0.8000
               s2 =    0.8944
                t =   10.0000
        ln(h2/h1) =   -0.6931
                N =        664
               p1 =    0.5000

Accrual and follow-up information:
         duration =   10.0000
        follow-up =    9.0000
          accrual =    1.0000   (uniform)

Estimated power:
            power =    0.9000
```

and obtain the estimate of power 0.9.

◁

For examples of how such information may be used to construct power curves, see [ST] **stpower** and example 7 in *Power and effect-size determination* of [ST] **stpower logrank**.

▷ Example 9: Using streg to perform the log hazard-ratio test

In this example we demonstrate the importance of sample-size computations to ensure a high power of a test to detect a difference between exponential survivor functions. We consider an asymptotic Wald (or normal z test) test to test the equality of the log of the hazard ratio to zero.

Continuing example 8, suppose that the investigators have only 100 subjects available for the study. As we see below, the power to detect a 50% risk reduction (the hazard ratio of 0.5) of the experimental group reduces from 90% to 24%:

```
. stpower exponential 0.8, t(10) n(100) aperiod(1) fperiod(9) loghazard unconditional
Note: input parameters are survival probabilities.

Estimated power for two-sample comparison of survivor functions
Exponential test, log-hazard difference, unconditional
Ho: ln(h2/h1) = 0

Input parameters:
            alpha =    0.0500   (two sided)
               s1 =    0.8000
               s2 =    0.8944
                t =   10.0000
        ln(h2/h1) =   -0.6931
                N =        100
               p1 =    0.5000

Accrual and follow-up information:
         duration =   10.0000
        follow-up =    9.0000
          accrual =    1.0000   (uniform)

Estimated power:
            power =    0.2414
```

To demonstrate the implication of this reduction, consider the following example. We generate the data according to the study from example 8 with the following code.

```
program simdata
        args n h1 h2 R
        set obs 'n'
        generate double entry = 'R'*uniform()
        generate double u = uniform()
        /* random allocation to two groups of equal sizes */
        generate double u1 = uniform()
        generate double u2 = uniform()
        sort u1 u2, stable
        generate byte drug = (_n<='n'/2)
        /* exponential failure times with rates h1 and h2 */
        generate double failtime = entry - ln(1-u)/'h1' if drug==0
        replace failtime = entry - ln(1-u)/'h2' if drug==1
end

. clear

. set seed 234

. quietly simdata 100 0.0223 0.0112 1
```

The entry times of subjects are generated from a uniform $[0, 1)$ distribution and stored in variable entry. The subjects are randomized to two groups of equal size of 50 subjects each. The survival times are generated from exponential distribution with the hazard rate of $-\ln(0.8)/10 = 0.0223$ in the control group, drug $= 0$, and the hazard rate of $0.5 \times 0.0223 = 0.0112$ in the experimental group, drug $= 1$, conditional on subjects' entry times in entry.

Before analyzing these survival data, we need to set it up properly using stset. The failure-time variable is failtime. The study terminates at $t = 10$, so we use exit(time 10) with stset to specify that all failure times past 10 are to be treated as censored. Since subjects enter the study at random times (entry) and become at risk of a failure upon entering the study, we also specify option origin(entry) to ensure that the analysis time is adjusted for the entry times. For more details, see [ST] **stset**.

```
. stset failtime, exit(time 10) origin(entry)

     failure event:  (assumed to fail at time=failtime)
obs. time interval:  (origin, failtime]
 exit on or before:  time 10
     t for analysis:  (time-origin)
             origin:  time entry

    100  total obs.
      0  exclusions

    100  obs. remaining, representing
     15  failures in single record/single failure data
891.5574  total analysis time at risk, at risk from t =          0
                             earliest observed entry t =          0
                                 last observed exit t =    9.99908
```

To perform the log hazard-ratio test, we fit an exponential regression model on drug by using streg (see [ST] **streg**). We can express the log of the hazard ratio in terms of regression coefficients as follows: $\ln(\Delta) = \ln(\lambda_2/\lambda_1) = \ln\{\exp(\beta_0 + \beta_1)/\exp(\beta_0)\} = \beta_1$, where β_0 and β_1 are the estimated coefficients for the constant and drug in the regression model. Then the test of H_o: $\ln(\Delta) = 0$ may be rewritten in terms of a coefficient on drug as H_o: $\beta_1 = 0$. This test is part of the standard output after streg.

```
. streg drug, distribution(exponential) nohr
         failure _d:  1 (meaning all fail)
   analysis time _t:  (failtime-origin)
             origin:  time entry
   exit on or before:  time 10
Iteration 0:   log likelihood = -54.114272
Iteration 1:   log likelihood = -53.090859
Iteration 2:   log likelihood = -53.053454
Iteration 3:   log likelihood = -53.053406
Iteration 4:   log likelihood = -53.053406
Exponential regression -- log relative-hazard form
No. of subjects =          100               Number of obs   =        100
No. of failures =           15
Time at risk    =  891.5574257
                                             LR chi2(1)      =       2.12
Log likelihood  =   -53.053406              Prob > chi2     =     0.1452
```

_t	Coef.	Std. Err.	z	P>|z|	[95% Conf. Interval]
drug	-.7729235	.5477226	-1.41	0.158	-1.84644 .300593
_cons	-3.756554	.3162278	-11.88	0.000	-4.376349 -3.136759

From the output table above, the *p*-value for a two-sided test of the coefficient for drug, 0.158, is greater than 0.05. On that basis, we do not have evidence to reject the null hypothesis of no difference between the two exponential survivor functions and therefore make an incorrect decision since we simulated the data with different group hazard rates. If we were to repeat this, say, 100 times, using different datasets simulated according to the alternative H_a: $\ln(\Delta) = \ln(0.5) = -0.6931$ (see [R] **simulate**), for roughly 76 of them we would have failed to reject the null hypothesis of no difference (a type II error). Therefore, more subjects are required to be able to detect the log of the hazard ratio of -0.4055 in this study.

◁

▷ **Example 10: Using results from streg to perform the Wald test of hazard difference**

We obtain the power of the test based on the difference between hazards for the study in the above example (omit option loghazard from the previous syntax).

```
. stpower exponential 0.8, t(10) n(100) aperiod(1) fperiod(9) unconditional
Note: input parameters are survival probabilities.

Estimated power for two-sample comparison of survivor functions
Exponential test, hazard difference, unconditional
Ho: h2-h1 = 0

Input parameters:
        alpha =    0.0500   (two sided)
           s1 =    0.8000
           s2 =    0.8944
            t =   10.0000
        h2-h1 =   -0.0112
            N =        100
           p1 =    0.5000
 Accrual and follow-up information:
     duration =   10.0000
    follow-up =    9.0000
       accrual =    1.0000   (uniform)
Estimated power:
        power =    0.2458
```

We obtain a power estimate of 0.2458, which is close to 0.2414 from example 9.

To test the difference between hazard rates by using the Wald test, we express this difference in terms of coefficients, $\lambda_2 - \lambda_1 = \exp(\beta_0)\{\exp(\beta_1) - 1\}$, and use `testnl` ([R] **testnl**) after `streg` to perform the nonlinear hypothesis test of H_o: $\exp(\beta_0)\{\exp(\beta_1) - 1\} = 0$.

```
. testnl exp(_b[_cons])*(exp(_b[drug])-1) = 0

 (1)  exp(_b[_cons])*(exp(_b[drug])-1) = 0

              chi2(1) =        2.03
          Prob > chi2 =      0.1540
```

We obtain the same conclusions from the Wald test based on the difference between hazards as in example 9. That is, based on the p-value of 0.1540 we fail to reject the null hypothesis of no difference between hazards of two groups (or miss the alternative H_a: $\delta = -0.0112$ corresponding to reduction in hazard from roughly 0.02 to 0.01) for the data from example 9.

◁

❏ Technical Note

Often in practice, to test the disparity in two exponential survivor functions the log-rank test is used instead of the hazard-difference test. Also, the Wald (or the score) test from the Cox model is used instead of the exponential log hazard-ratio test. Refer to [ST] **sts test** and [ST] **stcox** for examples on how to perform these tests (also see [ST] **stpower logrank** and [ST] **stpower cox**).

❏

❏ Technical Note

Sometimes the estimates of sample size and power obtained under the assumption of the exponential model are used as an approximation to the results used in a more general context of the log-rank test or the Cox proportional hazards model. Refer to Lachin (2000, 409–410) for the rationale behind this. Also see Lakatos and Lan (1992) for a discussion of the circumstances under which sample-size estimates obtained assuming the exponential model may be inaccurate when used with more general proportional hazards models.

❏

Saved Results

`stpower exponential` saves the following in `r()`:

Scalars

r(power)	power of test
r(alpha)	significance level of test
r(hratio)	hazard ratio
r(onesided)	1 if one-sided test, 0 otherwise
r(h1)	hazard in the control group (if specified)
r(h2)	hazard in the experimental group
r(t)	reference survival time (if t() is specified)
r(p1)	proportion of subjects in the control group
r(fperiod)	length of the follow-up period (if specified)
r(aperiod)	length of the accrual period (if specified)
r(ashape)	shape parameter (if aperiod() is specified)
r(lh1)	loss hazard in the control group (if specified)
r(lh2)	loss hazard in the experimental group (if specified)
r(lt)	reference loss to follow-up time (if losstime() is specified)

Macros
    r(method)   type of method (hazard difference or log-hazard difference)
    r(accrual)   type of entry distribution (uniform or exponential) (if requested)
    r(type)   type of approach (conditional or unconditional)

Matrices
    r(N) 1×3 matrix of required sample sizes
    r(Pr) 1×4 matrix of probabilities of an event (when computed)
    r(Ea) 1×3 matrix of expected number of events under the alternative (when computed)
    r(Eo) 1×3 matrix of expected number of events under the null (when computed)
    r(La) 1×3 matrix of expected number of losses under the alternative (when computed)
    r(Lo) 1×3 matrix of expected number of losses under the null (when computed)

Methods and Formulas

stpower exponential is implemented as an ado-file.

In addition to the notation given in *Introduction*, denote N, N_1, and N_2 to be the total number of subjects required for the study, the number of subjects in the control group, and the number of subjects in the experimental group, respectively. Let $p_1 = N_1/N$ and $p_2 = N_2/N = 1 - p_1$ be the proportions of subjects allocated to the control and the experimental groups; γ be the shape parameter of the truncated exponential distribution with p.d.f. $g(z) = \gamma \exp(-\gamma z)/\{1 - \exp(-\gamma R)\}$, $0 \leq z \leq R$, $\gamma \neq 0$; η_1 and η_2 be the loss hazards in the control and the experimental groups; and $z_{(1-\alpha/k)}$ and $z_{(1-\beta)}$ be the $(1 - \alpha/k)$th and the $(1 - \beta)$th quantiles of the standard normal distribution, with $k = 1$ for the one-sided test and $k = 2$ for the two-sided test. Denote $\overline{\lambda} = p_1 \lambda_1 + p_2 \lambda_2$. Recall that the difference between hazards is denoted by $\delta = \lambda_2 - \lambda_1$ and the hazard ratio is denoted by $\Delta = \lambda_2/\lambda_1$.

If survival probabilities $S_1(t)$ and $S_2(t)$ at a fixed time t are specified rather than hazard rates, the hazard rates are computed as $\lambda_i = -\ln\{S_i(t)\}/t$, $i = 1, 2$. If loss to follow-up probabilities $L_1(t)$ and $L_2(t)$ at a fixed time t are given instead of loss to follow-up hazard rates, the loss hazard rates are computed as $\eta_i = -\ln\{1 - L_i(t)\}/t$, $i = 1, 2$.

All formulas below are derived under the assumption of exponential survival distributions with hazard rates in the control and the experimental groups λ_1 and λ_2, respectively, and rely on large-sample properties of the maximum likelihood estimates of λ_1 and λ_2.

Denote $\xi_o = \zeta(\overline{\lambda}, \gamma, \eta_1) p_1^{-1} + \zeta(\overline{\lambda}, \gamma, \eta_2) p_2^{-1}$ and $\xi_a = \zeta(\lambda_1, \gamma, \eta_1) p_1^{-1} + \zeta(\lambda_2, \gamma, \eta_2) p_2^{-1}$.

The formula for the sample-size calculation using the conditional approach is

$$N = \frac{\left(z_{1-\alpha/k} \xi_o^{1/2} + z_{1-\beta} \xi_a^{1/2} \right)^2}{\psi^2}$$

and using the unconditional approach is

$$N = \frac{(z_{1-\alpha/k} + z_{1-\beta})^2 \xi_a}{\psi^2}$$

where $\zeta(\lambda, \gamma, \eta) = \lambda^2/p_E$ if $\psi = \delta$, $\zeta(\lambda, \gamma, \eta) = 1/p_E$ if $\psi = \ln(\Delta)$, and p_E is to be defined later. λ and η denote a failure hazard rate and a loss to follow-up hazard rate.

In the absence of censoring, the overall probability of an event (failure), p_E, is set to 1. Here the resulting formula for the sample size for the log hazard-ratio test depends only on the ratio of hazards and not on the individual group hazard rates. The resulting sample size formula for the test of the difference may also be rewritten as a function of the ratio of hazards only. Therefore, under no censoring, for a fixed value of the hazard ratio $\Delta = \lambda_2/\lambda_1$ the estimates of the sample size (or power) will be constant with respect to varying hazard rates λ_1 and λ_2.

In the presence of censoring, when each subject is followed up for a fixed period $f = T$,

$$p_E = p_E(\lambda, \eta) = \frac{\lambda}{\lambda + \eta}[1 - \exp\{-(\lambda + \eta)T\}]$$

In the presence of an accrual period, the probability of an event is defined as

$$p_E = p_E(\lambda, \eta) = \frac{\lambda}{(\lambda + \eta)}\left[1 - \frac{\exp\{-(\lambda + \eta)(T - R)\} - \exp\{-(\lambda + \eta)T\}}{(\lambda + \eta)R}\right]$$

or

$$p_E = p_E(\lambda, \gamma, \eta) = \frac{\lambda}{(\lambda + \eta)}\left(1 + \frac{\gamma \exp\{-(\lambda + \eta)T\}[1 - \exp\{(\lambda + \eta - \gamma)R\}]}{(\lambda + \eta - \gamma)\{1 - \exp(-\gamma R)\}}\right)$$

under uniform or truncated exponential accrual with shape γ over $[0, R]$, respectively. Uniform accrual is assumed for $|\gamma| < 10^{-6}$.

The formulas are obtained from Lachin (1981), Lachin and Foulkes (1986), and Lakatos and Lan (1992). To avoid division by 0 in the case $\lambda + \eta = \gamma$, the probability of an event is taken to be the limit of the above expression, $p_E = \lim_{\lambda + \eta \to \gamma} p_E(\lambda, \gamma, \eta)$.

The final estimate of the sample size is rounded up to the nearest even integer under the equal-group allocation and rounded up to the nearest integer otherwise. The number of subjects required to be recruited in each group is obtained as $N_1 = \pi_1 N$ and $N_2 = N - N_1$ where N_1 is rounded down to the nearest integer.

The expected number of events and losses to follow-up are computed as suggested by Lachin and Foulkes (1986). Under the null hypothesis

$$E_{H_o} = N_1 p_E(\overline{\lambda}, \gamma, \eta_1) + N_2 p_E(\overline{\lambda}, \gamma, \eta_2)$$
$$L_{H_o} = N_1(\eta_1/\overline{\lambda})p_E(\overline{\lambda}, \gamma, \eta_1) + N_2(\eta_2/\overline{\lambda})p_E(\overline{\lambda}, \gamma, \eta_2)$$

and under the alternative hypothesis

$$E_{H_a} = N_1 p_E(\lambda_1, \gamma, \eta_1) + N_2 p_E(\lambda_2, \gamma, \eta_2)$$
$$L_{H_a} = N_1(\eta_1/\lambda_1)p_E(\lambda_1, \gamma, \eta_1) + N_2(\eta_2/\lambda_2)p_E(\lambda_2, \gamma, \eta_2)$$

For unconditional tests, the expected number of events and losses to follow-up under the null is computed by setting $\overline{\lambda} = \lambda_1$. The estimates of the expected number of events and losses to follow-up in each group are rounded to the nearest integer.

To obtain the estimate of the power, $1 - \beta$, the formulas for the sample size are solved for $z_{(1-\beta)}$ and the normal cumulative distribution function is used to obtain the corresponding probability $1 - \beta$.

To obtain the unknown shape parameter γ of a truncated exponential entry distribution, an iterative procedure is used to solve the equation

$$\pi = G(t^*) = \frac{1 - \exp\left(-\gamma t^*\right)}{1 - \exp\left(-\gamma R\right)}$$

for a given proportion of subjects π recruited at a given time t^* for $t^* \in [0, R]$.

References

Chow, S.-C., J. Shao, and H. Wang. 2003. *Sample Size Calculations in Clinical Research.* New York: Marcel Dekker.

Freedman, L. S. 1982. Tables of the number of patients required in clinical trials using the logrank test. *Statistics in Medicine* 1: 121–129.

George, S. L., and M. M. Desu. 1974. Planning the size and duration of a clinical trial studying the time to some critical event. *Journal of Chronic Diseases* 27: 15–24.

Lachin, J. M. 1981. Introduction to sample size determination and power analysis for clinical trials. *Controlled Clinical Trials* 2: 93–113.

——. 2000. *Biostatistical Methods: The Assessment of Relative Risks.* New York: Wiley.

Lachin, J. M., and M. A. Foulkes. 1986. Evaluation of sample size and power for analysis of survival with allowance for nonuniform patient entry, losses to follow-up, noncompliance, and stratification. *Biometrics* 42: 507–519.

Lakatos, E., and K. K. G. Lan. 1992. A comparison of sample size methods for the logrank statistic. *Statistics in Medicine* 11: 179–191.

Rubinstein, L. V., M. H. Gail, and T. J. Santner. 1981. Planning the duration of a comparative clinical trial with loss to follow-up and a period of continued observation. *Journal of Chronic Diseases* 34: 469–479.

Schoenfeld, D. 1981. The asymptotic properties of nonparametric tests for comparing survival distributions. *Biometrika* 68: 316–319.

Also see [ST] **stpower**.

Also See

[ST] **stpower** — Sample-size, power, and effect-size determination for survival analysis

[ST] **stpower logrank** — Sample size, power, and effect size for the log-rank test

[ST] **stpower cox** — Sample size, power, and effect size for the Cox proportional hazards model

[R] **sampsi** — Sample size and power determination

[ST] **streg** — Fit parametric survival models

[R] **test** — Test linear hypotheses after estimation

[ST] **glossary** — Glossary of terms

Title

> **stpower logrank** — Sample size, power, and effect size for the log-rank test

Syntax

Sample-size determination

> stpower logrank $\left[\, surv_1 \,\left[\, surv_2 \,\right]\,\right]$ $\left[\,,\ options\,\right]$

Power determination

> stpower logrank $\left[\, surv_1 \,\left[\, surv_2 \,\right]\,\right]$, n(*numlist*) $\left[\, options \,\right]$

Effect-size determination

> stpower logrank $\left[\, surv_1 \,\right]$, n(*numlist*) { power(*numlist*) | beta(*numlist*) } $\left[\, options \,\right]$

where

$surv_1$ is the survival probability in the control group at the end of the study t^*;

$surv_2$ is the survival probability in the experimental group at the end of the study t^*.

$surv_1$ and $surv_2$ may each be specified either as one number or as a list of values (see [U] **11.1.8 numlist**) enclosed in parentheses.

options	description
Main	
*alpha(*numlist*)	significance level; default is alpha(0.05)
*power(*numlist*)	power; default is power(0.8)
*beta(*numlist*)	probability of type II error; default is beta(0.2)
*n(*numlist*)	sample size; required to compute power or effect size
*hratio(*numlist*)	hazard ratio (effect size) of the experimental to the control group; default is hratio(0.5)
onesided	one-sided test; default is two sided
*p1(*numlist*)	proportion of subjects in the control group; default is p1(0.5) meaning equal group sizes
*nratio(*numlist*)	ratio of sample sizes, N_2/N_1; default is nratio(1) meaning equal group sizes
schoenfeld	use the formula based on the log hazard ratio in calculations; default is to use the formula based on the hazard ratio
parallel	treat number lists in starred options as parallel (do not enumerate all possible combinations of values) when multiple values per option are specified

Censoring

simpson(# # # | *matname*)	survival probabilities in the control group at three specific time points to compute the probability of an event (failure), using Simpson's rule under uniform accrual
st1(*varname_s varname_t*)	variables *varname_s*, containing survival probabilities in the control group, and *varname_t*, containing respective time points, to compute the probability of an event (failure), using numerical integration under uniform accrual
wdprob(#)	the proportion of subjects anticipated to withdraw from the study; default is wdprob(0)

Reporting

table	display results in a table with default columns
columns(*colnames*)	display results in a table with specified *colnames* columns
notitle	suppress table title
nolegend	suppress table legend
colwidth(# [# ...])	column widths; default is colwidth(9)
separator(#)	draw a horizontal separator line every # lines; default is separator(0) meaning no separator lines
saving(*filename* [, replace])	save the table data to *filename*; use replace to overwrite existing *filename*
†noheader	suppress table header; seldom used
†continue	draw a continuation border in the table output; seldom used

Starred options may be specified either as one number or as a list of values (see [U] **11.1.8 numlist**).

†noheader and continue are not shown in the dialog box.

colnames	description
alpha	significance level
power	power
beta	type II error probability
n	total number of subjects
n1	number of subjects in the control group
n2	number of subjects in the experimental group
e	total number of events (failures)
hr	hazard ratio
loghr	log of the hazard ratio
s1	survival probability in the control group
s2	survival probability in the experimental group
p1	proportion of subjects in the control group
nratio	ratio of sample sizes, experimental to control
w	proportion of withdrawals

By default, the following *colnames* are displayed:

> power, n, n1, n2, e, and alpha are always displayed;
>
> hr is displayed, unless the schoenfeld option is specified, in which case, loghr is displayed;
>
> s1 and s2 if survival probabilities are specified; and
>
> w if withdrawal proportion (wdprob() option) is specified.

Description

stpower logrank estimates required sample size, power, and effect size for survival analysis comparing survivor functions in two groups by using the log-rank test. It also reports the number of events (failures) required to be observed in a study. This command supports two methods to obtain the estimates, those according to Freedman (1982) and Schoenfeld (1981). The command provides options to take into account unequal allocation of subjects between the two groups and possible withdrawal of subjects from the study (loss to follow-up). Optionally, the estimates can be adjusted for uniform accrual of subjects into the study. Also, the minimal effect size (minimal detectable value of the hazard ratio or the log hazard ratio) may be obtained for given power and sample size.

You can use stpower logrank to

1. calculate required number of events and sample size when you know power and effect size (expressed as a hazard ratio) for uncensored and censored survival data,

2. calculate power when you know sample size (number of events) and effect size (expressed as a hazard ratio) for uncensored and censored survival data, and

3. calculate effect size (hazard ratio or log hazard ratio if option schoenfeld is specified) when you know sample size (number of events) and power for uncensored and censored survival data.

stpower logrank's input parameters *surv*$_1$ and *surv*$_2$ are the values of survival probabilities in the control group (or the less favorable of the two groups), s_1, and in the experimental group, s_2, at the end of the study t^*.

Options

> ┌─── Main ───
───

alpha(*numlist*) sets the significance level of the test. The default is alpha(0.05).

power(*numlist*) sets the power of the test. The default is power(0.8). If beta() is specified, this value is set to be 1−beta(). Only one of power() or beta() may be specified.

beta(*numlist*) sets the probability of a type II error of the test. The default is beta(0.2). If power() is specified, this value is set to be 1−power(). Only one of beta() or power() may be specified.

n(*numlist*) specifies the number of subjects in the study to be used to compute the power of the test or the minimal effect size (minimal detectable value of the hazard ratio or log hazard ratio) if power() or beta() is also specified.

hratio(*numlist*) specifies the hazard ratio (effect size) of the experimental group to the control group. The default is hratio(0.5). This value defines the clinically significant improvement of the experimental procedure over the control desired to be detected by the log-rank test, with a certain power specified in power(). If both arguments *surv*$_1$ and *surv*$_2$ are specified, hratio() is not allowed and the hazard ratio is instead computed as $\ln(surv_2)/\ln(surv_1)$.

onesided indicates a one-sided test. The default is two sided.

p1(*numlist*) specifies the proportion of subjects in the control group. The default is p1(0.5), meaning equal allocation of subjects to the control and the experimental groups. Only one of p1() or nratio() may be specified.

nratio(*numlist*) specifies the sample-size ratio of the experimental group relative to the control group, N_2/N_1. The default is nratio(1), meaning equal allocation between the two groups. Only one of nratio() or p1() may be specified.

schoenfeld requests calculations using the formula based on the log hazard ratio, according to Schoenfeld (1981). The default is to use the formula based on the hazard ratio, according to Freedman (1982).

parallel reports results sequentially (in parallel) over the list of numbers supplied to options allowing *numlist*. By default, results are computed over all combinations of the number lists in the following order of nesting: alpha(), p1() or nratio(), list of arguments $surv_1$ and $surv_2$, hratio(), power() or beta(), and n(). This option requires that options with multiple values each contain the same number of elements.

Censoring

simpson(*# # #* | *matname*) specifies survival probabilities in the control group at three specific time points, in order to compute the probability of an event (failure) using Simpson's rule, under the assumption of uniform accrual. Either the actual values or a 1×3 matrix *matname* containing these values can be specified. By default, the probability of an event is approximated as an average of the failure probabilities $1-s_1$ and $1-s_2$; see *Methods and Formulas*. simpson() may not be combined with st1() and may not be used if arguments $surv_1$ or $surv_2$ are specified.

st1(*varname$_s$ varname$_t$*) specifies variables *varname$_s$*, containing survival probabilities in the control group, and *varname$_t$*, containing respective time points, to compute the probability of an event (failure) using numerical integration, under the assumption of uniform accrual; see [R] **dydx**. The minimum and the maximum values of *varname$_t$* must be the length of the follow-up period and the duration of the study, respectively. By default, the probability of an event is approximated as an average of the failure probabilities $1-s_1$ and $1-s_2$; see *Methods and Formulas*. st1() may not be combined with simpson() and may not be used if arguments $surv_1$ or $surv_2$ are specified.

wdprob(*#*) specifies the proportion of subjects anticipated to withdraw from the study. The default is wdprob(0). wdprob() may not be combined with n().

Reporting

table displays results in a tabular format and is implied if any number list contains more than one element. This option is useful if you are producing results one case at a time and wish to construct your own custom table using a forvalues loop.

columns(*colnames*) specifies results in a table with specified *colnames* columns. The order of the columns in the output table is the same as the order of *colnames* specified in columns(). Column names in columns() must be space separated.

notitle prevents the table title from displaying.

nolegend prevents the table legend from displaying and column headers from being marked.

colwidth(*#* [*# ...*]) specifies column widths. The default is 9 for all columns. The number of specified values may not exceed the number of columns in the table. A missing value (.) may be specified for any column to indicate the default width (9). If fewer widths are specified than the number of columns in the table, the last width specified is used for the remaining columns.

separator(#) specifies how often separator lines should be drawn between rows of the table. The default is separator(0), meaning that no separator lines should be displayed.

saving(*filename*[, replace]) creates a Stata data file (.dta file) containing the table values with variable names corresponding to the displayed *colnames*. replace indicates that *filename* be overwritten, if it exists. saving() is only appropriate with tabular output.

The following options are available with stpower logrank but are not shown in the dialog box:

noheader prevents the table header from displaying. This option is useful when the command is issued repeatedly, such as within a loop. noheader implies notitle.

continue draws a continuation border at the bottom of the table. This option is useful when the command is issued repeatedly within a loop.

Remarks

Remarks are presented under the following headings:

Introduction
Computing sample size in the absence of censoring
Computing sample size in the presence of censoring
Withdrawal of subjects from the study
Including information about subject accrual
Power and effect-size determination
Performing the analysis using the log-rank test

Introduction

Consider a survival study comparing the survivor functions in two groups using the log-rank test. Let $S_1(t)$ and $S_2(t)$ denote the survivor functions of the control and the experimental groups, respectively. The key assumption of the log-rank test is that the hazard functions are proportional. That is, $h_2(t) = \Delta h_1(t)$ for any t or, equivalently, $S_2(t) = \{S_1(t)\}^\Delta$, where Δ is the hazard ratio. If $\Delta < 1$, the survival in the experimental group is higher relative to the survival in the control group; the new treatment is superior to the standard treatment. If $\Delta > 1$, then the standard treatment is superior to the new treatment. Under the proportional-hazards assumption, the test of the equality of the two survivor functions H_o: $S_1(t) = S_2(t)$ versus H_a: $S_1(t) \neq S_2(t)$ is equivalent to the test H_o: $\Delta = 1$ versus H_a: $\Delta \neq 1$ or H_o: $\ln(\Delta) = 0$ versus H_a: $\ln(\Delta) \neq 0$.

The methods implemented in stpower logrank for sample-size or power determination relate the power of the log-rank test directly to the number of events observed in the study. Depending on whether censoring occurs in a study, the required number of subjects is either equal to the number of events or is computed using the estimates of the number of events and the combined probability of an event (failure). Thus, in the presence of censoring, in addition to the number of events, the probability of a subject not being censored (failing) needs to be estimated to obtain the final estimate of the required number of subjects in the study.

To determine the required number of events, the investigator must specify the size or significance level α and the clinically significant difference between the two treatments (effect size) to be detected by the log-rank test, H_a: $\Delta = \Delta_a$, with prespecified power, $1 - \beta$. The significance level α represents the probability of a *type I error*, a rejection of the numll hypothesis when it is true. β represents the probability of a *type II error*, a failure to reject the null hypothesis when the alternative hypothesis is true. The significance level is often set to 0.05 and values for power() usually vary from 0.8 to 0.95. By default, stpower logrank uses power(0.8) or, equivalently, beta(0.2), and alpha(0.05).

The effect size, a difference between the two treatments, is usually expressed as a hazard ratio, Δ_a, using option hratio(). Under an unequal allocation of subjects between the two groups, the proportion of subjects in the control group may be specified in p1() or the ratio of sample sizes may be supplied to nratio(). Optionally, results for the one-sided log-rank test may be requested by using onesided.

When all subjects fail by the end of the study (no censoring), a *type I study*, the information above is sufficient to obtain the number of subjects required in the study. Often in practice not all subjects fail by the end of the study, in which case censoring of subjects occurs (a *type II study*). Here the estimates of the survival probabilities in the control and experimental groups are necessary to estimate the probability of an event and, then, the required sample size.

By default, stpower logrank performs computations for the uncensored data (a type I study). It uses the hazard ratio specified in hratio() or the default hazard ratio of 0.5 to obtain required sample size or power. For censored data (a type II study), under administrative censoring, the value of the survival probability in the control group (supplied as argument $surv_1$ or, in the presence of an accrual period, in option simpson() or st1()) must be specified. If the value of the survival probability in the experimental group, $surv_2$, is omitted, $surv_1$ and the value of the hazard ratio in hratio() are used to compute the survival probability in the experimental group, s_2. If both arguments $surv_1$ and $surv_2$ are specified, the hazard ratio, Δ_a, is computed using these values and option hratio() is not allowed.

If power determination is desired, sample size n() must be specified. If both n() and power() (or beta()) are specified, the minimal effect size (minimal value of the hazard ratio or log hazard ratio) that can be detected by the log-rank test with requested power and fixed sample size is computed.

stpower logrank supports two methods, those of Freedman (1982) and Schoenfeld (1981), to obtain the estimates of the number of events or power (see also Marubini and Valsecchi 1997, 127, 134 and Collett 2003, 301, 306). The latter is used if option schoenfeld is specified. The final estimates of the sample size are based on the approximation of the probability of an event due to Freedman (1982), the default, or, for uniform accrual, due to Schoenfeld (1983) (also see Collett 2003) if option simpson() is specified.

Optionally, the results may be displayed in a table by using table or columns() as demonstrated in [ST] **stpower**. Refer to [ST] **stpower** and to example 7 in *Power and effect-size determination* to see how to obtain a graph of a power curve.

Computing sample size in the absence of censoring

We demonstrate several examples of how to use stpower logrank to obtain the estimates of sample size and number of events using Freedman (1982) and Schoenfeld (1981) methods for uncensored data, a type I study (when no censoring of subjects occurs).

▷ Example 1: Number of events (failures)

Consider a survival study to be conducted to compare the survivor function of subjects receiving a treatment (the experimental group) to the survivor function of those receiving a placebo or no treatment (the control group) using the log-rank test. Suppose that the study continues until all subjects fail (no censoring). The investigator wants to know how many events need to be observed in the study to achieve a power of 80% of a two-sided log-rank test with $\alpha = 0.05$, to detect a 50% reduction in the hazard of the experimental group ($\Delta_a = 0.5$). Since the default settings of stpower logrank are power(0.8), alpha(0.05), and hratio(0.5), to obtain the estimate of the required number of events for the above study using the Freedman method (the default), we simply type

```
. stpower logrank
Estimated sample sizes for two-sample comparison of survivor functions
Log-rank test, Freedman method
Ho: S1(t) = S2(t)

Input parameters:
        alpha =    0.0500  (two sided)
       hratio =    0.5000
        power =    0.8000
           p1 =    0.5000
Estimated number of events and sample sizes:
          E =        72
          N =        72
         N1 =        36
         N2 =        36
```

From the output, a total of 72 events (failures) must be observed to achieve the required power of 80%. Since all subjects experience an event by the end of the study, the number of subjects required to be recruited to the study is equal to the number of events. That is, the investigator needs to recruit a total of 72 subjects (36 per group) to the study.

We can request the Schoenfeld method by specifying option schoenfeld:

```
. stpower logrank, schoenfeld
Estimated sample sizes for two-sample comparison of survivor functions
Log-rank test, Schoenfeld method
Ho: S1(t) = S2(t)

Input parameters:
        alpha =    0.0500  (two sided)
   ln(hratio) =   -0.6931
        power =    0.8000
           p1 =    0.5000
Estimated number of events and sample sizes:
          E =        66
          N =        66
         N1 =        33
         N2 =        33
```

We obtain a slightly smaller estimate, 66, of the total number of events.   ◁

❏ Technical Note

Freedman (1982) and Schoenfeld (1981) derive the formulas for the number of events based on the asymptotic distribution of the log-rank test statistic. Freedman (1982) uses the asymptotic mean and variance of the log-rank test statistic expressed as a function of the true hazard ratio Δ, whereas Schoenfeld (1981) (see also Collett 2003, 302) bases the derivation on the asymptotic mean of the log-rank test statistic as a function of the true log hazard ratio $\ln(\Delta)$. We label the corresponding approaches as "Freedman method" and "Schoenfeld method" in the output.

For values of the hazard ratio close to one, the two methods tend to give similar results. In general, the Freedman method gives higher estimates than the Schoenfeld method. The performance of the Freedman method was studied by Lakatos and Lan (1992) and was found to slightly overestimate the sample size under the assumption of proportional hazards. Hsieh (1992) investigates the performance of the two methods under the unequal allocation and concludes that Freedman's formula predicts the highest power for the log-rank test when the sample-size ratio of the two groups equals the reciprocal of the hazard ratio. Schoenfeld's formula predicts highest powers when sample sizes in the two groups are equal.

❏

Computing sample size in the presence of censoring

Because of limited costs and time, it is often infeasible to continue the study until all subjects experience an event. Instead, the study terminates at some prespecified point in time. As a result, some subjects may not experience an event by the end of the study; that is, administrative censoring of subjects occurs. This increases the requirement on the number of subjects in the study to ensure that a certain number of events is observed.

In the presence of censoring (for a type II study) Freedman (1982) assumes the following. The analysis occurs at a fixed time t^* after the last patient was accrued and all information about subject follow-up beyond time t^* is excluded. To minimize an overestimation of the sample size because of neglecting this information, the author suggests choosing t^* as the minimum follow-up time f beyond which the frequency of occurrence of events is low (the time at which, say, 85% of the total events expected are observed). Under this assumption, the number of required subjects does not depend on the rates of accrual and occurrence of events but only on the proportions of patients in the two treatment groups, s_1 and s_2, surviving after the minimum follow-up time f. See *Including information about subject accrual* about how to compute the sample size in the presence of a long accrual.

If censoring of subjects occurs, the probability of a subject not being censored needs to be estimated to obtain an accurate estimate of the required sample size. The assumption above justifies a simple procedure, suggested by Freedman (1982) and used by default by stpower logrank, to compute this probability using the estimates of survival probabilities at the end of the study in the control and the experimental groups. Therefore, for a type II study (under administrative censoring), these probabilities must be supplied to stpower logrank.

There are three ways of providing the information about survival of subjects in two groups. The first way is to supply both survival probabilities as arguments *surv*$_1$ and *surv*$_2$. The second way is to specify the survival probability in the control group as *surv*$_1$ and a hazard ratio in hratio(). Finally, the third way is to supply survival in the control group *surv*$_1$ only and rely on the default hratio(0.5). Below we demonstrate the first way.

▷ Example 2: Sample size in the presence of censoring

Consider an example from Machin et al. (1997, 181) of a study of patients with resectable colon cancer. The goal of the study was to compare the efficacy of the drug levamisole against a placebo with respect to relapse-free survival, using a one-sided log-rank test with a significance level of 5%. The investigators anticipated a 10% increase (from 50% to 60%, with respective hazard ratio of 0.737) in the survival of the experimental group with respect to the survival of the control (placebo) group at the end of the study. They wanted to detect this increase with a power of 80%. To obtain the required sample size, we enter the survival probabilities 0.5 and 0.6 as arguments and specify option onesided to request a one-sided test.

```
. stpower logrank 0.5 0.6, onesided

Estimated sample sizes for two-sample comparison of survivor functions
Log-rank test, Freedman method
Ho: S1(t) = S2(t)

Input parameters:
        alpha =    0.0500  (one sided)
           s1 =    0.5000
           s2 =    0.6000
        hratio =   0.7370
        power =    0.8000
           p1 =    0.5000

Estimated number of events and sample sizes:
          E =         270
          N =         600
         N1 =         300
         N2 =         300
```

From the above output, the investigators would have to observe a total of 270 events (relapses) to detect a 26% decrease in the hazard ($\Delta_a = 0.737$) of the experimental group relative to the hazard of the control group with a power of 80% using a one-sided log-rank test with $\alpha = 0.05$. They would have to recruit a total of 600 patients (300 per group) to observe that many events. In the absence of censoring, only 270 subjects would have been required to detect a decrease in hazard corresponding to $\Delta_a = 0.737$:

```
. stpower logrank, hratio(0.737) onesided

Estimated sample sizes for two-sample comparison of survivor functions
Log-rank test, Freedman method
Ho: S1(t) = S2(t)

Input parameters:
        alpha =    0.0500  (one sided)
        hratio =   0.7370
        power =    0.8000
           p1 =    0.5000

Estimated number of events and sample sizes:
          E =         270
          N =         270
         N1 =         135
         N2 =         135
```

Similarly, using the Schoenfeld method,

```
. stpower logrank 0.5 0.6, onesided schoenfeld
  (output omitted )
```

we find that 590 subjects are required in the study to observe a total of 266 events to ensure a power of a test of 80%.

◁

Although all examples demonstrated above assume equal-group sizes, the information about the unequal allocation of subjects between the two groups may be provided by using p1() or nratio().

(Continued on next page)

Withdrawal of subjects from the study

Under administrative censoring, the subject is known to have experienced either of the two outcomes by the end of the study: survival or failure. Often in practice, subjects may withdraw from the study before it terminates and therefore may not experience an event by the end of the study (or be censored), but for reasons other than administrative. Withdrawal of subjects from a study may greatly affect the estimate of the sample size and must be accounted for in the computations. Refer to [ST] **stpower** and [ST] **glossary** for a formal definition of withdrawal.

Freedman (1982) suggests a conservative adjustment for the estimate of the sample size in the presence of withdrawal. Withdrawal is assumed to be independent of failure (event) times and administrative censoring.

The proportion of subjects anticipated to withdraw from a study may be specified by using wdprob().

▷ Example 3: Withdrawal of subjects from the study

Continuing example 2, suppose that a withdrawal rate of 10% is expected in the study of colon cancer patients. To account for this, we also specify wdprob(0.1):

```
. stpower logrank 0.5 0.6, onesided wdprob(0.1)
Estimated sample sizes for two-sample comparison of survivor functions
Log-rank test, Freedman method
Ho: S1(t) = S2(t)

Input parameters:
          alpha =    0.0500   (one sided)
             s1 =    0.5000
             s2 =    0.6000
         hratio =    0.7370
          power =    0.8000
             p1 =    0.5000
     withdrawal =      10.00%

Estimated number of events and sample sizes:
              E =       270
              N =       666
             N1 =       333
             N2 =       333
```

The estimate of the total sample size using the Freedman method increases from 600 to 666 when the withdrawal rate is assumed to be 10%. The adjustment of the estimate of the sample size for the withdrawal of subjects is conservative. It assumes equal withdrawals from each group; that is, 10% of subjects are lost by the end of the study in each group. This adjustment affects only the estimates of the sample sizes but not the number of events. The reasons for this are the following. Withdrawal is assumed to be independent of event times and the ratio of subjects surviving until the end of the study in the two groups does not change under equal withdrawals.

◁

We could use the alternative syntax and specify the survival probability in the control group, 0.5, with the value of the hazard ratio 0.737 in hratio() instead of supplying the two survival probabilities:

```
. stpower logrank 0.5, hratio(0.737) onesided wdprob(0.1)
```
(output omitted)

Including information about subject accrual

Many clinical studies have an accrual period of R, during which the subjects are recruited to the study and a follow-up period of $f = T - R$, during which the subjects are followed up until the end of the study, T, and no new subjects enter the study. The information about the duration of an accrual and a follow-up periods affects the probability of a subject failing during the study.

Freedman (1982) suggests approximating the combined event-free probability as an average of the survival probabilities in the control and the experimental groups at the minimum follow-up time $t^* = f$ (the default approach used in stpower logrank). However, for a long accrual of subjects, this approach may overestimate the required number of subjects, often seriously, because it does not take into account the information about subject follow-up beyond time f. Here Freedman (1982) proposes to use the survival probabilities at the *average follow-up time*, defined as $t^* = (f + T)/2 = f + 0.5R$, instead of the minimum follow-up time f.

Alternatively, Schoenfeld (1983) (see also Collett 2003, 306) presents a formula for the required number of subjects allowing for uniform entry (accrual, recruitment) over $[0, R]$ and a follow-up period, f. This information is incorporated into the formula for the probability of a failure. The formula involves the integrals of the survivor functions of the control and the experimental groups. Schoenfeld (1983) suggests approximating the integral by using Simpson's rule, which requires the estimates of the survivor function at three specific time points, f, $0.5R + f$, and $T = R + f$. It is sufficient to provide the estimates of these three survival probabilities, $S_1(f)$, $S_1(0.5R + f)$, and $S_1(T)$, for the control group only. The corresponding survival probabilities of the experimental group are automatically computed using the value of the hazard ratio in hratio() and the proportional-hazards assumption.

The three estimates of the survival probabilities of the control group may be supplied by using option simpson() to adjust the estimates of the sample size or power for uniform entry and a follow-up period. If the estimate of the survivor function over an array of values in the range $[f, T]$ is available from a previous study, it can be supplied using option st1() to form a more accurate approximation of the probability of an event using numerical integration (see [R] **dydx**). Here the value of the length of the accrual period is needed for the computation. It is computed as the difference between the maximum and the minimum values of the time variable *varname$_t$*, supplied using st1(), that is $R = T - f = \max(varname_t) - \min(varname_t)$.

▷ Example 4: Sample size in the presence of accrual and follow-up periods

Consider an example described in Collett (2003, 309) of a survival study of chronic active hepatitis. A new treatment is to be compared to a standard treatment with respect to the survival times of the patients with this disease. The investigators desire to detect a change in a hazard ratio of 0.57 with 90% power and a 5% two-sided significance level. Also, subjects are to be entered into the study uniformly over a period of 18 months and then followed up for 24 months. From the Kaplan–Meier estimate of the survivor function available for the control group, the survival probabilities at $f = 24$, $0.5R + f = 33$, and $T = 42$ months are 0.70, 0.57, and 0.45, respectively.

(Continued on next page)

```
. stpower logrank, hratio(0.57) power(0.9) schoenfeld simpson(0.7 0.57 0.45)
Note: probability of an event is computed using Simpson's rule with
      S1(f) = 0.70, S1(f+R/2) = 0.57, S1(T) = 0.45
      S2(f) = 0.82, S2(f+R/2) = 0.73, S2(T) = 0.63

Estimated sample sizes for two-sample comparison of survivor functions
Log-rank test, Schoenfeld method
Ho: S1(t) = S2(t)

Input parameters:

        alpha =    0.0500   (two sided)
   ln(hratio) =   -0.5621
        power =    0.9000
           p1 =    0.5000

Estimated number of events and sample sizes:

          E =          134
          N =          380
         N1 =          190
         N2 =          190
```

Collett (2003, 305) reports the required number of events to be 133 which, apart from roundoff errors, agrees with our estimate of 134. In a later example, Collett (2003, 309) uses the number of events, rounded to 140, to compute the required sample size as $140/0.35 = 400$, where 0.35 is the estimate of the combined probability of an event. By hand, without rounding the number of events, we compute the required sample size as $133/0.35 = 380$ and obtain the same estimate of the total sample size as in the output.

Using the average follow-up time suggested by Freedman (1982), we obtain the following:

```
. stpower logrank 0.57, hratio(0.57) power(0.9) schoenfeld

Estimated sample sizes for two-sample comparison of survivor functions
Log-rank test, Schoenfeld method
Ho: S1(t) = S2(t)

Input parameters:

        alpha =    0.0500   (two sided)
           s1 =    0.5700
           s2 =    0.7259
   ln(hratio) =   -0.5621
        power =    0.9000
           p1 =    0.5000

Estimated number of events and sample sizes:

          E =          134
          N =          378
         N1 =          189
         N2 =          189
```

We specify the survival probability in the control group at $t^* = 0.5R + f = 0.5 \times 18 + 24 = 33$ as $S_1(33) = 0.57$ and the hazard ratio of 0.57 (coincidentally). The respective survival probability in the experimental group is $S_2(33) = S_1(33)^\Delta = 0.57^{0.57} = 0.726$. Here we obtain the estimate, 378, of the sample size, which is close to the estimate of 380 computed using the more complicated approximation. In this example, the two approximations produce similar results, but this may not always be the case.

◁

❏ Technical Note

The approximation suggested by Schoenfeld (1983) and Collett (2003) is considered to be more accurate since it takes into account information about the patient survival beyond the average follow-up time. In general, the Freedman and Schoenfeld approximations will tend to give similar results when $\{\widetilde{S}(f) + \widetilde{S}(T)\}/2 \approx \widetilde{S}(0.5R + f)$; see *Methods and Formulas* for a formal definition of $\widetilde{S}(\cdot)$.

❏

If we use the survival probability in the control group, $S_1(24) = 0.7$, at a follow-up time $t^* = f = 24$ instead of the average follow-up time $t^* = 33$ in the presence of an accrual period,

```
. stpower logrank 0.7, hratio(0.57) power(0.9) schoenfeld
(output omitted )
```

we obtain the estimate of the total sample size of 550, which is significantly greater than the previously estimated sample sizes of 380 and 378.

Power and effect-size determination

Sometimes the number of subjects available for the enrollment into the study is limited. In such cases, the researchers may want to investigate with what power they can detect a desired treatment effect for a given sample size.

▷ Example 5: Using stpower logrank to compute power

Recall the colon cancer study described in example 2. Suppose that only 100 subjects are available to be recruited to the study. We find out how this affects the power to detect a hazard ratio of 0.737.

```
. stpower logrank 0.5, hratio(0.737) onesided n(100)

Estimated power for two-sample comparison of survivor functions
Log-rank test, Freedman method
Ho: S1(t) = S2(t)

Input parameters:

         alpha =    0.0500   (one sided)
            s1 =    0.5000
            s2 =    0.6000
         hratio =   0.7370
             N =       100
            p1 =    0.5000

Estimated number of events and power:

             E =        46
         power =    0.2646
```

The power to detect an alternative H_a: $\Delta = 0.737$ decreased from 0.8 to 0.2646 when the sample size decreased from 600 to 100 (the number of events decreased from 270 to 46).

◁

▷ Example 6: Using stpower logrank to compute effect size

Continuing above example, we can find that the value of the hazard ratio which can be detected for a fixed sample size of 100 with 80% power is approximately 0.42, corresponding to an increase in survival probability from 0.5 to roughly 0.75.

```
. stpower logrank 0.5, n(100) power(0.8) onesided

Estimated hazard ratio for two-sample comparison of survivor functions
Log-rank test, Freedman method
Ho: S1(t) = S2(t)

Input parameters:
        alpha =    0.0500   (one sided)
           s1 =    0.5000
           s2 =    0.7455
            N =       100
        power =    0.8000
           p1 =    0.5000

Estimated number of events and hazard ratio:
            E =        38
        hratio =    0.4237
```

◁

▷ Example 7: Plotting power curves

Here we demonstrate how to produce a graph of power curves over a range of hazard-ratio values. Continuing example 5, we visualize the effect of reducing the sample size from 600 to 100 on a power of the log-rank test to detect a hazard ratio of 0.737 by plotting two power curves for the sample sizes $N = 100$ and $N = 600$.

First, we generate a dataset named `mypower` containing the table values by using the `saving()` option. We request to compute the power for each of the two sample sizes over 100 values of the hazard ratio from 0.01 to 0.99 with 0.01 step size by supplying number lists 100, 600, and 0.01(0.01)0.99 to options `n()` and `hratio()`, respectively. The values of hazard ratios, sample sizes, and powers are saved in variables `hr`, `n`, and `power`, respectively.

```
. quietly stpower logrank 0.5, hratio(0.01(0.01)0.99) n(100 600) onesided saving(mypower)
```

Next we generate the graph:

```
. use mypower

. twoway (line power hr if n==100) (line power hr if n==600) ,
    yline( .8, lstyle(foreground) lwidth(vvthin))
    xline(.42, lstyle(foreground) lwidth(vvthin))
    yline(.26, lstyle(foreground) lwidth(vvthin))
    xline(.74, lstyle(foreground) lwidth(vvthin))
    legend(label(1 "N = 100") label(2 "N = 600"))
    text(.85 .5 "(.42, .8)" .3 .81 "(.74, .26)" .85 .81 "(.74, .8)")
    title("Power curves") note("s1 = .5, alpha = .05 (one sided)")
    xtitle("Hazard ratio") ytitle("Power")
```

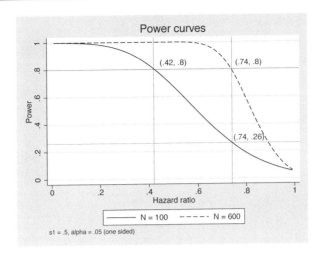

❏ Technical Note

The decrease in sample size reduces the number of events observed in the study and therefore changes the estimates of the power. If the number of events were fixed, power would have been independent of the sample size, provided that all other parameters were held constant, because the formulas relate power directly to the number of events and not the number of subjects.

❏

Examples 5 and 7 demonstrate that a significant reduction in a sample size (a number of events) greatly reduces the power of the log-rank test to detect a desired change in survival of the two groups. Indeed, we examine this further in the next section.

Performing the analysis using the log-rank test

▷ Example 8: Using the log-rank test to detect a change in survival for a fixed sample size

Continuing example 5, consider the generated dataset `drug.dta`, consisting of variables `drug`, a drug type, and `failtime`, a time to failure.

```
. use http://www.stata-press.com/data/r10/drug
(Patient Survival in Drug Trial)
. tabulate drug
```

Treatment type	Freq.	Percent	Cum.
Placebo	50	33.33	33.33
Drug A	50	33.33	66.67
Drug B	50	33.33	100.00
Total	150	100.00	

. by drug, sort: summarize failtime

-> drug = Placebo

Variable	Obs	Mean	Std. Dev.	Min	Max
failtime	50	1.03876	.5535538	.1687701	2.382302

-> drug = Drug A

Variable	Obs	Mean	Std. Dev.	Min	Max
failtime	50	1.191802	.5927507	.2366922	2.277536

-> drug = Drug B

Variable	Obs	Mean	Std. Dev.	Min	Max
failtime	50	1.717314	.8350659	.5511715	3.796102

Failure times of the control group (Placebo) were generated from the Weibull distribution with $\lambda_w = 0.693$ and $p = 2$ (see [ST] **streg**); failure times of the two experimental groups, Drug A and Drug B, were generated from Weibull distributions with hazard functions proportional to the hazard of the control group in ratios 0.737 and 0.42, respectively. The Weibull family of survival distributions is chosen arbitrarily, and the Weibull parameter λ_w is chosen such that the survival at 1 year, $t = 1$, is roughly equal to 0.5. Subjects are randomly allocated to one of the three groups in equal proportions. Subjects with failure times greater than $t = 1$ will be censored at $t = 1$.

Before analyzing these survival data, we need to set it up using stset. After that, we can use sts test, logrank to test the survivor functions separately for Drug A against Placebo and Drug B against Placebo by using the log-rank test. See [ST] **stset** and [ST] **sts test** for more information about these two commands.

. stset failtime, exit(time 1)

```
     failure event:  (assumed to fail at time=failtime)
obs. time interval:  (0, failtime]
 exit on or before:  time 1
```

```
      150  total obs.
        0  exclusions

      150  obs. remaining, representing
       59  failures in single record/single failure data
 128.9845  total analysis time at risk, at risk from t =          0
                              earliest observed entry t =          0
                                  last observed exit t =          1
```

. sts test drug if drug!=2, logrank

```
        failure _d:  1 (meaning all fail)
  analysis time _t:  failtime
 exit on or before:  time 1
```

Log-rank test for equality of survivor functions

drug	Events observed	Events expected
Placebo	25	22.17
Drug A	21	23.83
Total	46	46.00

```
            chi2(1) =     0.70
            Pr>chi2 =     0.4028
```

```
. sts test drug if drug!=1, logrank

        failure _d:  1 (meaning all fail)
  analysis time _t:  failtime
  exit on or before:  time 1
```

Log-rank test for equality of survivor functions

drug	Events observed	Events expected
Placebo	25	16.61
Drug B	13	21.39
Total	38	38.00

$$\text{chi2(1)} = 7.55$$
$$\text{Pr>chi2} = 0.0060$$

From the results from `sts test` for the `Drug A` group, we fail to reject the null hypothesis of no difference between the survivor functions in the two groups; the test made a type II error. On the other hand, for the `Drug B` group the one-sided p-value of 0.003, computed as $0.006/2 = 0.003$, suggests that the null hypothesis of nonsuperiority of the experimental treatment be rejected at the 0.005 significance level. We correctly conclude that the data provide the evidence that `Drug B` is superior to the `Placebo`.

Results from `sts test, logrank` for the two experimental groups agree with findings from examples 5 and 7. For the sample size of 100, the power of the log-rank test to detect the hazard ratio of 0.737 (10% increase in survival) is low (26%), whereas this sample size is sufficient for the test to detect a change in a hazard of 0.42 (25% increase in survival) with approximately 80% power.

Here we simulated our data from the alternative hypothesis and therefore can determine whether the correct decision or a type II error was made by the test. In practice, however, there is no way of determining the accuracy of the decision from the test. All we know is that in a long series of trials there is a 5% chance that a particular test will incorrectly reject the null hypothesis and a 74% and a 20% chance that the test will miss the alternatives $H_a: \Delta = 0.737$ and $H_a: \Delta = 0.42$, respectively. ◁

Saved Results

`stpower logrank` saves the following in `r()`:

Scalars

`r(E)`	total number of events (failures)
`r(power)`	power of test
`r(alpha)`	significance level of test
`r(hratio)`	hazard ratio
`r(onesided)`	type of test (0 if two-sided test, 1 if one-sided test)
`r(s1)`	survival probability in the control group (if specified)
`r(s2)`	survival probability in the experimental group (if specified)
`r(p1)`	proportion of subjects in the control group
`r(w)`	proportion of withdrawals (if specified)
`r(Pr_E)`	probability of an event (failure) (when computed)

Macros

`r(method)`	type of method (Freedman or Schoenfeld)

Matrices

`r(N)`	1×3 matrix of required sample sizes

Methods and Formulas

stpower logrank is implemented as an ado-file.

Let $S_1(t)$ and $S_2(t)$ denote the survivor functions of the control and the experimental groups and $\Delta(t) = \ln\{S_2(t)\}/\ln\{S_1(t)\}$ denote the hazard ratio at time t of the experimental to the control groups. Thus, for a given constant hazard ratio Δ, the survivor function of the experimental group at any time $t > 0$ may be computed as $S_2(t) = \{S_1(t)\}^\Delta$ under the assumption of proportional hazards. Define E and N to be the total number of events and the total number of subjects required for the study; w to be the proportion of subjects withdrawn from the study (lost to follow-up); $z_{(1-\alpha/k)}$ and $z_{(1-\beta)}$ to be the $(1 - \alpha/k)$th and the $(1 - \beta)$th quantiles of the standard normal distribution, with $k = 1$ for the one-sided test and $k = 2$ for the two-sided test. Let λ be the allocation ratio to the experimental group with respect to the control group, i.e., $N_2 = \lambda N_1$. If π_1 is the proportion of subjects allocated to the control group, then $\lambda = (1 - \pi_1)/\pi_1$.

The total number of events required to be observed in a study to ensure a power of $1 - \beta$ of the log-rank test to detect the hazard ratio Δ with significance level α, according to Freedman (1982) is

$$E = \frac{1}{\lambda}(z_{1-\alpha/k} + z_{1-\beta})^2 \left(\frac{\lambda\Delta + 1}{\Delta - 1}\right)^2$$

and according to Schoenfeld (1983) and Collett (2003, 301) is

$$E = \frac{(z_{1-\alpha/k} + z_{1-\beta})^2}{\pi_1(1 - \pi_1)\ln^2(\Delta)} = \frac{1}{\lambda}(z_{1-\alpha/k} + z_{1-\beta})^2 \left\{\frac{1 + \lambda}{\ln(\Delta)}\right\}^2$$

Both formulas are approximations and rely on a set of assumptions such as distinct failure times, all subjects completing the course of the study (no withdrawal), and a constant ratio, λ, of subjects at risk in two groups at each failure time.

The total sample size required to observe the total number of events E is given by

$$N = \frac{E}{p_E}$$

The estimate of the sample size is rounded up to the nearest even integer, for an equal allocation, or rounded up to the nearest integer otherwise. The number of subjects required to be recruited in each group is obtained as $N_1 = \pi_1 N$ and $N_2 = N - N_1$, where N_1 is rounded down to the nearest integer.

By default, the probability of an event (failure), p_E, is approximated as suggested by Freedman (1982):

$$p_E = 1 - \frac{S_1(t^*) + \lambda S_2(t^*)}{1 + \lambda}$$

where t^* is the minimum follow-up time f or, in the presence of an accrual period, the average follow-up time $(f + T)/2 = f + 0.5R$.

If simpson() is specified, the probability of an event is approximated using Simpson's rule as suggested by Schoenfeld (1983):

$$p_E = 1 - \frac{1}{6}\left\{\widetilde{S}(f) + 4\widetilde{S}(0.5R + f) + \widetilde{S}(T)\right\}$$

where $\widetilde{S}(t) = \{S_1(t) + \lambda S_2(t)\}/(1 + \lambda)$ and f, R, and $T = f + R$ are the follow-up period, the accrual period, and the total duration of the study, respectively.

The methods do not incorporate time explicitly but rather use it to determine values of the survival probabilities $S_1(t)$ and $S_2(t)$ used in the computations.

If st1() is used, the integral in the expression for the probability of an event

$$p_{\mathrm{E}} = 1 - \frac{1}{R} \int_f^T \widetilde{S}(t) dt$$

is computed numerically using cubic splines ([R] **dydx**). The value of R is computed as the difference between the maximum and the minimum values of $varname_t$ in st1(), $R = T - f = \max(varname_t) - \min(varname_t)$.

To account for the proportion of subjects, w, withdrawn from the study (lost to follow-up), a conservative adjustment to the total sample size is applied as follows:

$$N_w = \frac{N}{1 - w}$$

Equal withdrawal rates are assumed in the adjustment of the group sample sizes for the withdrawal of subjects. Equal withdrawals do not affect the estimates of the number of events, provided that withdrawal is independent of event times and the ratio of subjects at risk in two groups remains constant at each failure time.

The power for each method is estimated using the formula

$$1 - \beta = \Phi\{|\psi|^{-1}(\lambda N p_{\mathrm{E}})^{1/2} - z_{1-\alpha/k}\}$$

where $\Phi(\cdot)$ is the standard normal cumulative distribution function; $\psi = (\lambda\Delta + 1)/(\Delta - 1)$ or $\psi = (1 + \lambda)/\ln(\Delta)$ if option schoenfeld is specified.

The estimate of the hazard ratio (or log hazard ratio) for fixed power and sample size is computed (iteratively for censoring) using the formulas for the sample size given above. The value of the hazard (log hazard) ratio corresponding to the reduction in a hazard of the experimental group relative to the control group is reported.

References

Collett, D. 2003. *Modelling Survival Data in Medical Research.* 2nd ed. London: Chapman & Hall/CRC.

Freedman, L. S. 1982. Tables of the number of patients required in clinical trials using the logrank test. *Statistics in Medicine* 1: 121–129.

Hsieh, F. Y. 1999. Comparing sample size formulae for trials with unbalanced allocation using the logrank test. *Statistics in Medicine* 11: 1091–1098.

Lakatos, E., and K. K. G. Lan. 1992. A comparison of sample size methods for the logrank statistic. *Statistics in Medicine* 11: 179–191.

Machin, D., M. Campbell, P. Fayers, and A. Pinol. 1997. *Sample Size Tables for Clinical Studies.* 2nd ed. Oxford: Blackwell Science.

Marubini, E., and M. G. Valsecchi. 1997. *Analysing Survival Data from Clinical Trials and Observational Studies.* Chichester, UK: Wiley.

Schoenfeld, D. 1981. The asymptotic properties of nonparametric tests for comparing survival distributions. *Biometrika* 68: 316–319.

——. 1983. Sample-size formula for the proportional-hazards regression model. *Biometrics* 39: 499–503.

Also see [ST] **stpower**.

Also See

[ST] **stpower** — Sample-size, power, and effect-size determination for survival analysis

[ST] **stpower cox** — Sample size, power, and effect size for the Cox proportional hazards model

[ST] **stpower exponential** — Sample size and power for the exponential test

[R] **sampsi** — Sample size and power determination

[ST] **sts test** — Test equality of survivor functions

[ST] **stcox** — Fit Cox proportional hazards model

[R] **test** — Test linear hypotheses after estimation

[ST] **glossary** — Glossary of terms

Title

> **stptime** — Calculate person-time, incidence rates, and SMR

Syntax

> stptime [*if*] [, *options*]

options	description
Main	
at(*numlist*)	compute person-time at specified intervals; default is to compute overall person-time and incidence rates
trim	exclude observations $\leq$ minimum or $>$ maximum of at()
by(*varname*)	compute incidence rates or SMRs by *varname*
Options	
per(#)	units to be used in reported rates
dd(#)	number of decimal digits to be displayed
smr(*groupvar ratevar*)	use *groupvar* and *ratevar* in using() dataset to calculate SMRs
using(*filename*)	specify filename to merge that contains smr() variables
level(#)	set confidence level; default is level(95)
noshow	do not show st setting information
Advanced	
jackknife	jackknife confidence intervals
title(*string*)	label output table with *string*
output(*filename* [, replace])	save summary dataset as *filename*; use replace to overwrite existing *filename*

You must stset your data before using stptime; see [ST] **stset**.

by is allowed; see [D] **by**.

fweights, iweights, and pweights may be specified using stset; see [ST] **stset**.

Description

stptime calculates person-time and incidence rates. stptime computes standardized mortality/morbidity ratios (SMRs) after merging the data with a suitable file of standard rates specified with the using() option.

Options

> **Main**

at(*numlist*) specifies intervals at which person-time is to be computed. The intervals are specified in analysis time t units. If at() is not specified, overall person-time and incidence rates are computed.

If, for example, you specify at(5(5)20) and the trim option is not specified, person-time is reported for the intervals $t = (0 - 5]$, $t = (5 - 10]$, $t = (10 - 15]$, and $t = (15 - 20]$.

trim specifies that observations less than or equal to the minimum or greater than the maximum value listed in at() be excluded from the computations.

by(*varname*) specifies a categorical variable by which incidence rates or SMR are to be computed.

_____| Options |_____

per(#) specifies the units to be used in reported rates. For example, if the analysis time is in years, specifying per(1000) results in rates per 1,000 person-years.

dd(#) specifies the maximum number of decimal digits to be reported for rates, ratios, and confidence intervals. This option affects only how values are displayed, not how they are calculated.

smr(*groupvar ratevar*) specifies two variables in the using() dataset. The *groupvar* identifies the age-group or calendar-period variable used to match the data in memory and the using() dataset. The *ratevar* variable contains the appropriate reference rates. stptime then calculates SMRs rather than incidence rates.

using(*filename*) specifies the filename that contains a file of standard rates that is to be merged with the data so that SMR can be calculated.

level(#) specifies the confidence level, as a percentage, for confidence intervals. The default is level(95) or as set by set level; see [U] **20.7 Specifying the width of confidence intervals**.

noshow prevents stptime from showing the key st variables. This option is seldom used since most people type stset, show or stset, noshow to set whether they want to see these variables mentioned at the top of the output of every st command; see [ST] **stset**.

_____| Advanced |_____

jackknife specifies that jackknife confidence intervals be produced. This is the default if pweights or iweights were specified when the dataset was stset.

title(*string*) replaces the default "person-time" label on the output table with *string*.

output(*filename*[, replace]) saves a summary dataset in *filename*. The file contains counts of failures and person-time, incidence rates (or SMRs), confidence limits, and categorical variables identifying the time intervals. This dataset could be used for further calculations or simply as input to the table command.

> replace indicates that *filename* be overwritten, if it exists. This option is not shown in the dialog box.

Remarks

stptime computes and tabulates the person-time and incidence rate (formed from the number of failures divided by the person-time). If you use the by() option, this will be calculated by different levels of one or more categorical explanatory variables specified by *varname*. Confidence intervals for the rate are also given. By default, the confidence intervals are calculated using the quadratic approximation to the Poisson log likelihood for the log-rate parameter. However, whenever the Poisson assumption is questionable, such as when pweights or iweights are used, jackknife confidence intervals can also be calculated.

stptime can also calculate and report SMRs if the data have been merged with a suitable file of reference rates.

If pweights or iweights were specified when the dataset was stset, stptime calculates jackknife confidence intervals by default.

The summary dataset can be saved to a file specified with the output() option for further analysis or a more elaborate graphical display.

▷ Example 1

We begin with a simple fictitious example from Clayton and Hills (1993, 42). Thirty subjects were monitored until the development of a particular disease. Here are the data for the first five subjects:

```
. use http://www.stata-press.com/data/r10/stptime
. list in 1/5
```

	id	year	fail
1.	1	19.6	1
2.	2	10.8	1
3.	3	14.1	1
4.	4	3.5	1
5.	5	4.8	1

The id variable identifies the subject, year records the time to failure in years, and fail is the failure indicator, which is one for all 30 subjects in the data. To use stptime, we must first stset the data.

```
. stset year, fail(fail) id(id)
                 id:  id
      failure event:  fail != 0 & fail < .
 obs. time interval:  (year[_n-1], year]
 exit on or before:   failure
```

```
        30  total obs.
         0  exclusions

        30  obs. remaining, representing
        30  subjects
        30  failures in single failure-per-subject data
     261.9  total analysis time at risk, at risk from t =          0
                            earliest observed entry t =           0
                               last observed exit t =          36.5
```

We can use stptime to obtain the overall person-time of observation and disease incidence rate.

```
. stptime, title(person-years)
         failure _d:  fail
    analysis time _t:  year
                 id:  id
```

Cohort	person-years	failures	rate	[95% Conf. Interval]	
total	261.9	30	.11454754	.08009	.1638299

The total 261.9 person-years reported by stptime matches what stset reported as total analysis time at risk. stptime computed an incidence rate of .11454754 per person-year. In epidemiology, incidence rates are often presented per 1,000 person-years. We can do this by specifying per(1000).

```
. stptime, title(person-years) per(1000)

        failure _d:  fail
  analysis time _t:  year
               id:   id
```

Cohort	person-years	failures	rate	[95% Conf. Interval]	
total	261.9	30	114.54754	80.09001	163.8299

More interesting would be to compare incidence rates at 10-year intervals. We will specify dd(4) to display rates to four decimal places.

```
. stptime,  per(1000) at(0(10)40) dd(4)

        failure _d:  fail
  analysis time _t:  year
               id:   id
```

Cohort	person-time	failures	rate	[95% Conf. Interval]	
(0 - 10]	188.8000	18	95.3390	60.0676	151.3215
(10 - 20]	55.1000	10	181.4882	97.6506	337.3044
(20 - 30]	11.5000	1	86.9565	12.2490	617.3106
> 30	6.5000	1	153.8462	21.6713	1092.1648
total	261.9000	30	114.5475	80.0900	163.8299

◁

▷ Example 2

Using the diet data (Clayton and Hills 1993) described in example 1 of [ST] **stsplit**, we will use stptime to tabulate age-specific person-years and CHD incidence rates. In this dataset, coronary heart disease (CHD) has been coded as fail = 1, 3, or 13.

We first stset the data: failure codes for CHD are specified; origin is set to date of birth, making age the analysis time; and the scale is set to 365.25, so analysis time is measured in years.

```
. use http://www.stata-press.com/data/r10/diet
(Diet data with dates)
. stset dox, origin(time dob) enter(time doe) id(id) scale(365.25)
> fail(fail==1 3 13)

              id:  id
   failure event:  fail == 1 3 13
obs. time interval:  (dox[_n-1], dox]
 enter on or after:  time doe
 exit on or before:  failure
   t for analysis:  (time-origin)/365.25
           origin:  time dob

─────────────────────────────────────────────────────────────

     337   total obs.
       0   exclusions

─────────────────────────────────────────────────────────────

     337   obs. remaining, representing
     337   subjects
      46   failures in single failure-per-subject data
4603.669   total analysis time at risk, at risk from t =         0
                          earliest observed entry t =   30.07529
                            last observed exit t =   69.99863
```

The incidence of CHD per 1,000 person-years can be tabulated in 10-year intervals.

```
. stptime, per(1000) at(40(10)70) trim
        failure _d:  fail == 1 3 13
  analysis time _t:  (dox-origin)/365.25
            origin:  time dob
  enter on or after:  time doe
                id:  id
              note:  _group<=40 trimmed
```

Cohort	person-time	failures	rate	[95% Conf. Interval]	
(40 - 50]	907.00616	6	6.6151701	2.971936	14.72457
(50 - 60]	2107.0418	18	8.5427828	5.382317	13.55906
(60 - 70]	1493.2923	22	14.732548	9.700656	22.37457
total	4507.3402	46	10.205575	7.644246	13.62512

◁

The SMR for a cohort is the ratio of the total number of observed deaths to the number expected from age-specific reference rates. This expected number can be found by multiplying the person-time in each cohort by the reference rate for that cohort. Using the `smr` option to define the cohort variable and reference rate variable in the `using()` dataset, `stptime` calculates SMRs and confidence intervals. You must specify the `per()` option. For example, if the reference rates were per 100,000, you would specify `per(100000)`.

▷ Example 3

In `smrchd.dta`, we have age-specific CHD rates per 1,000 person-years for a reference population. We can merge these data with our current data and use `stptime` to obtain SMRs and confidence intervals.

```
. stptime, smr(ageband rate) using(http://www.stata-press.com/data/r10/smrchd)
> per(1000) at(40(10)70) trim
        failure _d:  fail == 1 3 13
  analysis time _t:  (dox-origin)/365.25
            origin:  time dob
  enter on or after:  time doe
                id:  id
              note:  _group<=40 trimmed
```

Cohort	person-time	observed failures	expected failures	SMR	[95% Conf. Interval]	
(40 - 50]	907.00616	6	5.62344	1.067	.4793445	2.374931
(50 - 60]	2107.0418	18	18.7527	.95986	.6047547	1.52349
(60 - 70]	1493.2923	22	22.8474	.96291	.6340298	1.46239
total	4507.3402	46	47.2235	.97409	.7296205	1.300477

The `stptime` command can also calculate person-time and incidence rates or SMRs by categories of the explanatory variable. In our diet data, the variable `hienergy` is coded 1 if the total energy consumption is more than 2.75 Mcal and 0 otherwise. We want to compute the person-years and incidence rates for these two levels of `hienergy`.

```
. stptime, by(hienergy) per(1000)
        failure _d:  fail == 1 3 13
  analysis time _t:  (dox-origin)/365.25
          origin:  time dob
   enter on or after:  time doe
              id:  id
```

hienergy	person-time	failures	rate	[95% Conf. Interval]	
0	2059.4305	28	13.595992	9.387478	19.69123
1	2544.2382	18	7.0748093	4.457431	11.2291
total	4603.6687	46	9.9920309	7.484296	13.34002

We can also compute the incidence rate for the two levels of `hienergy` and the three previously defined age cohorts:

```
. stptime, by(hienergy) per(1000) at(40(10)70) trim
        failure _d:  fail == 1 3 13
  analysis time _t:  (dox-origin)/365.25
          origin:  time dob
   enter on or after:  time doe
              id:  id
```

hienergy	person-time	failures	rate	[95% Conf. Interval]	
0					
(40 - 50]	346.87474	2	5.76577	1.442006	23.05407
(50 - 60]	979.34018	12	12.253148	6.958681	21.57587
> 60	699.13758	14	20.024671	11.85966	33.81104
1					
(40 - 50]	560.13142	4	7.1411813	2.680213	19.02702
(50 - 60]	1127.7016	6	5.3205566	2.390317	11.84292
> 60	794.15469	8	10.073604	5.037786	20.14327
total	4507.3402	46	10.205575	7.644246	13.62512

or compute the corresponding SMR.

```
. stptime, smr(ageband rate) using(http://www.stata-press.com/data/r10/smrchd)
> by(hienergy) per(1000) at(40(10)70) trim
        failure _d:  fail == 1 3 13
  analysis time _t:  (dox-origin)/365.25
          origin:  time dob
   enter on or after:  time doe
              id:  id
```

hienergy	person-time	observed failures	expected failures	SMR	[95% Conf. Interval]	
0						
(40 - 50]	346.87474	2	2.15062	.9299629	.2325815	3.718399
(50 - 60]	979.34018	12	8.71613	1.376758	.7818743	2.424256
> 60	699.13758	14	10.6968	1.308802	.7751411	2.209872
1						
(40 - 50]	560.13142	4	3.47281	1.151803	.4322924	3.068875
(50 - 60]	1127.7016	6	10.0365	.5978154	.2685749	1.330665
> 60	794.15469	8	12.1506	.6584055	.329267	1.316554
total	4507.3402	46	47.2235	.9740917	.7296205	1.300477

Saved Results

stptime saves the following in r():

Scalars

r(ptime)	person–time
r(failures)	observed failures
r(expected)	expected number of failures
r(smr)	standardized mortality ratio
r(lb)	lower bound for SMR
r(ub)	upper bound for SMR

Methods and Formulas

stptime is implemented as an ado-file.

Reference

Clayton, D. G., and M. Hills. 1993. *Statistical Models in Epidemiology*. Oxford: Oxford University Press.

Also See

[ST] **strate** — Tabulate failure rates and rate ratios

[ST] **stci** — Confidence intervals for means and percentiles of survival time

[ST] **stir** — Report incidence-rate comparison

[ST] **stset** — Declare data to be survival-time data

[ST] **stsplit** — Split and join time-span records

[ST] **epitab** — Tables for epidemiologists

Title

> **strate** — Tabulate failure rates and rate ratios

Syntax

Tabulate failure rates

> strate [*varlist*] [*if*] [*in*] [, *strate_options*]

Calculate rate ratios with the Mantel–Haenszel method

> stmh *varname* [*varlist*] [*if*] [*in*] [, *options*]

Calculate rate ratios with the Mantel–Cox method

> stmc *varname* [*varlist*] [*if*] [*in*] [, *options*]

strate_options	description
Main	
per(*#*)	units to be used in reported rates
smr(*varname*)	use *varname* as reference-rate variable to calculate SMRs
cluster(*varname*)	cluster variable to be used by the jackknife
jackknife	report jackknife confidence intervals
missing	include missing values as extra categories
level(*#*)	set confidence level; default is level(95)
output(*filename*[, replace])	save summary dataset as *filename*; use replace to overwrite existing *filename*
nolist	suppress listed output
graph	graph rates against exposure category
nowhisker	omit confidence intervals from the graph
Plot	
marker_options	change look of markers (color, size, etc.)
marker_label_options	add marker labels; change look or position
cline_options	affect rendition of the plotted points
CI plot	
ciopts(*rspike_options*)	affect rendition of the confidence intervals (whiskers)
Add plots	
addplot(*plot*)	add other plots to the generated graph
Y axis, X axis, Titles, Legend, Overall	
twoway_options	any options other than by() documented in [G] *twoway_options*

options	description
Main	
by(*varlist*)	tabulate rate ratio on *varlist*
<u>compare</u>(*num1*,*den2*)	compare categories of exposure variable
<u>missing</u>	include missing values as extra categories
<u>level</u>(#)	set confidence level; default is level(95)

You must stset your data before using strate, stmh, and stmc; see [ST] **stset**.

by is allowed with stmh and stmc; see [D] **by**.

fweights, iweights, and pweights may be specified using stset; see [ST] **stset**.

Description

strate tabulates rates by one or more categorical variables declared in *varlist*. You can also save an optional summary dataset, which includes event counts and rate denominators, for further analysis or display. The combination of the commands stsplit and strate implements most, if not all, the functions of the special-purpose person-years programs in widespread use in epidemiology. See Clayton and Hills (1993) and [ST] **stsplit**. If your interest is solely in calculating person-years, see [ST] **stptime**.

stmh calculates stratified rate ratios and significance tests by using a Mantel–Haenszel-type method.

stmc calculates rate ratios that are stratified finely by time by using the Mantel–Cox method. The corresponding significance test (the log-rank test) is also calculated.

Both stmh and stmc can estimate the failure rate ratio for two categories of the explanatory variable specified by the first argument of *varlist*. You can define categories to be compared by specifying them with the compare() option. The remaining variables in *varlist* before the comma are categorical variables, which are to be "controlled for" using stratification. Strata are defined by cross-classification of these variables.

You can also use stmh and stmc to carry out trend tests for a metric explanatory variable. Here a one-step Newton approximation to the log-linear Poisson regression coefficient is computed.

Options for strate

> **Main**

per(#) specifies the units to be used in reported rates. For example, if the analysis time is in years, specifying per(1000) results in rates per 1,000 person-years.

smr(*varname*) specifies a reference-rate variable. strate then calculates SMRs rather than rates. This option will usually follow stsplit to separate the follow-up records by age bands and possibly calendar periods.

cluster(*varname*) defines a categorical variable that indicates clusters of data to be used by the jackknife. If the jackknife option is selected and this option is not specified, the cluster variable is taken as the id variable defined in the st data. Specifying cluster() implies jackknife.

jackknife specifies that jackknife confidence intervals be produced. This is the default if weights were specified when the dataset was stset.

missing specifies that missing values of the explanatory variables be treated as extra categories. The default is to exclude such observations.

level(*#*) specifies the confidence level, as a percentage, for confidence intervals. The default is level(95) or as set by set level; see [U] **20.7 Specifying the width of confidence intervals**.

output(*filename*[, replace]) saves a summary dataset in *filename*. The file contains counts of failures and person-time, rates (or SMRs), confidence limits, and all the categorical variables in the *varlist*. This dataset could be used for further calculations or simply as input to the table command.

> replace indicates that *filename* be overwritten, if it exists. This option is not shown in the dialog box.

nolist suppresses the output. This is used only when saving results to a file specified by output().

graph produces a graph of the rate against the numerical code used for the categories of *varname*.

nowhisker omits the confidence intervals from the graph.

___

Plot

marker_options affect the rendition of markers drawn at the plotted points, including their shape, size, color, and outline; see [G] ***marker_options***.

marker_label_options specify if and how the markers are to be labeled; see [G] ***marker_label_options***.

cline_options affect whether lines connect the plotted points and the rendition of those lines; see [G] ***cline_options***.

___

CI plot

ciopts(*rspike_options*) affects the rendition of the confidence intervals (whiskers); see [G] ***rspike_options***.

___

Add plots

addplot(*plot*) provides a way to add other plots to the generated graph; see [G] ***addplot_option***.

___

Y axis, X axis, Titles, Legend, Overall

twoway_options are any of the options documented in [G] ***twoway_options***, excluding by(). These include options for titling the graph (see [G] ***title_options***) and for saving the graph to disk (see [G] ***saving_option***).

Options for stmh and stmc

___

Main

by(*varlist*) specifies categorical variables by which the rate ratio is to be tabulated.

> A separate rate ratio is produced for each category or combination of categories of *varlist*, and a test for unequal rate ratios (effect modification) is displayed.

compare(*num1*,*den2*) specifies the categories of the exposure variable to be compared. The first code defines the numerator categories, and the second defines the denominator categories.

> When compare is absent and there are only two categories, the larger is compared with the smaller; when there are more than two categories, compare analyzes log-linear trend.

missing specifies that missing values of the explanatory variables be treated as extra categories. The default is to exclude such observations.

level(#) specifies the confidence level, as a percentage, for confidence intervals. The default is level(95) or as set by set level; see [U] **20.7 Specifying the width of confidence intervals**.

Remarks

Remarks are presented under the following headings:

Tabulation of rates by using strate
Stratified rate ratios using stmh
Log-linear trend test for metric explanatory variables using stmh
Controlling for age with fine strata by using stmc

Tabulation of rates by using strate

strate tabulates the rate, formed from the number of failures divided by the person-time, by different levels of one or more categorical explanatory variables specified by *varlist*. Confidence intervals for the rate are also given. By default, the confidence intervals are calculated using the quadratic approximation to the Poisson log likelihood for the log-rate parameter. However, whenever the Poisson assumption is questionable, jackknife confidence intervals can also be calculated. The jackknife option also allows for multiple records for the same cluster (usually subject).

strate can also calculate and report SMRs if the data have been merged with a suitable file of reference rates.

You can save the summary dataset saved to a file specified with the output() option for further analysis or more elaborate graphical display.

If weights were specified when the dataset was stset, strate calculates jackknife confidence intervals by default.

▷ Example 1

Using the diet data (Clayton and Hills 1993) described in example 1 of [ST] **stsplit**, we will use strate to tabulate age-specific CHD. In this dataset, coronary heart disease (CHD) has been coded as fail = 1, 3, or 13.

We first stset the data: failure codes for CHD are specified; origin is set to date of birth, making age analysis time; and the scale is set to 365.25, so analysis time is measured in years.

(Continued on next page)

```
. use http://www.stata-press.com/data/r10/diet
(Diet data with dates)

. stset dox, origin(time doe) id(id) scale(365.25) fail(fail==1 3 13)
                id:  id
     failure event:  fail == 1 3 13
obs. time interval:  (dox[_n-1], dox]
 exit on or before:  failure
    t for analysis:  (time-origin)/365.25
            origin:  time doe
```

```
      337  total obs.
        0  exclusions
```

```
      337  obs. remaining, representing
      337  subjects
       46  failures in single failure-per-subject data
 4603.669  total analysis time at risk, at risk from t =          0
                              earliest observed entry t =          0
                                last observed exit t =   20.04107
```

Now we stsplit the data into 10-year age bands.

```
. stsplit ageband, at(40(10)70) after(time=dob) trim
(26 + 0 obs. trimmed due to lower and upper bounds)
(418 observations (episodes) created)
```

stsplit added 418 observations to the dataset in memory and generated a new variable, ageband, which identifies each observation's age group.

The CHD rate per 1,000 person-years can now be tabulated for categories of ageband:

```
. strate ageband, per(1000) graph
        failure _d:  fail == 1 3 13
   analysis time _t:  (dox-origin)/365.25
            origin:  time doe
                id:  id
              note:  ageband<=40 trimmed
```

Estimated rates (per 1000) and lower/upper bounds of 95% confidence intervals
(729 records included in the analysis)

ageband	D	Y	Rate	Lower	Upper
40	6	0.9070	6.6152	2.9719	14.7246
50	18	2.1070	8.5428	5.3823	13.5591
60	22	1.4933	14.7325	9.7007	22.3746

Since we specified the `graph` option, `strate` also generated a plot of the estimated rates and confidence intervals. ◁

The SMR for a cohort is the ratio of the total number of observed deaths to the number expected from age-specific reference rates. This expected number can be found by first expanding on age, using `stsplit`, and then multiplying the person-years in each age band by the reference rate for that band. `merge` (see [D] **merge**) can be used to add the reference rates to the dataset. Using the `smr` option to define the variable containing the reference rates, `strate` calculates SMRs and confidence intervals. You must specify the `per()` option. For example, if the reference rates were per 100,000, you would specify `per(100000)`. When reference rates are available by age and calendar period, you must call `stsplit` twice to expand on both time scales before merging the data with the reference-rate file.

▷ Example 2

In `smrchd.dta` we have age-specific CHD rates per 1,000 person-years for a reference population. We can merge these data with our current data and use `strate` to obtain SMRs and confidence intervals.

(Continued on next page)

```
. sort ageband

. merge ageband using http://www.stata-press.com/data/r10/smrchd
variable ageband does not uniquely identify observations in the master data
ageband was byte now float

. strate ageband, per(1000) smr(rate)
        failure _d:  fail == 1 3 13
   analysis time _t:  (dox-origin)/365.25
           origin:  time doe
               id:  id
             note:  ageband<=40 trimmed
Estimated SMRs and lower/upper bounds of 95% confidence intervals
(729 records included in the analysis)
```

ageband	D	E	SMR	Lower	Upper
40	6	5.62	1.0670	0.4793	2.3749
50	18	18.75	0.9599	0.6048	1.5235
60	22	22.85	0.9629	0.6340	1.4624

◁

Stratified rate ratios using stmh

The stmh command is used for estimating rate ratios, controlled for confounding, using stratification. You can use it to estimate the ratio of the rates of failure for two categories of the explanatory variable. Categories to be compared may be defined by specifying the codes of the levels with compare().

The first variable listed on the command line after stmh is the explanatory variable used in comparing rates, and any remaining variables, if any, are categorical variables, which are to be controlled for using stratification.

▷ Example 3

To illustrate this command, let us return to the diet data. The variable hienergy is coded 1 if the total energy consumption is more than 2.75 Mcal and 0 otherwise. We want to compare the rate for hienergy level 1 with the rate for level 0, controlled for ageband.

To do this, we first stset and stsplit the data into age bands as before, and then we use stmh:

```
. use http://www.stata-press.com/data/r10/diet, clear
(Diet data with dates)

. stset dox, origin(time dob) enter(time doe) id(id) scale(365.25)
> fail(fail==1 3 13)
  (output omitted )

. stsplit ageband, at(40(10)70) after(time=dob) trim
(26 + 0 obs. trimmed due to lower and upper bounds)
(418 observations (episodes) created)
```

```
. stmh hienergy, by(ageband)
        failure _d:  fail == 1 3 13
  analysis time _t:  (dox-origin)/365.25
            origin:  time dob
 enter on or after:  time doe
                id:  id
              note:  ageband<=40 trimmed
Maximum likelihood estimate of the rate ratio
  comparing hienergy==1 vs. hienergy==0
  by ageband
RR estimate, and lower and upper 95% confidence limits
```

ageband	RR	Lower	Upper
40	1.24	0.23	6.76
50	0.43	0.16	1.16
60	0.50	0.21	1.20

```
Overall estimate controlling for ageband
```

RR	chi2	P>chi2	[95% Conf. Interval]	
0.534	4.36	0.0369	0.293	0.972

```
Approx test for unequal RRs (effect modification): chi2(2) =    1.19
                                                   Pr>chi2 =  0.5514
```

Since the RR estimates are approximate, the test for unequal rate ratios is also approximate.

We can also compare the effect of hienergy between jobs, controlling for ageband.

```
. stmh hienergy ageband, by(job)
        failure _d:  fail == 1 3 13
  analysis time _t:  (dox-origin)/365.25
            origin:  time dob
 enter on or after:  time doe
                id:  id
              note:  ageband<=40 trimmed
Mantel-Haenszel estimate of the rate ratio
  comparing hienergy==1 vs. hienergy==0
  controlling for ageband
  by job
RR estimate, and lower and upper 95% confidence limits
```

job	RR	Lower	Upper
0	0.42	0.13	1.33
1	0.64	0.22	1.87
2	0.51	0.21	1.26

```
Overall estimate controlling for ageband job
```

RR	chi2	P>chi2	[95% Conf. Interval]	
0.521	4.88	0.0271	0.289	0.939

```
Approx test for unequal RRs (effect modification): chi2(2) =    0.28
                                                   Pr>chi2 =  0.8695
```

◁

Log-linear trend test for metric explanatory variables using stmh

stmh may also be used to carry out trend tests for a metric explanatory variable. A one-step Newton approximation to the log-linear Poisson regression coefficient is also computed.

The diet dataset contains the height for each patient recorded in the variable height. We can test for a trend of heart disease rates with height controlling for age band by typing

```
. stmh height ageband
         failure _d:  fail == 1 3 13
   analysis time _t:  (dox-origin)/365.25
            origin:  time dob
    enter on or after:  time doe
                id:  id
              note:  ageband<=40 trimmed
Score test for trend of rates with height
  with an approximate estimate of the
  rate ratio for a one unit increase in height
  controlling for ageband

RR estimate, and lower and upper 95% confidence limits
```

RR	chi2	P>chi2	[95% Conf. Interval]	
0.906	18.60	0.0000	0.866	0.948

stmh tested for trend of heart disease rates with height within age bands and provided a rough estimate of the rate ratio for a 1-cm increase in height—this estimate is a one-step Newton approximation to the maximum likelihood estimate. It is not consistent, but it does provide a useful indication of the size of the effect.

The rate ratio is significantly less than 1, so there is clear evidence for a decreasing rate with increasing height (about 9% decrease in rate per centimeter increase in height).

Controlling for age with fine strata by using stmc

The stmc (Mantel–Cox) command is used to control for variation of rates on a time scale by breaking up time into short intervals, or *clicks*.

Usually this approach is used only to calculate significance tests, but the rate ratio estimated remains just as useful as in the coarsely stratified analysis from stmh. The method may be viewed as an approximate form of Cox regression.

The rate ratio produced by stmc is controlled for analysis time separately for each level of the variables specified with by() and then combined to give a rate ratio controlled for both time and the by() variables.

▷ Example 4

For example, to obtain the effect of high energy controlled for age by stratifying finely, we first stset the data specifying the date of birth, dob, as the origin (so analysis time is age), and then we use stmc:

```
. stset dox, origin(time dob) enter(time doe) id(id) scale(365.25)
> fail(fail==1 3 13)
  (output omitted )
```

```
. stmc hienergy
           failure _d:  fail == 1 3 13
     analysis time _t:  (dox-origin)/365.25
              origin:  time dob
   enter on or after:  time doe
                  id:  id
```

Mantel-Cox comparisons

Mantel-Haenszel estimates of the rate ratio
     comparing hienergy==1 vs. hienergy==0
     controlling for time (by clicks)

Overall Mantel-Haenszel estimate, controlling for time from dob

RR	chi2	P>chi2	[95% Conf. Interval]	
0.537	4.20	0.0403	0.293	0.982

The rate ratio of 0.537 is close to that obtained with `stmh` when controlling for age by using 10-year age bands. ◁

Saved Results

`stmh` and `stmc` save the following in `r()`:

Scalars
     `r(RR)`   overall rate ratio

Methods and Formulas

`strate`, `stmh`, and `stmc` are implemented as ado-files.

Nathan Mantel (1919–2002) was an American biostatistician who grew up in New York. He worked at the National Cancer Institute from 1947 to 1974 on a wide range of medical problems and was also later affiliated with George Washington University and the American University in Washington.

William M. Haenszel (1910–1998) was an American biostatistician and epidemiologist who graduated from the University of Buffalo. He also worked at the National Cancer Institute and later at the University of Illinois.

Acknowledgments

The original versions of `strate`, `stmh`, and `stmc` were written by David Clayton, Cambridge Institute for Medical Research, and Michael Hills, London School of Hygiene and Tropical Medicine (retired).

References

Clayton, D. G., and M. Hills. 1993. *Statistical Models in Epidemiology*. Oxford: Oxford University Press.

——. 1995. ssa7: Analysis of follow-up studies. *Stata Technical Bulletin* 27: 19–26. Reprinted in *Stata Technical Bulletin Reprints*, vol. 5, pp. 219–227.

——. 1997. ssa10: Analysis of follow-up studies with Stata 5.0. *Stata Technical Bulletin* 40: 27–39. Reprinted in *Stata Technical Bulletin Reprints*, vol. 7, pp. 253–268.

Gail, M. H. 1997. A conversation with Nathan Mantel. *Statistical Science* 12: 88–97.

Hankey, B. 1997. A conversation with William M. Haenszel. *Statistical Science* 12: 108–112.

Also See

[ST] **stci** — Confidence intervals for means and percentiles of survival time

[ST] **stir** — Report incidence-rate comparison

[ST] **stptime** — Calculate person-time, incidence rates, and SMR

[ST] **stset** — Declare data to be survival-time data

Title

> **streg** — Fit parametric survival models

Syntax

streg $\left[\,varlist\,\right]\,\left[\,if\,\right]\,\left[\,in\,\right]\,\left[\,,\ options\,\right]$

options	description
Model	
<u>noc</u>onstant	suppress constant term
<u>d</u>istribution(<u>e</u>xponential)	exponential survival distribution
<u>d</u>istribution(<u>g</u>ompertz)	Gompertz survival distribution
<u>d</u>istribution(<u>logl</u>ogistic)	log-logistic survival distribution
<u>d</u>istribution(<u>ll</u>ogistic)	synonym for distribution(loglogistic)
<u>d</u>istribution(<u>w</u>eibull)	Weibull survival distribution
<u>d</u>istribution(<u>logn</u>ormal)	lognormal survival distribution
<u>d</u>istribution(<u>ln</u>ormal)	synonym for distribution(lognormal)
<u>d</u>istribution(<u>gamma</u>)	generalized gamma survival distribution
<u>f</u>railty(<u>gamma</u>)	gamma frailty distribution
<u>f</u>railty(<u>invg</u>aussian)	inverse Gaussian distribution
<u>t</u>ime	use accelerated failure-time metric
Model 2	
<u>str</u>ata(*varname*)	strata ID variable
<u>off</u>set(*varname*)	include *varname* in model with coefficient constrained to 1
<u>sh</u>ared(*varname*)	shared frailty ID variable
<u>anc</u>illary(*varlist*)	use *varlist* to model the first ancillary parameter
anc2(*varlist*)	use *varlist* to model the second ancillary parameter
<u>constr</u>aints(*constraints*)	apply specified linear constraints
<u>col</u>linear	keep collinear variables
SE/Robust	
vce(*vcetype*)	*vcetype* may be oim, <u>r</u>obust, <u>c</u>luster *clustvar*, opg, <u>boot</u>strap, or <u>jack</u>knife
Reporting	
<u>l</u>evel(#)	set confidence level; default is level(95)
nohr	do not report hazard ratios
tr	report time ratios
<u>nos</u>how	do not show st setting information
<u>nohe</u>ader	suppress header from coefficient table
<u>nolr</u>test	do not perform the likelihood-ratio test
Max options	
maximize_options	control the maximization process; seldom used

You must stset your data before using streg; see [ST] **stset**.

bootstrap, by, jackknife, nestreg, statsby, stepwise, svy, and xi are allowed; see [U] **11.1.10 Prefix commands**.

shared(), vce(), and noheader are not allowed with the svy prefix.

fweights, iweights, and pweights may be specified using stset; see [ST] **stset**. However, weights may not be specified if you are using the bootstrap prefix with the streg command.

See [U] **20 Estimation and postestimation commands** for more capabilities of estimation commands.

Description

streg performs maximum likelihood estimation for parametric regression survival-time models. streg can be used with single- or multiple-record or single- or multiple-failure st data. Survival models currently supported are exponential, Weibull, Gompertz, lognormal, log-logistic, and generalized gamma. Parametric frailty models and shared-frailty models are also fitted using streg.

Also see [ST] **stcox** for proportional hazards models.

Options

> ⌐ Model └

noconstant; see [ST] **estimation options**.

distribution(*distname*) specifies the survival model to be fitted. A specified distribution() is remembered from one estimation to the next when distribution() is not specified.

For instance, typing streg x1 x2, distribution(weibull) fits a Weibull model. Subsequently, you do not need to specify distribution(weibull) to fit other Weibull regression models.

The currently supported distributions are listed in the options table, but new ones may have been added since this manual was printed. Type help streg for an up-to-date list.

All Stata estimation commands, including streg, redisplay results when you type the command name without arguments. To fit a model with no explanatory variables, type streg, distribution(*distname*)....

frailty(gamma | invgaussian) specifies the assumed distribution of the frailty, or heterogeneity. The estimation results, in addition to the standard parameter estimates, will contain an estimate of the variance of the frailties and a likelihood-ratio test of the null hypothesis that this variance is zero. When this null hypothesis is true, the model reduces to the model with frailty(*distname*) not specified.

A specified frailty() is remembered from one estimation to the next when distribution() is not specified. When you specify distribution(), the previously remembered specification of frailty() is forgotten.

time specifies that the model be fitted in the accelerated failure-time metric rather than in the log relative-hazard metric. This option is valid only for the exponential and Weibull models since they have both a proportional hazards and an accelerated failure-time parameterization. Regardless of metric, the likelihood function is the same, and models are equally appropriate viewed in either metric; it is just a matter of changing the interpretation.

time must be specified at estimation.

Model 2

strata(*varname*) specifies the stratification ID variable. Observations with equal values of the variable are assumed to be in the same stratum. Stratified estimates (with equal coefficients across strata but intercepts and ancillary parameters unique to each stratum) are then obtained. This option is not available if frailty(*distname*) is specified.

offset(*varname*); see [ST] **estimation options**.

shared(*varname*) is valid with frailty() and specifies a variable defining those groups over which the frailty is shared, analogous to a random-effects model for panel data where *varname* defines the panels. frailty() specified without shared() treats the frailties as occurring at the observation level.

A specified shared() is remembered from one estimation to the next when distribution() is not specified. When you specify distribution(), the previously remembered specification of shared() is forgotten.

shared() may not be used with distribution(gamma), vce(robust), vce(cluster *clustvar*), vce(opg), or the svy prefix.

If shared() is specified without frailty() and there is no remembered frailty() from the previous estimation, frailty(gamma) is assumed to provide behavior analogous to stcox; see [ST] **stcox**.

ancillary(*varlist*) specifies that the ancillary parameter for the Weibull, lognormal, Gompertz, and log-logistic distributions and that the first ancillary parameter (sigma) of the generalized log-gamma distribution be estimated as a linear combination of *varlist*. This option may not be used with frailty(*distname*).

When an ancillary parameter is constrained to be strictly positive, the logarithm of the ancillary parameter is modeled as a linear combination of *varlist*.

anc2(*varlist*) specifies that the second ancillary parameter (kappa) for the generalized log-gamma distribution be estimated as a linear combination of *varlist*. This option may not be used with frailty(*distname*).

constraints(*constraints*), collinear; see [ST] **estimation options**.

SE/Robust

vce(*vcetype*) specifies the type of standard error reported, which includes types that are derived from asymptotic theory, that are robust to some kinds of misspecification, that allow for intragroup correlation, and that use bootstrap or jackknife methods; see [R] **vce_option**.

Reporting

level(*#*) specifies the confidence level, as a percentage, for confidence intervals. The default is level(95) or as set by set level; see [U] **20.7 Specifying the width of confidence intervals**.

nohr, which may be specified at estimation or upon redisplaying results, specifies that coefficients rather than exponentiated coefficients be displayed, i.e., that coefficients rather than hazard ratios be displayed. This option affects only how coefficients are displayed, not how they are estimated.

This option is valid only for models with a natural proportional-hazards parameterization: exponential, Weibull, and Gompertz. These three models, by default, report hazard ratios (exponentiated coefficients).

tr specifies that exponentiated coefficients be displayed, which are interpreted as time ratios. tr is appropriate only for the log-logistic, lognormal, and gamma models, or for the exponential and Weibull models when fitted in the accelerated failure-time metric.

tr may be specified at estimation or upon replay.

noshow prevents streg from showing the key st variables. This option is rarely used since most people type stset, show or stset, noshow to set once and for all whether they want to see these variables mentioned at the top of the output of every st command; see [ST] **stset**.

noheader suppresses the output header, either at estimation or upon replay.

nolrtest is valid only with frailty models, in which case it suppresses the likelihood-ratio test for significant frailty.

⌐‾‾‾‾‾‾⌐ Max options ⌐

maximize_options: difficult, technique(*algorithm_spec*), iterate(*#*), [no]log, trace, gradient, showstep, hessian, shownrtolerance, tolerance(*#*), ltolerance(*#*), gtolerance(*#*), nrtolerance(*#*), nonrtolerance, from(*init_specs*); see [R] **maximize**. These options are seldom used.

Setting the optimization type to technique(bhhh) resets the default *vcetype* to vce(opg).

Remarks

Remarks are presented under the following headings:

> *Introduction*
> *Distributions*
> > *Weibull and exponential models*
> > *Gompertz model*
> > *Lognormal and log-logistic models*
> > *Generalized gamma model*
> *Examples*
> *Parameterization of ancillary parameters*
> *Stratified estimation*
> *(Unshared-) frailty models*
> *Shared-frailty models*

Introduction

What follows is a brief summary of what you can do with streg. For a complete tutorial, see Cleves, Gould, and Gutierrez (2004), which devotes four chapters to this topic.

Two often-used models for adjusting survivor functions for the effects of covariates are the accelerated failure-time (AFT) model and the multiplicative or proportional hazards (PH) model. In the AFT model, the natural logarithm of the survival time $\ln t$ is expressed as a linear function of the covariates, yielding the linear model

$$\ln t_j = \mathbf{x}_j \boldsymbol{\beta} + z_j$$

where $\mathbf{x}_j$ is a vector of covariates, $\boldsymbol{\beta}$ is a vector of regression coefficients, and z_j is the error with density $f()$. The distributional form of the error term determines the regression model. If we let $f()$ be the normal density, the lognormal regression model is obtained. Similarly, by letting $f()$ be the logistic density, the log-logistic regression is obtained. Setting $f()$ equal to the extreme-value density yields the exponential and the Weibull regression models.

The effect of the AFT model is to change the time scale by a factor of $\exp(-\mathbf{x}_j\boldsymbol{\beta})$. Depending on whether this factor is greater or less than 1, time is either accelerated or decelerated (degraded). That is, if a subject at baseline experiences a probability of survival past time t equal to $S(t)$, then a subject with covariates $\mathbf{x}_j$ would have probability of survival past time t equal to $S()$ evaluated at the point $\exp(-\mathbf{x}_j\boldsymbol{\beta})t$, instead. Thus accelerated failure time does not imply a positive acceleration of time with the increase of a covariate but instead implies a deceleration of time, or equivalently an increase in the expected waiting time for failure.

In the PH model, the concomitant covariates have a multiplicative effect on the hazard function

$$h(t_j) = h_0(t)g(\mathbf{x}_j)$$

for some $h_0(t)$, and for $g(\mathbf{x}_j)$ a nonnegative function of the covariates. A popular choice, and the one adopted here, is to let $g(\mathbf{x}_j) = \exp(\mathbf{x}_j\boldsymbol{\beta})$. The function $h_0(t)$ may either be left unspecified, yielding the Cox proportional hazard model (see [ST] **stcox**), or take a specific parametric form. For the **streg** command, $h_0(t)$ is assumed to be parametric. Three regression models are currently implemented as PH models: the exponential, Weibull, and Gompertz models. The exponential and Weibull models are implemented as both AFT and PH models, and the Gompertz model is implemented only in the PH metric.

The above model allows for the presence of an intercept term, β_0, within $\mathbf{x}_j\boldsymbol{\beta}$. Thus what is commonly referred to as the *baseline hazard function*—the hazard when all covariates are zero—is actually equal to $h_0(t)\exp(\beta_0)$. That is, the intercept term serves to scale the baseline hazard. Of course, specifying noconstant suppresses the intercept or equivalently constrains β_0 to equal zero.

streg is suitable only for data that have been stset. By stsetting your data, you define the variables _t0, _t, and _d, which serve as the trivariate response variable (t_0, t, d). Each response corresponds to a period under observation, $(t_0, t]$, resulting in either failure $(d = 1)$ or right-censoring $(d = 0)$ at time t. As a result, **streg** is appropriate for data exhibiting delayed entry, gaps, time-varying covariates, and even multiple-failure data.

Distributions

Six parametric survival distributions are currently supported by **streg**. The parameterization and ancillary parameters for each distribution are summarized in table 1:

Table 1. Parametric survival distributions supported by **streg**

Distribution	Metric	Survival function	Parameterization	Ancillary parameters
Exponential	PH	$\exp(-\lambda_j t_j)$	$\lambda_j = \exp(\mathbf{x}_j\boldsymbol{\beta})$	
Exponential	AFT	$\exp(-\lambda_j t_j)$	$\lambda_j = \exp(-\mathbf{x}_j\boldsymbol{\beta})$	
Weibull	PH	$\exp(-\lambda_j t_j^p)$	$\lambda_j = \exp(\mathbf{x}_j\boldsymbol{\beta})$	p
Weibull	AFT	$\exp(-\lambda_j t_j^p)$	$\lambda_j = \exp(-p\mathbf{x}_j\boldsymbol{\beta})$	p
Gompertz	PH	$\exp\{-\lambda_j\gamma^{-1}(e^{\gamma t_j} - 1)\}$	$\lambda_j = \exp(\mathbf{x}_j\boldsymbol{\beta})$	γ
Lognormal	AFT	$1 - \Phi\left\{\frac{\ln(t_j) - \mu_j}{\sigma}\right\}$	$\mu_j = \mathbf{x}_j\boldsymbol{\beta}$	σ
Log-logistic	AFT	$\{1 + (\lambda_j t_j)^{1/\gamma}\}^{-1}$	$\lambda_j = \exp(-\mathbf{x}_j\boldsymbol{\beta})$	γ
Generalized gamma				
if $\kappa > 0$	AFT	$1 - I(\gamma, u)$	$\mu_j = \mathbf{x}_j\boldsymbol{\beta}$	σ, κ
if $\kappa = 0$	AFT	$1 - \Phi(z)$	$\mu_j = \mathbf{x}_j\boldsymbol{\beta}$	σ, κ
if $\kappa < 0$	AFT	$I(\gamma, u)$	$\mu_j = \mathbf{x}_j\boldsymbol{\beta}$	σ, κ

where PH $=$ proportional hazards, AFT $=$ accelerated failure time, and $\Phi(z)$ is the standard normal cumulative distribution. For the generalized gamma, $\gamma = |\kappa|^{-2}$, $u = \gamma \exp(|\kappa|z)$, $I(a, x)$ is the incomplete gamma function, and $z = \text{sign}(\kappa)\{\ln(t_j) - \mu_j\}/\sigma$.

Plotted in figure 1 are example hazard functions for five of the six distributions. The exponential hazard (not separately plotted) is a special case of the Weibull hazard when the Weibull ancillary parameter $p = 1$. The generalized gamma (not plotted) is extremely flexible and therefore can take many shapes.

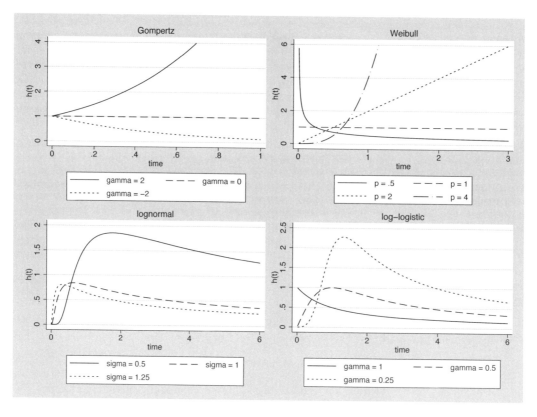

Figure 1. Example plots of hazard functions

Weibull and exponential models

The Weibull and exponential models are parameterized as both PH and AFT models. The Weibull distribution is suitable for modeling data with monotone hazard rates that either increase or decrease exponentially with time, whereas the exponential distribution is suitable for modeling data with constant hazard (see figure 1).

For the PH model, $h_0(t) = 1$ for exponential regression, and $h_0(t) = p\,t^{p-1}$ for Weibull regression, where p is the shape parameter to be estimated from the data. Some authors refer not to p but to $\sigma = 1/p$.

The AFT model is written as

$$\ln(t_j) = \mathbf{x}_j \boldsymbol{\beta}^* + z_j$$

where z_j has an extreme-value distribution scaled by σ. Let $\boldsymbol{\beta}$ be the vector of regression coefficients derived from the PH model, so that $\boldsymbol{\beta}^* = -\sigma\boldsymbol{\beta}$. This relationship holds only if the ancillary parameter p is a constant; it does not hold when the ancillary parameter is parameterized in terms of covariates.

streg uses, by default, for the exponential and Weibull models, the proportional-hazards metric simply because it eases comparison with those results produced by stcox. You can, however, specify option time to choose the accelerated failure-time parameterization.

The Weibull hazard and survivor functions are

$$h(t) = p\lambda t^{p-1}$$

$$S(t) = \exp(-\lambda t^p)$$

where λ is parameterized as described in table 1. If $p = 1$, these functions reduce to those of the exponential.

Gompertz model

The Gompertz regression is parameterized only as a PH model. First described in 1825, this model has been extensively used by medical researchers and biologists modeling mortality data. The Gompertz distribution implemented is the two-parameter function as described in Lee and Wang (2003) with the following hazard and survivor functions:

$$h(t) = \lambda \exp(\gamma t)$$

$$S(t) = \exp\{-\lambda\gamma^{-1}(e^{\gamma t} - 1)\}$$

The model is implemented by parameterizing $\lambda_j = \exp(\mathbf{x}_j\boldsymbol{\beta})$, implying that $h_0(t) = \exp(\gamma t)$, where γ is an ancillary parameter to be estimated from the data.

This distribution is suitable for modeling data with monotone hazard rates that either increase or decrease exponentially with time (see figure 1).

When γ is positive, the hazard function increases with time; when γ is negative, the hazard function decreases with time; and when γ is zero, the hazard function is equal to λ for all t, so the model reduces to an exponential.

Some recent survival analysis texts, such as Klein and Moeschberger (2003), restrict γ to be strictly positive. If $\gamma < 0$, then as t goes to infinity, the survivor function $S(t)$ exponentially decreases to a nonzero constant, implying that there is a nonzero probability of never failing (living forever). That is, there is always a nonzero hazard rate, yet it decreases exponentially. By restricting γ to be positive, we know that the survivor function always goes to zero as t tends to infinity.

Although the above argument may be desirable from a mathematical perspective, in Stata's implementation, we took the more traditional approach of not restricting γ. We did this because in survival studies subjects are not monitored forever—there is a date when the study ends, and in many investigations, specifically in medical research, an exponentially decreasing hazard rate is clinically appealing.

Lognormal and log-logistic models

The lognormal and log-logistic models are implemented in only the AFT form. These two distributions are similar and tend to produce comparable results. For the lognormal distribution, the natural logarithm of time follows a normal distribution; for the log-logistic distribution, the natural logarithm of time follows a logistic distribution.

The lognormal survivor and density functions are

$$S(t) = 1 - \Phi\left\{\frac{\ln(t) - \mu}{\sigma}\right\}$$

$$f(t) = \frac{1}{t\sigma\sqrt{2\pi}} \exp\left[\frac{-1}{2\sigma^2}\left\{\ln(t) - \mu\right\}^2\right]$$

where $\Phi(z)$ is the standard normal cumulative distribution function.

The lognormal regression is implemented by setting $\mu_j = \mathbf{x}_j\boldsymbol{\beta}$ and treating the standard deviation σ as an ancillary parameter to be estimated from the data.

The log-logistic regression is obtained if z_j has a logistic density. The log-logistic survivor and density functions are

$$S(t) = \left\{1 + (\lambda t)^{1/\gamma}\right\}^{-1}$$

$$f(t) = \frac{\lambda^{1/\gamma}t^{1/\gamma-1}}{\gamma\left\{1 + (\lambda t)^{1/\gamma}\right\}^2}$$

This model is implemented by parameterizing $\lambda_j = \exp(-\mathbf{x}_j\boldsymbol{\beta})$ and treating the scale parameter γ as an ancillary parameter to be estimated from the data.

Unlike the exponential, Weibull, and Gompertz distributions, the lognormal and the log-logistic distributions are indicated for data exhibiting nonmonotonic hazard rates, specifically initially increasing and then decreasing rates (figure 1).

Generalized gamma model

The generalized gamma model is implemented only in the AFT form. The three-parameter generalized gamma survivor and density functions are

$$S(t) = \begin{cases} 1 - I(\gamma, u), & \text{if } \kappa > 0 \\ 1 - \Phi(z), & \text{if } \kappa = 0 \\ I(\gamma, u), & \text{if } \kappa < 0 \end{cases}$$

$$f(t) = \begin{cases} \frac{\gamma^\gamma}{\sigma t \sqrt{\gamma}\Gamma(\gamma)} \exp(z\sqrt{\gamma} - u), & \text{if } \kappa \neq 0 \\ \frac{1}{\sigma t\sqrt{2\pi}} \exp(-z^2/2), & \text{if } \kappa = 0 \end{cases}$$

where $\gamma = |\kappa|^{-2}$, $z = \text{sign}(\kappa)\{\ln(t) - \mu\}/\sigma$, $u = \gamma \exp(|\kappa|z)$, $\Phi(z)$ is the standard normal cumulative distribution function, and $I(a, x)$ is the incomplete gamma function. See the `gammap(a,x)` entry in [D] **functions** to see how the incomplete gamma function is implemented in Stata.

This model is implemented by parameterizing $\mu_j = \mathbf{x}_j\boldsymbol{\beta}$ and treating the parameters κ and σ as ancillary parameters to be estimated from the data.

The hazard function of the generalized gamma distribution is extremely flexible, allowing for many possible shapes, including as special cases the Weibull distribution when $\kappa = 1$, the exponential when $\kappa = 1$ and $\sigma = 1$, and the lognormal distribution when $\kappa = 0$. The generalized gamma model is, therefore, commonly used for evaluating and selecting an appropriate parametric model for the data. The Wald or likelihood-ratio test can be used to test the hypotheses that $\kappa = 1$ or that $\kappa = 0$.

Examples

▷ Example 1

The Weibull distribution provides a good illustration of `streg` since this distribution is parameterized as both AFT and PH and serves to compare and contrast the two approaches.

We wish to analyze an experiment testing the ability of emergency generators with new-style bearings to withstand overloads. This dataset is described in [ST] **stcox**. This time, we wish to fit a Weibull model:

```
. use http://www.stata-press.com/data/r10/kva
(Generator experiment)

. streg load bearings, distribution(weibull)

        failure _d:  1 (meaning all fail)
   analysis time _t:  failtime

Fitting constant-only model:

Iteration 0:   log likelihood = -13.666193
Iteration 1:   log likelihood = -9.7427276
Iteration 2:   log likelihood = -9.4421169
Iteration 3:   log likelihood = -9.4408287
Iteration 4:   log likelihood = -9.4408286

Fitting full model:

Iteration 0:   log likelihood = -9.4408286
Iteration 1:   log likelihood =  -2.078323
Iteration 2:   log likelihood =  5.2226016
Iteration 3:   log likelihood =  5.6745808
Iteration 4:   log likelihood =  5.6934031
Iteration 5:   log likelihood =  5.6934189
Iteration 6:   log likelihood =  5.6934189
```

(Continued on next page)

```
Weibull regression -- log relative-hazard form
No. of subjects =          12              Number of obs   =          12
No. of failures =          12
Time at risk    =         896
                                           LR chi2(2)      =       30.27
Log likelihood  =    5.6934189             Prob > chi2     =      0.0000
```

_t	Haz. Ratio	Std. Err.	z	P>|z|	[95% Conf. Interval]
load	1.599315	.1883807	3.99	0.000	1.269616 2.014631
bearings	.1887995	.1312109	-2.40	0.016	.0483546 .7371644
/ln_p	2.051552	.2317074	8.85	0.000	1.597414 2.505691
p	7.779969	1.802677			4.940241 12.25202
1/p	.1285352	.0297826			.0816192 .2024193

Since we did not specify otherwise, the estimation took place in the hazard metric, which is the default for distribution(weibull). The estimates are directly comparable to those produced by stcox: stcox estimated a hazard ratio of 1.526 for load and .0636 for bearings.

However, we estimated the baseline hazard function as well, assuming that it is Weibull. The estimates are the full maximum-likelihood estimates. The shape parameter is fitted as $\ln p$, but streg then reports p and $1/p = \sigma$ so that you can think about the parameter however you wish.

We find that p is greater than 1, which means that the hazard of failure increases with time and, here, increases dramatically. After 100 hours, the bearings are more than 1 million times more likely to fail per second than after 10 hours (or, to be precise, $(100/10)^{7.78-1}$). From our knowledge of generators, we would expect this; it is the accumulation of heat due to friction that causes bearings to expand and seize.

◁

❏ Technical Note

Regression results are often presented in a metric other than the natural regression coefficients, i.e., as hazard ratios, relative risk ratios, odds ratios, etc. In those cases, standard errors are calculated using the delta method.

However, the Z test and p-values given are calculated from the natural regression coefficients and standard errors. Although a test based on, say, a hazard ratio and its standard error would be asymptotically equivalent to that based on a regression coefficient, in real samples a hazard ratio will tend to have a more skewed distribution since it is an exponentiated regression coefficient. Also, it is more natural to think of these tests as testing whether a regression coefficient is nonzero, rather than testing whether a transformed regression coefficient is unequal to some nonzero value (one for a hazard ratio).

Finally, the confidence intervals given are obtained by transforming the endpoints of the corresponding confidence interval for the untransformed regression coefficient. This ensures that, say, strictly positive quantities such as hazard ratios have confidence intervals that do not overlap zero.

❏

▷ Example 2

The previous estimation took place in the PH metric, and exponentiated coefficients—hazard ratios—were reported. If we want to see the unexponentiated coefficients, we could redisplay results and specify the `nohr` option:

```
. streg, nohr
Weibull regression -- log relative-hazard form
No. of subjects =          12                Number of obs   =         12
No. of failures =          12
Time at risk    =         896
                                             LR chi2(2)      =      30.27
Log likelihood  =    5.6934189               Prob > chi2     =     0.0000
```

_t	Coef.	Std. Err.	z	P>|z|	[95% Conf. Interval]	
load	.4695753	.1177884	3.99	0.000	.2387143	.7004363
bearings	-1.667069	.6949745	-2.40	0.016	-3.029194	-.3049443
_cons	-45.13191	10.60663	-4.26	0.000	-65.92053	-24.34329
/ln_p	2.051552	.2317074	8.85	0.000	1.597414	2.505691
p	7.779969	1.802677			4.940241	12.25202
1/p	.1285352	.0297826			.0816192	.2024193

◁

▷ Example 3

We could just as well have fitted this model in the AFT metric:

```
. streg load bearings, d(weibull) time nolog
        failure _d:  1 (meaning all fail)
   analysis time _t:  failtime

Weibull regression -- accelerated failure-time form
No. of subjects =          12                Number of obs   =         12
No. of failures =          12
Time at risk    =         896
                                             LR chi2(2)      =      30.27
Log likelihood  =    5.6934189               Prob > chi2     =     0.0000
```

_t	Coef.	Std. Err.	z	P>|z|	[95% Conf. Interval]	
load	-.060357	.0062214	-9.70	0.000	-.0725507	-.0481632
bearings	.2142771	.0746451	2.87	0.004	.0679753	.3605789
_cons	5.80104	.1752301	33.11	0.000	5.457595	6.144485
/ln_p	2.051552	.2317074	8.85	0.000	1.597414	2.505691
p	7.779969	1.802677			4.940241	12.25202
1/p	.1285352	.0297826			.0816192	.2024193

This is the same model we previously fitted, but it is presented in a different metric. Calling the previous coefficients b, these coefficients are $-\sigma b = -b/p$. For instance, in the previous example, the coefficient on `load` was reported as .4695753, and $-.4695753/7.779969 = -.06035696$. `d()` is a convenient shorthand for `distribution()`.

◁

▷ Example 4

streg may also be applied to more complicated data. Below we have multiple records per subject on a failure that can occur repeatedly:

```
. use http://www.stata-press.com/data/r10/mfail3
. stdescribe
```

Category	total	mean	per subject min	median	max
no. of subjects	926				
no. of records	1734	1.87257	1	2	4
(first) entry time		0	0	0	0
(final) exit time		470.6857	1	477	960
subjects with gap	6				
time on gap if gap	411	68.5	16	57.5	133
time at risk	435444	470.2419	1	477	960
failures	808	.8725702	0	1	3

In this dataset, subjects have up to four records—most have two—and have up to three failures—most have one—and, although you cannot tell from the above output, the data have time-varying covariates, as well. There are even six subjects with gaps in their histories, meaning that, for a while, they went unobserved. Although we could estimate in the AFT metric, it is easier to interpret results in the PH metric (or the log relative-hazard metric, as it is also known):

```
. streg x1 x2, d(weibull) vce(robust)
Fitting constant-only model:

Iteration 0:   log pseudolikelihood = -1398.2504
Iteration 1:   log pseudolikelihood = -1382.8224
Iteration 2:   log pseudolikelihood = -1382.7457
Iteration 3:   log pseudolikelihood = -1382.7457

Fitting full model:

Iteration 0:   log pseudolikelihood = -1382.7457
Iteration 1:   log pseudolikelihood = -1328.4186
Iteration 2:   log pseudolikelihood = -1326.4483
Iteration 3:   log pseudolikelihood = -1326.4449
Iteration 4:   log pseudolikelihood = -1326.4449

Weibull regression -- log relative-hazard form
```

No. of subjects	=	926	Number of obs	=	1734
No. of failures	=	808			
Time at risk	=	435444			
			Wald chi2(2)	=	154.45
Log pseudolikelihood =	-1326.4449		Prob > chi2	=	0.0000

(Std. Err. adjusted for 926 clusters in id)

_t	Haz. Ratio	Robust Std. Err.	z	P>|z|	[95% Conf. Interval]	
x1	2.240069	.1812848	9.97	0.000	1.911504	2.625111
x2	.3206515	.0504626	-7.23	0.000	.2355458	.436507
/ln_p	.1771265	.0310111	5.71	0.000	.1163458	.2379071
p	1.193782	.0370205			1.123384	1.268591
1/p	.8376738	.0259772			.7882759	.8901674

A one-unit change in x1 approximately doubles the hazard of failure, whereas a one-unit change in x2 cuts the hazard to one-third. We also see that these data are close to being exponentially distributed; p is nearly 1.

Above we mentioned that interpreting results in the PH metric is easier, though regression coefficients are not difficult to interpret in the AFT metric. A positive coefficient means that time is decelerated by a unit increase in the covariate in question. This may seem awkward, but think of this instead as a unit increase in the covariate causing a delay in failure and thus *increasing* the expected time until failure.

The difficulty that arises with the AFT metric is merely that it places an emphasis on log(time-to-failure) rather than risk (hazard) of failure. With this emphasis usually comes a desire to predict the time to failure, and therein lies the difficulty with complex survival data. Predicting the log(time to failure) with `predict` assumes that the subject is at risk from time 0 until failure and has a fixed covariate pattern over this period. With these data, such assumptions produce predictions having little to do with the test subjects, who exhibit not only time-varying covariates but also multiple failures.

Predicting time to failure with complex survival data is difficult regardless of the metric under which estimation took place. Those who estimate in the PH metric are probably used to dealing with results from Cox regression, of which predicted time to failure is typically not the focus.

◁

▷ Example 5

The multiple-failure data above are close enough to exponentially distributed that we will reestimate using exponential regression:

```
. streg x1 x2, d(exp) vce(robust)
Iteration 0:   log pseudolikelihood = -1398.2504
Iteration 1:   log pseudolikelihood = -1343.6083
Iteration 2:   log pseudolikelihood = -1341.5932
Iteration 3:   log pseudolikelihood = -1341.5893
Iteration 4:   log pseudolikelihood = -1341.5893
Exponential regression -- log relative-hazard form
No. of subjects     =          926        Number of obs   =       1734
No. of failures     =          808
Time at risk        =       435444
                                           Wald chi2(2)    =     166.92
Log pseudolikelihood =  -1341.5893         Prob > chi2     =     0.0000
                            (Std. Err. adjusted for 926 clusters in id)
```

_t	Haz. Ratio	Robust Std. Err.	z	P>|z|	[95% Conf. Interval]	
x1	2.19065	.1684399	10.20	0.000	1.884186	2.54696
x2	.3037259	.0462489	-7.83	0.000	.2253552	.4093511

◁

❏ Technical Note

For our "complex" survival data, we specified `vce(robust)` when fitting the Weibull and exponential models. This was because these data were `stset` with an `id()` variable, and given the time-varying covariates and multiple failures, it is important not to assume that the observations within each subject are independent. When we specified `vce(robust)`, it was implicit that we were "clustering" on the groups defined by the `id()` variable.

You might sometimes have multiple observations per subject, which exist merely as a result of the data-organization mechanism and are not used to record gaps, time-varying covariates, or multiple failures. Such data could be collapsed into single-observation-per-subject data with no loss of information. In these cases, we refer to splitting the observations to form multiple observations per subject as *noninformative*. When the episode-splitting is noninformative, the model-based (nonrobust) standard errors produced will be the same as those produced when the data are collapsed into single records per subject. Thus for these type of data, clustering of these multiple observations that results from specifying vce(robust) is not critical.

❏

▷ Example 6

A reasonable question to ask is, "Given that we have several possible parametric models, how can we select one?" When parametric models are nested, the likelihood-ratio or Wald test can be used to discriminate between them. This can certainly be done for Weibull versus exponential or gamma versus Weibull or lognormal. When models are not nested, however, these tests are inappropriate, and the task of discriminating between models becomes more difficult. A common approach to this problem is to use the Akaike information criterion (AIC). Akaike (1974) proposed penalizing each log likelihood to reflect the number of parameters being estimated in a particular model and then comparing them. Here the AIC can be defined as

$$\text{AIC} = -2(\log \text{ likelihood}) + 2(c + p + 1)$$

where c is the number of model covariates and p is the number of model-specific ancillary parameters listed in Table 1. Although the best-fitting model is the one with the largest log likelihood, the preferred model is the one with the smallest AIC value. The AIC value may be obtained by using the estat ic postestimation command.

Using the cancer.dta distributed with Stata, let's first fit a generalized gamma model and test the hypothesis that $\kappa = 0$ (test for the appropriateness of the lognormal) and then test the hypothesis that $\kappa = 1$ (test for the appropriateness of the Weibull).

```
. use http://www.stata-press.com/data/r10/cancer
(Patient Survival in Drug Trial)
. stset studytime, failure(died)
 (output omitted )
. replace drug = drug==2 | drug==3        // 0, placebo : 1, nonplacebo
(48 real changes made)
```

```
. streg drug age, d(gamma) nolog

        failure _d:  died
    analysis time _t:  studytime

Gamma regression -- accelerated failure-time form

No. of subjects =          48          Number of obs    =          48
No. of failures =          31
Time at risk    =         744
                                        LR chi2(2)       =       36.07
Log likelihood  =   -42.452006          Prob > chi2      =      0.0000
```

_t	Coef.	Std. Err.	z	P>|z|	[95% Conf. Interval]
drug	1.394658	.2557198	5.45	0.000	.893456	1.895859
age	-.0780416	.0227978	-3.42	0.001	-.1227245	-.0333587
_cons	6.456091	1.238457	5.21	0.000	4.02876	8.883421
/ln_sig	-.3793632	.183707	-2.07	0.039	-.7394222	-.0193041
/kappa	.4669252	.5419478	0.86	0.389	-.595273	1.529123
sigma	.684297	.1257101			.4773897	.980881

The Wald test of the hypothesis that $\kappa = 0$ (test for the appropriateness of the lognormal) is reported in the output above. The p-value is 0.389, suggesting that lognormal might be an adequate model for these data.

The Wald test for $\kappa = 1$ is

```
. test [kappa]_cons = 1

 ( 1)  [kappa]_cons = 1

        chi2(  1) =      0.97
      Prob > chi2 =    0.3253
```

providing some support against rejecting the Weibull model.

We now fit the exponential, Weibull, log-logistic, and lognormal models separately. To directly compare coefficients, we will ask Stata to report the exponential and Weibull models in AFT form by specifying the time option. The output from fitting these models and the results from the generalized gamma model are summarized in table 2.

Table 2. Results obtained from streg, using cancer.dta with drug as indicator

Parameter	Exponential	Weibull	Lognormal	Log-logistic	Generalized gamma
Age	−.0886715	−.0714323	−.0833996	−.0803289	−.078042
Drug	1.682625	1.305563	1.445838	1.420237	1.394658
Constant	7.146218	6.289679	6.580887	6.446711	6.456091
Ancillary		1.682751	0.751136	0.429276	0.684297
Kappa					0.466925
Log-likelihood	−48.397094	−42.931335	−42.800864	−43.21698	−42.452006
AIC	102.7942	93.86267	93.60173	94.43396	94.90401

The largest log likelihood was obtained for the generalized gamma model; however, the lognormal model is preferred by the AIC.

◁

Parameterization of ancillary parameters

By default, all ancillary parameters are estimated as being constant. For example, the ancillary parameter, p, of the Weibull distribution is assumed to be a constant that is not dependent on any covariates. streg's ancillary() and anc2() options allow for complete parameterization of parametric survival models. By specifying, for example,

    . streg x1 x2, d(weibull) ancillary(x2 z1 z2)

both λ and the ancillary parameter, p, are parameterized in terms of covariates.

Ancillary parameters are usually restricted to be strictly positive, in which case the logarithm of the ancillary parameter is modeled using a linear predictor, which can assume any value on the real line.

▷ Example 7

Consider a dataset in which we model the time until hip fracture as Weibull for patients on the basis of age, sex, and whether the patient wears a hip-protective device (variable protect). We believe that the hazard is scaled according to sex and the presence of the device but believe the hazards for both sexes to be of different *shapes*.

    . use http://www.stata-press.com/data/r10/hip3, clear
    (hip fracture study)

    . streg protect age, d(weibull) ancillary(male) nolog

             failure _d: fracture
       analysis time _t: time1
                     id: id

    Weibull regression -- log relative-hazard form

    No. of subjects =   148   Number of obs   =   206
    No. of failures =   37
    Time at risk   =   1703

                                                      LR chi2(2)   =   39.80
    Log likelihood =   -69.323532   Prob > chi2   =   0.0000

_t	Coef.	Std. Err.	z	P>|z|	[95% Conf. Interval]	
_t						
protect	-2.130058	.3567005	-5.97	0.000	-2.829178	-1.430938
age	.0939131	.0341107	2.75	0.006	.0270573	.1607689
_cons	-10.17575	2.551821	-3.99	0.000	-15.17722	-5.174269
ln_p						
male	-.4887189	.185608	-2.63	0.008	-.8525039	-.1249339
_cons	.4540139	.1157915	3.92	0.000	.2270667	.6809611

From our estimation results, we see that $\widehat{\ln(p)} = 0.454$ for females and $\widehat{\ln(p)} = 0.454 - 0.489 = -0.035$ for males. Thus $\hat{p} = 1.57$ for females and $\hat{p} = 0.97$ for males. When we combine this with the main equation in the model, the estimated hazards are then

$$\widehat{h}(t_j|\mathbf{x}_j) = \begin{cases} \exp\left(-10.18 - 2.13\text{protect}_j + 0.09\text{age}_j\right) 1.57 t_j^{0.57} & \text{if female} \\ \exp\left(-10.18 - 2.13\text{protect}_j + 0.09\text{age}_j\right) 0.97 t_j^{-0.03} & \text{if male} \end{cases}$$

If we believe this model, we would say that the hazard for males given age and protect is almost constant over time.

Contrast this with what we obtain if we type

```
. streg protect age if male, d(weibull)
. streg protect age if !male, d(weibull)
```

which is completely general, because not only will the shape parameter p differ over both sexes, but the regression coefficients will as well.

◁

The `anc2()` option is for use only with the gamma regression model, as it contains two ancillary parameters—`anc2()` is used to parametrize κ.

Stratified estimation

When we type

```
. streg xvars, d(distname) strata(varname)
```

we are asking that a completely stratified model be fitted. By *completely stratified*, we mean that both the model's intercept and any ancillary parameters are allowed to vary for each level of the strata variable. That is, we are constraining the coefficients on the covariates to be the same across strata but allowing the intercept and ancillary parameters to vary.

▷ Example 8

We demonstrate this by fitting a stratified lognormal model to the cancer data, with variable `drug` left in its original state: `drug==1` refers to the placebo, and `drug==2` and `drug==3` correspond to two alternative treatments.

```
. use http://www.stata-press.com/data/r10/cancer
(Patient Survival in Drug Trial)
. stset studytime died
 (output omitted )
. streg age, d(weibull) strata(drug) nolog
         failure _d:  died
   analysis time _t:  studytime
Weibull regression -- log relative-hazard form
No. of subjects =          48                Number of obs   =        48
No. of failures =          31
Time at risk    =         744
                                             LR chi2(3)      =     16.58
Log likelihood  =   -41.113074               Prob > chi2     =    0.0009
```

_t	Coef.	Std. Err.	z	P>|z|	[95% Conf. Interval]	
_t						
age	.1212332	.0367538	3.30	0.001	.049197	.1932694
_Sdrug_2	-4.561178	2.339448	-1.95	0.051	-9.146411	.0240556
_Sdrug_3	-3.715737	2.595986	-1.43	0.152	-8.803776	1.372302
_cons	-10.36921	2.341022	-4.43	0.000	-14.95753	-5.780896
ln_p						
_Sdrug_2	.4872195	.332019	1.47	0.142	-.1635257	1.137965
_Sdrug_3	.2194213	.4079989	0.54	0.591	-.5802418	1.019084
_cons	.4541282	.1715663	2.65	0.008	.1178645	.7903919

◁

Completely stratified models are fitted by first generating stratum-specific indicator variables (dummy variables) and then adding these as independent variables in the model and as covariates in the ancillary parameter. The strata() option is thus merely a shorthand method for generating the indicator variables from the drug categories and then placing these indicators in *both* the main equation and the ancillary equation(s).

We associate the term *stratification* with this process by noting that the intercept term of the main equation is a component of the baseline hazard (or baseline survivor) function. By allowing this intercept, as well as the ancillary shape parameter, to vary with respect to the strata, we allow the baseline functions to completely vary over the strata, analogous to a stratified Cox model.

▷ Example 9

We can produce a less-stratified model by combining xi (see [R] **xi**) with the ancillary() option.

```
. xi: streg age, d(weibull) ancillary(i.drug) nolog
i.drug              _Idrug_1-3          (naturally coded; _Idrug_1 omitted)

        failure _d:  died
   analysis time _t:  studytime

Weibull regression -- log relative-hazard form

No. of subjects =          48                Number of obs    =          48
No. of failures =          31
Time at risk    =         744
                                             LR chi2(1)       =        9.61
Log likelihood  =   -44.596379              Prob > chi2      =      0.0019
```

_t	Coef.	Std. Err.	z	P>|z|	[95% Conf. Interval]
_t					
age	.1126419	.0362786	3.10	0.002	.0415373 .1837466
_cons	-10.95772	2.308489	-4.75	0.000	-15.48227 -6.433162
ln_p					
_Idrug_2	-.3279568	.11238	-2.92	0.004	-.5482176 -.107696
_Idrug_3	-.4775351	.1091141	-4.38	0.000	-.6913948 -.2636755
_cons	.6684086	.1327284	5.04	0.000	.4082657 .9285514

By doing this, we are restricting not only the coefficients on the covariates to be the same across "strata" but also the intercept, while allowing only the ancillary parameter to differ.

◁

By using ancillary() or strata(), we may thus consider a wide variety of models, depending on what we believe about the effect of the covariate(s) in question. For example, when fitting a Weibull PH model to the cancer data, we may choose from many models, depending on what we want to assume is the effect of the categorical variable drug. For all models considered below, we assume implicitly that the effect of age is proportional on the hazard function.

1. drug has no effect:

        . streg age, d(weibull)

2. The effect of drug is proportional on the hazard (scale), and the effect of age is the same for each level of drug:

        . xi: streg age i.drug, d(weibull)

3. drug affects the shape of the hazard, and the effect of age is the same for each level of drug:

> . xi: streg age, d(weibull) ancillary(i.drug)

4. drug affects both the scale and shape of the hazard, and the effect of age is the same for each level of drug:

> . streg age, d(weibull) strata(drug)

5. drug affects both the scale and shape of the hazard, and the effect of age is different for each level of drug:

> . xi: streg i.drug*age, d(weibull) strata(drug)

These models may be compared using Wald or likelihood-ratio tests when the models in question are nested (such as 3 nested within 4) or by using the AIC for nonnested models.

Everything we said regarding the modeling of ancillary parameters and stratification applies to AFT models as well, for which interpretations may be stated in terms of the baseline survivor function, i.e., the unaccelerated probability of survival past time t.

❑ Technical Note

When fitting PH models as we have done in the previous three examples, streg will, by default, display the exponentiated regression coefficients, labeled as hazard ratios. However, in our previous examples using ancillary() and strata(), the regression outputs displayed the untransformed coefficients instead. This change in behavior has to do with the modeling of the ancillary parameter. When we use one or more covariates from the main equation to model an ancillary parameter, hazard ratios (and time ratios for AFT models) lose their interpretation. streg, as a precaution, disallows the display of hazard/time ratios when ancillary(), anc2(), or strata() is specified.

Keep this in mind when comparing results across various model specifications. For example, when comparing a stratified Weibull PH model to a standard Weibull PH model, be sure that the latter is displayed using the nohr option.

❑

(Unshared) frailty models

A frailty model is a survival model with unobservable heterogeneity, or *frailty*. At the observation level, frailty is introduced as an unobservable multiplicative effect, α, on the hazard function, such that

$$h(t|\alpha) = \alpha h(t)$$

where $h(t)$ is a nonfrailty hazard function, say, the hazard function of any of the six parametric models supported by streg described earlier in this entry. The frailty, α, is a random positive quantity and, for model identifiability, is assumed to have mean one and variance θ.

Exploiting the relationship between the cumulative hazard function and survivor function yields the expression for the survivor function, given the frailty

$$S(t|\alpha) = \exp\left\{-\int_0^t h(u|\alpha)du\right\} = \exp\left\{-\alpha\int_0^t \frac{f(u)}{S(u)}du\right\} = \{S(t)\}^\alpha$$

where $S(t)$ is the survivor function that corresponds to $h(t)$.

Since α is unobservable, it must be integrated out of $S(t|\alpha)$ to obtain the unconditional survivor function. Let $g(\alpha)$ be the probability density function of α, in which case an estimable form of our frailty model is achieved as

$$S_\theta(t) = \int_0^\infty S(t|\alpha)g(\alpha)d\alpha = \int_0^\infty \{S(t)\}^\alpha g(\alpha)d\alpha$$

Given the unconditional survivor function, we can obtain the unconditional hazard and density in the usual way:

$$f_\theta(t) = -\frac{d}{dt}S_\theta(t) \qquad h_\theta(t) = \frac{f_\theta(t)}{S_\theta(t)}$$

Hence, an unshared-frailty model is merely a typical parametric survival model, with the additional estimation of an overdispersion parameter, θ. In a standard survival regression, the likelihood calculations are based on $S(t)$, $h(t)$, and $f(t)$. In an unshared-frailty model, the likelihood is based analogously on $S_\theta(t)$, $h_\theta(t)$, and $f_\theta(t)$.

At this stage, the only missing piece is the choice of frailty distribution $g(\alpha)$. In theory, any continuous distribution supported on the positive numbers that has expectation one and finite variance θ is allowed here. For mathematical tractability, however, we limit the choice to either the gamma$(1/\theta, \theta)$ distribution or the inverse-Gaussian distribution with parameters one and $1/\theta$, denoted as IG$(1, 1/\theta)$. The gamma(a, b) distribution has probability density function

$$g(x) = \frac{x^{a-1}e^{-x/b}}{\Gamma(a)b^a}$$

and the IG(a, b) distribution has density

$$g(x) = \left(\frac{b}{2\pi x^3}\right)^{1/2} \exp\left\{-\frac{b}{2a}\left(\frac{x}{a} - 2 + \frac{a}{x}\right)\right\}$$

Therefore, performing the integrations described above will show that specifying `frailty(gamma)` will result in the frailty survival model (in terms of the nonfrailty survivor function $S(t)$)

$$S_\theta(t) = [1 - \theta \ln\{S(t)\}]^{-1/\theta}$$

Specifying `frailty(invgaussian)` will give

$$S_\theta(t) = \exp\left\{\frac{1}{\theta}\left(1 - [1 - 2\theta \ln\{S(t)\}]^{1/2}\right)\right\}$$

Regardless of the choice of frailty distribution, $\lim_{\theta \to 0} S_\theta(t) = S(t)$, and thus the frailty model reduces to $S(t)$ when there is no heterogeneity present.

When using frailty models, distinguish between the hazard faced by the individual (subject), $\alpha h(t)$, and the "average" hazard for the population, $h_\theta(t)$. Similarly, an individual will have probability of survival past time t equal to $\{S(t)\}^\alpha$, whereas $S_\theta(t)$ will measure the proportion of the population surviving past time t. You specify $S(t)$ as before with `distribution(`*distname*`)`, and the list of possible parametric forms for $S(t)$ is given in table 1. Thus when you specify `distribution()` you are specifying a model for an individual with frailty equal to one. Specifying `frailty(`*distname*`)` determines which of the two above forms for $S_\theta(t)$ is used.

The output of the estimation remains unchanged from the nonfrailty version, except for the additional estimation of θ and a likelihood-ratio test of H_0: $\theta = 0$. For more information on frailty models, Hougaard (1986) offers an excellent introduction. For a Stata-specific overview, see Gutierrez (2002).

▷ Example 10

Consider as an example a survival analysis of data on women with breast cancer. Our hypothetical dataset consists of analysis times on 80 women with covariates age, smoking, and dietfat, which measures the average weekly calories from fat ($\times 10^3$) in the patient's diet over the course of the study.

```
. use http://www.stata-press.com/data/r10/bc
. list in 1/12
```

	age	smoking	dietfat	t	dead
1.	30	1	4.919	14.2	0
2.	50	0	4.437	8.21	1
3.	47	0	5.85	5.64	1
4.	49	1	5.149	4.42	1
5.	52	1	4.363	2.81	1
6.	29	0	6.153	35	0
7.	49	1	3.82	4.57	1
8.	27	1	5.294	35	0
9.	47	0	6.102	3.74	1
10.	59	0	4.446	2.29	1
11.	35	0	6.203	15.3	0
12.	26	0	4.515	35	0

The data are well fitted by a Weibull model for the distribution of survival time conditional on age, smoking, and dietary fat. By omitting the variable dietfat from the model, we hope to introduce unobserved heterogeneity.

```
. stset t, fail(dead)
  (output omitted )
. streg age smoking, d(weibull) frailty(gamma)

        failure _d:  dead
   analysis time _t:  t

Fitting Weibull model:

Fitting constant-only model:

Iteration 0:   log likelihood = -137.15363
Iteration 1:   log likelihood =  -136.3927
Iteration 2:   log likelihood = -136.01557
Iteration 3:   log likelihood = -136.01202
Iteration 4:   log likelihood = -136.01201

Fitting full model:

Iteration 0:   log likelihood = -85.933969
Iteration 1:   log likelihood =  -73.61173
Iteration 2:   log likelihood = -68.999447
Iteration 3:   log likelihood = -68.340858
Iteration 4:   log likelihood = -68.136187
Iteration 5:   log likelihood = -68.135804
Iteration 6:   log likelihood = -68.135804
```

```
Weibull regression -- log relative-hazard form
              Gamma frailty
No. of subjects =              80          Number of obs   =          80
No. of failures =              58
Time at risk    =         1257.07
                                           LR chi2(2)      =      135.75
Log likelihood  =      -68.135804          Prob > chi2     =      0.0000
```

_t	Haz. Ratio	Std. Err.	z	P>|z|	[95% Conf. Interval]	
age	1.475948	.1379987	4.16	0.000	1.228811	1.772788
smoking	2.788548	1.457031	1.96	0.050	1.00143	7.764894
/ln_p	1.087761	.222261	4.89	0.000	.6521376	1.523385
/ln_the	.3307466	.5250758	0.63	0.529	-.698383	1.359876
p	2.967622	.6595867			1.91964	4.587727
1/p	.3369701	.0748953			.2179729	.520931
theta	1.392007	.7309092			.4973889	3.895711

```
Likelihood-ratio test of theta=0: chibar2(01) =    22.57 Prob>=chibar2 = 0.000
```

We could also use an inverse-Gaussian distribution to model the heterogeneity.

```
. streg age smoking, dist(weibull) frailty(invgauss) nolog
        failure _d: dead
   analysis time _t: t
Weibull regression -- log relative-hazard form
              Inverse-Gaussian frailty
No. of subjects =              80          Number of obs   =          80
No. of failures =              58
Time at risk    =         1257.07
                                           LR chi2(2)      =      125.44
Log likelihood  =      -73.838578          Prob > chi2     =      0.0000
```

_t	Haz. Ratio	Std. Err.	z	P>|z|	[95% Conf. Interval]	
age	1.284133	.0463256	6.93	0.000	1.196473	1.378217
smoking	2.905409	1.252785	2.47	0.013	1.247892	6.764528
/ln_p	.7173904	.1434382	5.00	0.000	.4362567	.9985241
/ln_the	.2374778	.8568064	0.28	0.782	-1.441832	1.916788
p	2.049079	.2939162			1.546906	2.714273
1/p	.4880241	.0700013			.3684228	.6464518
theta	1.268047	1.086471			.2364941	6.799082

```
Likelihood-ratio test of theta=0: chibar2(01) =    11.16 Prob>=chibar2 = 0.000
```

The results are similar with respect to the choice of frailty distribution, with the gamma frailty model producing a slightly higher likelihood. Both models show a statistically significant level of unobservable heterogeneity since the p-value for the LR test of H_0: $\theta = 0$ is virtually zero in both cases.

❏ Technical Note

With gamma- or inverse-Gaussian–distributed frailty, hazard ratios decay over time in favor of the *frailty effect*, and thus the displayed "Haz. Ratio" in the above output is actually the hazard ratio only for $t = 0$. The degree of decay depends on θ. Should the estimated θ be close to zero, the hazard ratios regain their usual interpretation. The rate of decay and the limiting hazard ratio differ between the gamma and inverse-Gaussian models; see Gutierrez (2002) for details.

For this reason, many researchers prefer fitting frailty models in the AFT metric since the interpretation of regression coefficients is unchanged by the frailty—the factors in question serve to either accelerate or decelerate the survival experience. The only difference is that, with frailty models, the unconditional probability of survival is described by $S_\theta(t)$ rather than $S(t)$.

❑

❑ Technical Note

The likelihood-ratio test of $\theta = 0$ is a boundary test and thus requires careful consideration concerning the calculation of its p-value. In particular, the null distribution of the likelihood-ratio test statistic is not the usual χ_1^2 but rather is a 50:50 mixture of a χ_0^2 (point mass at zero) and a χ_1^2, denoted as $\bar{\chi}_{01}^2$. See Gutierrez et al. (2001) for more details.

❑

To verify that the significant heterogeneity is caused by the omission of dietfat, we now refit the Weibull/inverse-Gaussian frailty model with dietfat included.

```
. streg age smoking dietfat, d(weibull) frailty(invgauss) nolog

        failure _d:  dead
   analysis time _t:  t

Weibull regression -- log relative-hazard form
               Inverse-Gaussian frailty

No. of subjects =          80              Number of obs    =          80
No. of failures =          58
Time at risk    =     1257.07
                                           LR chi2(3)       =      246.41
Log likelihood  =    -13.352142            Prob > chi2      =      0.0000
```

_t	Haz. Ratio	Std. Err.	z	P>|z|	[95% Conf. Interval]	
age	1.74928	.0985245	9.93	0.000	1.566453	1.953446
smoking	5.203549	1.70494	5.03	0.000	2.737815	9.889978
dietfat	9.229841	2.219329	9.24	0.000	5.761315	14.78655
/ln_p	1.431742	.0978844	14.63	0.000	1.239892	1.623592
/ln_the	-14.42724	2863.942	-0.01	0.996	-5627.651	5598.796
p	4.185986	.409743			3.455242	5.071276
1/p	.2388923	.0233838			.197189	.2894154
theta	5.42e-07	.0015534			0	.

```
Likelihood-ratio test of theta=0: chibar2(01) =      0.00 Prob>=chibar2 = 1.000
```

The estimate of the frailty variance component θ is near zero and the p-value of the test of H_0: $\theta = 0$ equals one, indicating negligible heterogeneity. A regular Weibull model could be fitted to these data (with dietfat included), producing almost identical estimates of the hazard ratios and ancillary parameter p, so such an analysis is omitted here.

Also, hazard ratios now regain their original interpretation. Thus, an increase in weekly calories from fat of 1,000 would increase the risk of death by more than ninefold.

◁

Shared-frailty models

A generalization of the frailty models considered in the previous section is the *shared-frailty* model, where the frailty is assumed to be group specific; this is analogous to a panel-data regression model. For observation j from the ith group, the hazard is

$$h_{ij}(t|\alpha_i) = \alpha_i h_{ij}(t)$$

for $i = 1, \ldots, n$ and $j = 1, \ldots, n_i$, where by $h_{ij}(t)$ we mean $h(t|\mathbf{x}_{ij})$, which is the individual hazard given covariates $\mathbf{x}_{ij}$.

Shared-frailty models are appropriate when you wish to model the frailties as being specific to groups of subjects, such as subjects within families. Here a shared-frailty model may be used to model the degree of correlation within groups; i.e., the subjects within a group are correlated because they share the same common frailty.

▷ Example 11

Consider the data from a study of 38 kidney dialysis patients, as described in McGilchrist and Aisbett (1991). The study is concerned with the prevalence of infection at the catheter-insertion point. Two recurrence times (in days) are measured for each patient, and each recorded time is the time from initial insertion (onset of risk) to infection or censoring.

```
. use http://www.stata-press.com/data/r10/catheter
(Kidney data, McGilchrist and Aisbett, Biometrics, 1991)

. list patient time infect age female in 1/10
```

	patient	time	infect	age	female
1.	1	16	1	28	0
2.	1	8	1	28	0
3.	2	13	0	48	1
4.	2	23	1	48	1
5.	3	22	1	32	0
6.	3	28	1	32	0
7.	4	318	1	31.5	1
8.	4	447	1	31.5	1
9.	5	30	1	10	0
10.	5	12	1	10	0

Each patient (`patient`) has two recurrence times (`time`) recorded, with each catheter insertion resulting in either infection (`infect==1`) or right-censoring (`infect==0`). Among the covariates measured are `age` and sex (`female==1` if female, `female==0` if male).

One subtlety to note concerns the use of the generic term *subjects*. In this example, the subjects are the individual catheter insertions, not the patients themselves. This is a function of how the data were recorded—the onset of risk occurs at catheter insertion (of which there are two for each patient) not, say, at the time of admission of the patient into the study. Thus we have two subjects (insertions) within each group (patient).

It is reasonable to assume independence of patients but unreasonable to assume that recurrence times within each patient are independent. One solution would be to fit a standard survival model, adjusting the standard errors of the parameter estimates to account for the possible correlation by specifying `vce(cluster patient)`.

We could also model the correlation by assuming that the correlation is the result of a latent patient-level effect, or frailty. That is, rather than fitting a standard model and specifying vce(cluster patient), we fit a frailty model and specify shared(patient). Assuming that the time-to-infection, given age and female, follows a Weibull distribution, and inverse-Gaussian distributed frailties, we get

```
. stset time, fail(infect)
 (output omitted )
. streg age female, d(weibull) frailty(invgauss) shared(patient) nolog

        failure _d:  infect
   analysis time _t:  time

Weibull regression --                        Number of obs     =        76
        log-relative hazard form             Number of groups  =        38
        Inverse-Gaussian shared frailty
Group variable: patient
                                             Obs per group: min =         2
No. of subjects =          76                               avg =         2
No. of failures =          58                               max =         2
Time at risk    =        7424
                                             LR chi2(2)        =      9.84
Log likelihood  =   -99.093527               Prob > chi2       =    0.0073
```

_t	Haz. Ratio	Std. Err.	z	P>|z|	[95% Conf. Interval]	
age	1.006918	.013574	0.51	0.609	.9806623	1.033878
female	.2331376	.1046382	-3.24	0.001	.0967322	.5618928
/ln_p	.1900625	.1315342	1.44	0.148	-.0677398	.4478649
/ln_the	.0357272	.7745362	0.05	0.963	-1.482336	1.55379
p	1.209325	.1590676			.9345036	1.564967
1/p	.8269074	.1087666			.638991	1.070087
theta	1.036373	.8027085			.2271066	4.729362

```
Likelihood-ratio test of theta=0: chibar2(01) =     8.70 Prob>=chibar2 = 0.002
```

Contrast this with what we obtain by assuming a subject-level lognormal model:

Benjamin Gompertz (1779–1865) came from a Jewish family who left Holland and settled in England. He was self-educated in mathematics and in 1824 was appointed as actuary and head clerk of the Alliance Assurance Company. He carried out pioneer work on the application of differential calculus to actuarial questions, particularly the dependence of mortality on age, and contributed to astronomy and the study of scientific instruments.

Ernst Hjalmar Waloddi Weibull (1887–1979) was a Swedish applied physicist most famous for his work on the statistics of material properties. He worked in Germany and Sweden as an inventor and a consulting engineer, publishing his first paper on the propagation of explosive waves in 1914, thereafter becoming a full professor at the Royal Institute of Technology in 1924. Weibull's ideas about the statistical distributions of material strength came to the attention of engineers in the late 1930s with the publication of two important papers: "Investigations into strength properties of brittle materials" and "The phenomenon of rupture in solids".

```
. streg age female, d(lnormal) frailty(invgauss) shared(patient) nolog
        failure _d:  infect
   analysis time _t:  time
```

Log-normal regression --

        accelerated failure-time form

        Inverse-Gaussian shared frailty

Group variable: patient

Number of obs =	76
Number of groups =	38

No. of subjects =	76
No. of failures =	58
Time at risk =	7424

Obs per group:	
min =	2
avg =	2
max =	2

Log likelihood = -97.614583

LR chi2(2) =	16.34
Prob > chi2 =	0.0003

_t	Coef.	Std. Err.	z	P>|z|	[95% Conf. Interval]	
age	-.0066762	.0099457	-0.67	0.502	-.0261694	.0128171
female	1.401719	.3334931	4.20	0.000	.7480844	2.055354
_cons	3.336709	.4972641	6.71	0.000	2.362089	4.311329
/ln_sig	.0625872	.1256185	0.50	0.618	-.1836205	.3087949
/ln_the	-1.606248	1.190775	-1.35	0.177	-3.940125	.7276282
sigma	1.064587	.1337318			.8322516	1.361783
theta	.2006389	.2389159			.0194458	2.070165

Likelihood-ratio test of theta=0: chibar2(01) =   1.53 Prob>=chibar2 = 0.108

The frailty effect is insignificant at the 10% level in the latter model yet highly significant in the former. We thus have two possible stories to tell concerning these data: if we believe the first model, we believe that the individual hazard of infection continually rises over time (Weibull), but there is a significant frailty effect causing the population hazard to begin falling after some time. If we believe the second model, we believe that the individual hazard first rises and then declines (lognormal), meaning that if a given insertion does not become infected initially, the chances that it will become infected begin to decrease after a certain point. Since the frailty effect is insignificant, the population hazard mirrors the individual hazard in the second model.

As a result, both models view the population hazard as rising initially and then falling past a certain point. The second version of our story corresponds to higher log likelihood, yet perhaps not significantly higher given the limited data. More investigation is required. One idea is to fit a more distribution-agnostic form of a frailty model, such as a piecewise exponential (Cleves, Gould, and Gutierrez, 2004, 296–298) or a Cox model with frailty; see [ST] **stcox**.

◁

Shared-frailty models are also appropriate when the frailties are subject specific yet there exist multiple records per subject. Here you would share frailties across the same id() variable previously stset. When you have subject-specific frailties and uninformative episode splitting, it makes no difference whether you fit a shared or an unshared frailty model. The estimation results will be the same. However, there is a distinction between unshared- and shared-frailty models for single-record-per-subject data with delayed entry; see Gutierrez (2002) for details.

Saved Results

streg saves the following in e():

Scalars

e(N)	number of observations	e(p_c)	significance, comparison model
e(N_sub)	number of subjects	e(chi2)	χ^2
e(N_fail)	number of failures	e(N_g)	number of groups
e(k)	number of parameters	e(g_max)	largest group size
e(k_eq)	number of equations	e(g_min)	smallest group size
e(k_eq_model)	number of equations in model Wald test	e(g_avg)	average group size
		e(p)	significance
e(k_aux)	number of auxiliary parameters	e(aux_p)	ancillary parameter (weibull)
e(k_dv)	number of dependent variables	e(gamma)	ancillary parameter (gompertz, loglogistic)
e(rank)	rank of e(V)	e(sigma)	ancillary parameter (gamma, lnormal)
e(rank0)	rank of e(V), constant-only model		
e(risk)	total time at risk	e(kappa)	ancillary parameter (gamma)
e(df_m)	model degrees of freedom	e(ll_c)	log likelihood, comparison model
e(ll)	log likelihood	e(ic)	number of iterations
e(ll_0)	log likelihood, constant-only model	e(rc)	return code
e(N_clust)	number of clusters	e(converged)	1 if converged, 0 otherwise
e(theta)	frailty parameter		
e(chi2_c)	χ^2, comparison model		

Macros

e(cmd)	model or regression name	e(frm2)	hazard or time
e(cmd2)	streg	e(chi2type)	Wald or LR; type of model χ^2 test
e(cmdline)	command as typed	e(offset1)	offset for main equation
e(dead)	_d	e(stcurve)	stcurve
e(depvar)	_t	e(diparm#)	display transformed parameter #
e(title)	title in estimation output	e(opt)	type of optimization
e(title2)	secondary title in estimation output	e(ml_method)	type of ml method
e(clustvar)	name of cluster variable	e(user)	name of likelihood-evaluator program
e(shared)	frailty grouping variable		
e(fr_title)	title in output identifying frailty	e(technique)	maximization technique
e(wtype)	weight type	e(crittype)	optimization criterion
e(wexp)	weight expression	e(properties)	b V
e(t0)	_t0	e(footnote)	program used to implement the footnote display
e(vce)	*vcetype* specified in vce()		
e(vcetype)	title used to label Std. Err.	e(predict)	program used to implement predict

Matrices

e(b)	coefficient vector	e(V)	variance–covariance matrix of the estimators
e(ilog)	iteration log (up to 20 iterations)		
e(gradient)	gradient vector		

Functions

e(sample)	marks estimation sample

Methods and Formulas

streg is implemented as an ado-file.

For an introduction to survival models, see Cleves, Gould, and Gutierrez (2004). For an introduction to survival analysis directed at social scientists, see Box-Steffensmeier and Jones (2004).

Consider for $j = 1, \ldots, n$ observations the trivariate response, (t_{0j}, t_j, d_j), representing a period of observation $(t_{0j}, t_j]$ ending in either failure ($d_j = 1$) or right-censoring ($d_j = 0$). This structure allows analysis of a wide variety of models and may be used to account for delayed entry, gaps, time-varying covariates, and multiple failures per subject. Regardless of the structure of the data, once they are stset, the data may be treated in a common manner by streg: the stset-created variable _t0 holds the t_{0j}, _t holds the t_j, and _d holds the d_j.

For a given survivor function, $S(t)$, the density function is obtained as

$$f(t) = -\frac{d}{dt} S(t)$$

and the hazard function (the instantaneous rate of failure) is obtained as $h(t) = f(t)/S(t)$. Available forms for $S(t)$ are listed in table 1. For a set of covariates from the jth observation, $\mathbf{x}_j$, define $S_j(t) = S(t|\mathbf{x} = \mathbf{x}_j)$, and similarly define $h_j(t)$ and $f_j(t)$. For example, in a Weibull PH model, $S_j(t) = \exp\{-\exp(\mathbf{x}_j\boldsymbol{\beta})t^p\}$.

Parameter estimation

In this command, $\boldsymbol{\beta}$ and the ancillary parameters are estimated via maximum likelihood. A subject known to fail at time t_j contributes to the likelihood function the value of the density at time t_j conditional on the entry time t_{0j}, $f_j(t_j)/S_j(t_{0j})$. A censored observation, known to survive only up to time t_j, contributes $S_j(t_j)/S_j(t_{0j})$, which is the probability of surviving beyond time t_j conditional on the entry time t_{0j}. The log likelihood is thus given by

$$\ln L = \sum_{j=1}^{n} \{d_j \ln f_j(t_j) + (1 - d_j) \ln S_j(t_j) - \ln S_j(t_{0j})\}$$

Implicit in the above log-likelihood expression are the regression parameters $\boldsymbol{\beta}$ and the ancillary parameters since both are components of the chosen $S_j(t)$ and its corresponding $f_j(t)$; see table 1. streg reports maximum likelihood estimates of $\boldsymbol{\beta}$ and of the ancillary parameters (if any for the chosen model). The reported log-likelihood value is $\ln L_r = \ln L + T$, where $T = \sum \ln(t_j)$ is summed over uncensored observations. This adjustment is made so that reported results match those of other statistical software. The adjustment removes the time units from $\ln L$. Whether the adjustment is made makes no difference to any test or result since such tests and results depend on differences in log-likelihood functions and/or their second derivatives.

Specifying ancillary(), anc2(), or strata() will parameterize the ancillary parameter(s) by using the linear predictor, $\mathbf{z}_j\boldsymbol{\alpha}_z$, where the covariates, $\mathbf{z}_j$, need not be distinct from $\mathbf{x}_j$. Here streg will report estimates of $\boldsymbol{\alpha}_z$ in addition to estimates of $\boldsymbol{\beta}$. The log likelihood here is simply the log likelihood given above, with $\mathbf{z}_j\boldsymbol{\alpha}_z$ substituted for the ancillary parameter. If the ancillary parameter is constrained to be strictly positive, its logarithm is parameterized instead; i.e., we substitute the linear predictor for the logarithm of the ancillary parameter in the above log likelihood. The gamma model has two ancillary parameters, σ and κ; we parameterize σ by using ancillary() and κ by using anc2(), and the linear predictors used for each may be distinct. Specifying strata() creates indicator variables for the strata, places these indicators in the main equation, and uses the indicators to parameterize any ancillary parameters that exist for the chosen model.

Unshared-frailty models have a log likelihood of the above form, with $S_\theta(t)$ and $f_\theta(t)$ substituted for $S(t)$ and $f(t)$, respectively. Equivalently, for gamma-distributed frailties,

$$\ln L = \sum_{j=1}^{n} \left[\theta^{-1} \ln \left\{ 1 - \theta \ln S_j(t_{0j}) \right\} - \left(\theta^{-1} + d_j \right) \ln \left\{ 1 - \theta \ln S_j(t_j) \right\} + d_j \ln h_j(t_j) \right]$$

and for inverse-Gaussian–distributed frailties,

$$\ln L = \sum_{j=1}^{n} \left[\theta^{-1} \left\{ 1 - 2\theta \ln S_j(t_{0j}) \right\}^{1/2} - \theta^{-1} \left\{ 1 - 2\theta \ln S_j(t_j) \right\}^{1/2} + \right.$$

$$\left. d_j \ln h_j(t_j) - \frac{1}{2} d_j \ln \left\{ 1 - 2\theta \ln S_j(t_j) \right\} \right]$$

In a shared-frailty model, the frailty is common to a group of observations. Thus to form an unconditional likelihood, the frailties must be integrated out at the group level. The data are organized as $i = 1, \ldots, n$ groups with the ith group comprising $j = 1, \ldots, n_i$ observations. The log likelihood is the sum of the log-likelihood contributions for each group. Define $D_i = \sum_j d_{ij}$ as the number of failures in the ith group. For gamma frailties, the log-likelihood contribution for the ith group is

$$\ln L_i = \sum_{j=1}^{n_i} d_{ij} \ln h_{ij}(t_{ij}) - (1/\theta + D_i) \ln \left\{ 1 - \theta \sum_{j=1}^{n_i} \ln \frac{S_{ij}(t_{ij})}{S_{ij}(t_{0ij})} \right\} +$$

$$D_i \ln \theta + \ln \Gamma(1/\theta + D_i) - \ln \Gamma(1/\theta)$$

For inverse-Gaussian frailties, define

$$C_i = \left\{ 1 - 2\theta \sum_{j=1}^{n_i} \ln \frac{S_{ij}(t_{ij})}{S_{ij}(t_{0ij})} \right\}^{-1/2}$$

The log-likelihood contribution for the ith group then becomes

$$\ln L_i = \theta^{-1}(1 - C_i^{-1}) + B(\theta C_i, D_i) + \sum_{j=1}^{n_i} d_{ij} \left\{ \ln h_{ij}(t_{ij}) + \ln C_i \right\}$$

The function $B(a, b)$ is related to the modified Bessel function of the third kind, commonly known as the BesselK function; see Wolfram (1996, 746). In particular,

$$B(a, b) = a^{-1} + \frac{1}{2} \left\{ \ln \left(\frac{2}{\pi} \right) - \ln a \right\} + \ln \text{BesselK} \left(\frac{1}{2} - b, a^{-1} \right)$$

For both unshared- and shared-frailty models, estimation of θ takes place jointly with the estimation of β and the ancillary parameters.

If the robust estimate of variance is requested, results are transformed as described in [U] **20.15 Obtaining robust variance estimates** and, in particular, in [P] **_robust**. If observations in the dataset represent repeated observations on the same subjects (that is, there are time-varying covariates), the assumption of independence of the observations is highly questionable, meaning that the conventional estimate of variance is not appropriate. We strongly advise that you use the vce(robust) and vce(cluster *clustvar*) options here. (streg knows to specify vce(cluster *clustvar*) if you specify vce(robust).) vce(robust) and vce(cluster *clustvar*) do not apply in shared-frailty models, where the correlation within groups is instead modeled directly.

References

Akaike, H. 1974. A new look at the statistical model identification. *IEEE Transaction and Automatic Control* AC-19: 716–723.

Box-Steffensmeier, J. M., and B. S. Jones. 2004. *Event History Modeling: A Guide for Social Scientists.* Cambridge: Cambridge University Press.

Cleves, M. A., W. W. Gould, and R. G. Gutierrez. 2004. *An Introduction to Survival Analysis Using Stata.* Rev. ed. College Station, TX: Stata Press.

Cox, D. R., and D. Oakes. 1984. *Analysis of Survival Data.* London: Chapman & Hall/CRC.

Crowder, M. J., A. C. Kimber, R. L. Smith, and T. J. Sweeting. 1991. *Statistical Analysis of Reliability Data.* London: Chapman & Hall/CRC.

Cui, J. 2005. Buckley–James method for analyzing censored data, with an application to a cardiovascular disease and an HIV/AIDS study. *Stata Journal* 5: 517–526.

Fisher, R. A., and L. H. C. Tippett. 1928. Limiting forms of the frequency distribution of the largest or smallest member of a sample. *Proceedings of the Cambridge Philosophical Society* 24: 180–190.

Gutierrez, R. G. 2002. Parametric frailty and shared frailty survival models. *Stata Journal* 2: 22–44.

Gutierrez, R. G., S. L. Carter, and D. M. Drukker. 2001. sg160: On boundary-value likelihood-ratio tests. *Stata Technical Bulletin* 60: 15–18. Reprinted in *Stata Technical Bulletin Reprints*, vol. 10, pp. 269–273.

Hooker, P. F. 1965. Benjamin Gompertz. *Journal of the Institute of Actuaries* 91: 203–212.

Hosmer, D. W., Jr., and S. Lemeshow. 1999. *Applied Survival Analysis: Regression Modeling of Time to Event Data.* New York: Wiley.

Hougaard, P. 1986. Survival models for heterogeneous populations derived from stable distributions. *Biometrika* 73: 387–396.

Kalbfleisch, J. D., and R. L. Prentice. 2002. *The Statistical Analysis of Failure Time Data.* 2nd ed. New York: Wiley.

Klein, J. P., and M. L. Moeschberger. 2003. *Survival Analysis: Techniques for Censored and Truncated Data.* 2nd ed. New York: Springer.

Lee, E. T., and J. W. Wang. 2003. *Statistical Methods for Survival Data Analysis.* 3rd ed. New York: Wiley.

McGilchrist, C. A., and C. W. Aisbett. 1991. Regression with frailty in survival analysis. *Biometrics* 47: 461–466.

Olshansky, S. J., and B. A. Carnes. 1997. Ever since Gompertz. *Demography* 34: 1–15.

Peto, R., and P. Lee. 1973. Weibull distributions for continuous-carcinogenesis experiments. *Biometrics* 29: 457–470.

Pike, M. C. 1966. A method of analysis of a certain class of experiments in carcinogenesis. *Biometrics* 22: 142–161.

Royston, P. 2006. Explained variation for survival models. *Stata Journal* 6: 83–96.

Schoenfeld, D. 1982. Partial residuals for the proportional hazards regression model. *Biometrika* 69: 239–241.

Scotto, M. G., and A. Tobias. 1998. sg83: Parameter estimation for the Gumbel distribution. *Stata Technical Bulletin* 43: 32–35. Reprinted in *Stata Technical Bulletin Reprints*, vol. 8, pp. 133–137.

———. 2000. sg146: Parameter estimation for the generalized extreme value distribution. *Stata Technical Bulletin* 56: 40–43. Reprinted in *Stata Technical Bulletin Reprints*, vol. 10, pp. 205–210.

Weibull, W. 1939. A statistical theory of the strength of materials. *Ingeniörs Vetenskaps Akademiens Handlingar*, no. 151. Stockholm: Generalstabens Litografiska Anstalts Förlag.

Wolfram, S. 1996. *The Mathematica Book.* 3rd ed. Champaign, IL: Wolfram Media.

Also See

[ST] **streg postestimation** — Postestimation tools for streg

[ST] **stcurve** — Plot survivor, hazard, or cumulative hazard function

[ST] **sts** — Generate, graph, list, and test the survivor and cumulative hazard functions

[ST] **stset** — Declare data to be survival-time data

[ST] **stcox** — Fit Cox proportional hazards model

[U] **20 Estimation and postestimation commands**

Title

Description

The following postestimation command is of special interest after `streg`:

command	description
stcurve	plots the survivor, hazard, and cumulative hazard functions

For information on `stcurve`, see [ST] **stcurve**.

The following standard postestimation commands are also available:

command	description
adjust	adjusted predictions of $\mathbf{x}\beta$ or $\exp(\mathbf{x}\beta)$
estat	AIC, BIC, VCE, and estimation sample summary
estat (svy)	postestimation statistics for survey data
estimates	cataloging estimation results
lincom	point estimates, standard errors, testing, and inference for linear combinations of coefficients
linktest	link test for model specification
lrtest[1]	likelihood-ratio test
mfx	marginal effects or elasticities
nlcom	point estimates, standard errors, testing, and inference for nonlinear combinations of coefficients
predict	predictions, residuals, influence statistics, and other diagnostic measures
predictnl	point estimates, standard errors, testing, and inference for generalized predictions
suest	seemingly unrelated estimation
test	Wald tests for simple and composite linear hypotheses
testnl	Wald tests of nonlinear hypotheses

[1] `lrtest` is not appropriate with `svy` estimation results.

See the corresponding entries in the *Stata Base Reference Manual* for details, but see [SVY] **estat** for details about `estat` (svy).

Special-interest postestimation command

`stcurve` is used after `streg` (or `stcox`) to plot the cumulative hazard, survivor, and hazard functions at the mean value of the covariates or at values specified by the `at()` options.

Syntax for predict

predict [*type*] *newvar* [*if*] [*in*] [, *statistic* oos <u>alpha1</u> <u>uncond</u>itional]

predict [*type*] { *stub** | *newvarlist* } [*if*] [*in*] , <u>sc</u>ores

statistic	description
Main	
<u>med</u>ian time	median survival time; the default
<u>med</u>ian <u>ln</u>time	median ln(survival time)
mean time	mean survival time
mean <u>ln</u>time	mean ln(survival time)
hazard	hazard
hr	hazard ratio, also known as the relative hazard
xb	linear prediction $\mathbf{x}_j\boldsymbol{\beta}$
stdp	standard error of the linear prediction; $\mathrm{SE}(\mathbf{x}_j\boldsymbol{\beta})$
<u>surv</u>	$S(t|t_0)$
csnell	(partial) Cox–Snell residuals
mgale	(partial) martingale-like residuals
*<u>deviance</u>	deviance residuals
*csurv	$S(t\,|\,\text{earliest } t_0 \text{ for subject})$
*ccsnell	cumulative Cox–Snell residuals
*cmgale	cumulative martingale-like residuals

Unstarred statistics are available both in and out of sample; type predict ... if e(sample) ... if wanted only for the estimation sample. Starred statistics are calculated for the estimation sample by default, but the oos option makes them available both in and out of sample.

When no option is specified, the predicted median survival time is calculated for all models. The predicted hazard ratio option hr is available only for the exponential, Weibull, and Gompertz models. The mean time and mean lntime options are not available for the Gompertz model. Unconditional estimates of mean time and mean lntime are not available when frailty() is specified.

Options for predict

> Main

median time calculates the predicted median survival time in analysis time units. This is the prediction from time 0 conditional on constant covariates. When no options are specified with predict, the predicted median survival time is calculated for all models.

median lntime calculates the natural logarithm of what median time produces.

mean time calculates the predicted mean survival time in analysis time units. This is the prediction from time 0 conditional on constant covariates. This option is not available for Gompertz regressions and is available only for frailty models if alpha1 is specified, in which case what you obtain is an estimate of the mean survival time conditional on a frailty effect of one.

mean lntime predicts the mean of the natural logarithm of time. This option is not available for Gompertz regression and is available only for frailty models if alpha1 is specified, in which case what you obtain is an estimate of the mean log-survival time conditional on a frailty effect of one.

hazard calculates the predicted hazard.

hr calculates the hazard ratio. This option is valid only for models having a proportional-hazards parameterization.

xb calculates the linear prediction from the fitted model. That is, you fit the model by estimating a set of parameters $\beta_0, \beta_1, \beta_2, \ldots, \beta_k$, and the linear prediction is $\widehat{y}_j = \widehat{\beta}_0 + \widehat{\beta}_1 x_{1j} + \widehat{\beta}_2 x_{2j} + \cdots + \widehat{\beta}_k x_{kj}$, often written in matrix notation as $\widehat{y}_j = \mathbf{x}_j \widehat{\boldsymbol{\beta}}$.

The $x_{1j}, x_{2j}, \ldots, x_{kj}$ used in the calculation are obtained from the data currently in memory and need not correspond to the data on the independent variables used in estimating β.

stdp calculates the standard error of the prediction, that is, the standard error of $\widehat{y}_j$.

surv calculates each observation's predicted survivor probability $S(t|t_0)$, where t_0 is _t0, the analysis time at which each record became at risk. For multiple-record data, see the csurv option below.

csnell calculates the (partial) Cox–Snell residual. If you have 1 observation per subject, csnell calculates the usual Cox–Snell residual. Otherwise, csnell calculates the additive contribution of this observation to the subject's overall Cox–Snell residual.

mgale calculates the (partial) martingale-like residual. The issues are the same as with csnell above.

deviance calculates the deviance residual. For multiple-record data, only one value per subject is calculated, and it is placed on the last record for the subject.

csurv calculates the predicted $S(t|\text{earliest } t_0)$ for each subject in multiple-record data by calculating the conditional survivor values $S(t|t_0)$ (see option surv above) and then multiplying them together.

What you obtain from surv will differ from what you obtain from csurv only if you have multiple records for that subject and delayed entry, gaps, or time-varying covariates.

ccsnell calculates the (cumulative) Cox–Snell residual in multiple-record data by calculating the partial Cox–Snell residuals (see option csnell above) and then summing them. Only one value per subject is recorded—the overall sum—and it is placed on the last record for the subject.

cmgale calculates the (cumulative) martingale-like residual in multiple-record data. This is based on calculating the partial martingale-like residuals (see option mgale above) and then summing them. Only one value per subject is recorded—the overall sum—and it is placed on the last record for the subject.

oos makes deviance, csurv, ccsnell, and cmgale available both in and out of sample.

alpha1, when used after fitting a frailty model, specifies that *statistic* be predicted conditional on a frailty value equal to one. This is the default for shared-frailty models.

unconditional, when used after fitting a frailty model, specifies that *statistic* be predicted unconditional on the frailty. That is, the prediction is averaged over the frailty distribution. This is the default for unshared-frailty models.

scores calculates equation-level score variables. The number of score variables created depends upon the chosen distribution.

The first new variable will always contain $\partial \ln L / \partial (\mathbf{x}_j \boldsymbol{\beta})$.

The subsequent new variables will contain the partial derivative of the log likelihood with respect to the ancillary parameters. For example, in the generalized gamma model, the second new variable will contain $\partial \ln L / \partial (\mathbf{z}_{1j} \boldsymbol{\sigma})$, and the third new variable will contain $\partial \ln L / \partial (\mathbf{z}_{2j} \boldsymbol{\kappa})$.

Remarks

predict after streg is used to generate a variable containing predicted values or residuals.

For a more detailed discussion on residuals, read *Cox regression residuals* in the [ST] **stcox** entry. Many of the concepts and ideas presented there also apply to streg models.

Regardless of the metric used, predict can generate predicted median survival times and median log-survival times for all models, and predicted mean times and mean log-survival times where available. Predicted survival, hazard, and residuals are also available for all models. The predicted hazard ratio can be calculated only for models with a proportional-hazards parameterization, i.e., the Weibull, exponential, and Gompertz models. However, the estimation need not take place in the log-hazard metric. You can perform, for example, a Weibull regression specifying the time option and then ask that hazard ratios be predicted.

After fitting a frailty model, you can use predict with the alpha1 option to generate predicted values based on $S(t)$ or use the unconditional option to generate predictions based on $S_\theta(t)$.

▷ Example 1

Let's return to example 1 of [ST] **streg** concerning the ability of emergency generators with new-style bearings to withstand overloads. Assume that, as before, we fit a proportional hazards Weibull model:

```
. use http://www.stata-press.com/data/r10/kva
(Generator experiment)
. streg load bearings, d(weibull) nolog
        failure _d:  1 (meaning all fail)
    analysis time _t:  failtime
Weibull regression -- log relative-hazard form
No. of subjects =          12                    Number of obs   =         12
No. of failures =          12
Time at risk    =         896
                                                 LR chi2(2)      =      30.27
Log likelihood  =     5.6934189                  Prob > chi2     =     0.0000
```

_t	Haz. Ratio	Std. Err.	z	P>|z|	[95% Conf. Interval]	
load	1.599315	.1883807	3.99	0.000	1.269616	2.014631
bearings	.1887995	.1312109	-2.40	0.016	.0483546	.7371644
/ln_p	2.051552	.2317074	8.85	0.000	1.597414	2.505691
p	7.779969	1.802677			4.940241	12.25202
1/p	.1285352	.0297826			.0816192	.2024193

Now we can predict both the median survival time and the log-median survival time for each observation:

```
. predict time, time
(option median time assumed; predicted median time)
. predict lntime, lntime
(option log median time assumed; predicted median log time)
. format time lntime %9.4f
```

```
. list failtime load bearings time lntime
```

	failtime	load	bearings	time	lntime
1.	100	15	0	127.5586	4.8486
2.	140	15	1	158.0407	5.0629
3.	97	20	0	94.3292	4.5468
4.	122	20	1	116.8707	4.7611
5.	84	25	0	69.7562	4.2450
6.	100	25	1	86.4255	4.4593
7.	54	30	0	51.5845	3.9432
8.	52	30	1	63.9114	4.1575
9.	40	35	0	38.1466	3.6414
10.	55	35	1	47.2623	3.8557
11.	22	40	0	28.2093	3.3397
12.	30	40	1	34.9504	3.5539

◁

▷ Example 2

Using the cancer data of example 6 in [ST] **streg**, again with `drug` remapped into a drug-treatment indicator, we can examine the various residuals that Stata produces. For a more detailed discussion on residuals, read *Cox regression residuals* in the [ST] **stcox** entry. Many of the concepts and ideas presented there also apply to **streg** models. For a more technical presentation of these residuals, see *Methods and Formulas.*

We will begin by requesting the generalized Cox–Snell residuals with the command `predict cs, csnell`. The `csnell` option causes `predict` to create a new variable, cs, containing the Cox–Snell residuals. If the model fits the data, these residuals should have a standard exponential distribution with $\lambda = 1$. One way to verify the fit is to calculate an empirical estimate of the cumulative hazard function—based, for example, on the Kaplan–Meier survival estimates or the Aalen–Nelson estimator, taking the Cox–Snell residuals as the time variable and the censoring variable as before—and plotting it against cs. If the model fits the data, the plot should be a straight line with a slope of 1.

To do this after fitting the model, we first `stset` the data, specifying cs as our new failure-time variable and `died` as the failure indicator. We then use the `sts generate` command to generate the variable km containing the Kaplan–Meier survival estimates. Last, we generate a new variable H (cumulative hazard) and plot it against the cs. The commands are

```
. use http://www.stata-press.com/data/r10/cancer, clear
(Patient Survival in Drug Trial)
. replace drug = drug==2 | drug==3          // 0, placebo : 1, nonplacebo
(48 real changes made)
. stset studytime, failure(died)
 (output omitted )
. qui streg age drug, d(exp)
. predict double cs, csnell
. qui stset cs, failure(died)
. qui sts generate km=s
. qui generate double H=-ln(km)
. line H cs cs, sort
```

We specified cs twice in the graph command so that a reference 45° line was plotted. We did this separately for each of four distributions. Results are plotted in figure 1:

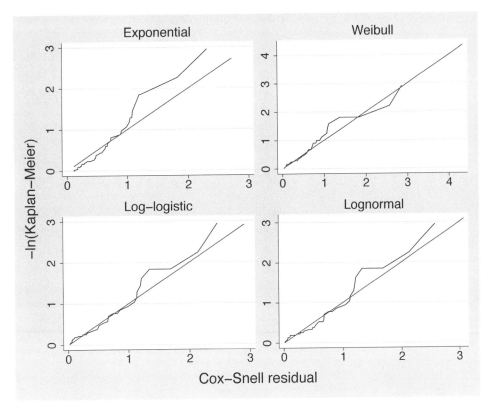

Figure 1. Cox–Snell residuals to evaluate model fit of four regression models

The plots indicate that the Weibull and lognormal models fit the data best and that the exponential model fits poorly. These results are consistent with our previous results based on Akaike's information criterion.

◁

▷ Example 3

Let's now look at the martingale-like and deviance residuals. We use the term "martingale-like" because, although these residuals do not arise naturally from martingale theory for parametric survival models as they do for the Cox proportional hazards model, they do share similar form. We can generate these residuals by using predict's mgale option. Martingale residuals take values between $-\infty$ and 1 and therefore are difficult to interpret. The deviance residuals are a rescaling of the martingale-like residuals so that they are symmetric about zero and thus more like residuals obtained from linear regression. Plots of either deviance residuals against the linear predictor (i.e., the log-relative hazard in PH models) or of deviance residuals against individual predictors can be useful in identifying aberrant observations and in assessing model fit. Continuing with our modified cancer data, we plot the deviance residual obtained after fitting a lognormal model:

```
. qui streg age drug, d(lnormal)
. predict dev, deviance
. scatter dev studytime, yline(0) m(o)
```

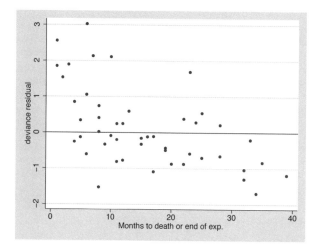

Figure 2. Deviance residuals to evaluate model fit of lognormal model

This plot shows the deviance residuals to be relatively well behaved.

◁

Methods and Formulas

All postestimation commands listed above are implemented as ado-files.

predict *newvar*, *options* may be used after streg to predict various quantities, according to the following *options*:

median time:
$$newvar_j = \{t : \widehat{S}_j(t) = 1/2\}$$

where $\widehat{S}_j(t)$ is $S_j(t)$ with the parameter estimates "plugged in".

median lntime:
$$newvar_j = \left\{y : \widehat{S}_j(e^y) = 1/2\right\}$$

mean time:
$$newvar_j = \int_0^\infty \widehat{S}_j(t)dt$$

mean lntime:
$$newvar_j = \int_{-\infty}^\infty y e^y \widehat{f}_j(e^y)dy$$

where $\widehat{f}_j(t)$ is $f_j(t)$ with the parameter estimates plugged in.

`hazard`:

$$newvar_j = \widehat{f}_j(t_j)/\widehat{S}_j(t_j)$$

`hr` (PH models only):

$$newvar_j = \exp(\mathbf{x}_j\widehat{\boldsymbol{\beta}})$$

`xb`:

$$newvar_j = \mathbf{x}_j\widehat{\boldsymbol{\beta}}$$

`stdp`:

$$newvar_j = \widehat{se}(\mathbf{x}_j\widehat{\boldsymbol{\beta}})$$

`surv` and `csurv`:

$$newvar_j = \widehat{S}_j(t_j)/\widehat{S}_j(t_{0j})$$

The above represents the probability of survival past time t_j given survival up until t_{0j} and represents what you obtain when you specify `surv`. If `csurv` is specified, these probabilities are multiplied (in time order) over a subject's multiple observations. What is obtained is then equal to the probability of survival past time t_j, given survival through the earliest observed t_{0j}, and given the subject's (possibly time-varying) covariate history. In single-record-per-subject data, `surv` and `csurv` are identical.

`csnell` and `ccsnell`:

$$newvar_j = -\ln\widehat{S}_j(t_j)$$

The Cox–Snell (1968) residual CS_j for observation j at time t_j is defined as $\widehat{H}_j(t_j) = -\ln\widehat{S}_j(t_j)$, which is the estimated cumulative hazard function obtained from the fitted model (Collett 2003, 111–112). Cox and Snell argued that if the correct model has been fitted to the data, these residuals are n observations from an exponential distribution with unit mean. Thus a plot of the cumulative hazard rate of the residuals against the residuals themselves should result in a straight line of slope 1. Cox–Snell residuals can never be negative and therefore are not symmetric about zero. The option `csnell` stores in each observation that observation's contribution to the subject's Cox–Snell residual, which we refer to as a partial Cox–Snell residual. The option `ccsnell` stores the subject's overall Cox–Snell residual in the last observation for that subject. If there is only 1 observation per subject, the Cox–Snell residuals stored by `ccsnell` and `csnell` are equal.

`mgale` and `cmgale`:

$$newvar_j = d_j - CS_j$$

Martingale residuals follows naturally from martingale theory for Cox proportional hazards, but their development does not carry over for parametric survival models. However, martingale-like residuals similar to those obtained for Cox can be derived from the Cox–Snell residuals: $M_j = d_j - CS_j$ where CS_j are the Cox–Snell residuals, as previously described.

Because martingale-like residuals are calculated from the Cox–Snell residuals, they also could be partial or not. Partial martingale residuals are generated with the option `mgale`, and overall martingale residuals are generated with the option `cmgale`.

Martingale residuals can be interpreted as the difference over time between the number of deaths in the data and the expected number from the fitted model. These residuals take values between $-\infty$ and 1 and have an expected value of zero, although like the Cox–Snell residuals, they are not symmetric about zero, making them difficult to interpret.

deviance:

$$newvar_j = \text{sign}(M_j)\left(-2\left\{M_j + d_j \ln(d_j - M_j)\right\}\right)$$

Deviance residuals are a scaling of the martingale-like residuals in an attempt to make them symmetric about zero. When the model fits the data, these residuals are symmetric about zero and thus can be more readily used to examine the data for outliers.

predict also allows two options for use after fitting frailty models: alpha1 and unconditional. If unconditional is specified, the above predictions are modified to be based on $S_\theta(t)$ and $f_\theta(t)$, rather than $S(t)$ and $f(t)$. If alpha1 is specified, the predictions are as described above.

References

Collett, D. 2003. *Modelling Survival Data in Medical Research.* 2nd ed. London: Chapman & Hall/CRC.

Cox, D. R., and E. J. Snell. 1968. A general definition of residuals (with discussion). *Journal of the Royal Statistical Society, Series B* 30: 248–275.

Also See

[ST] **streg** — Fit parametric survival models

[ST] **stcurve** — Plot survivor, hazard, or cumulative hazard function

[U] **20 Estimation and postestimation commands**

Title

sts — Generate, graph, list, and test the survivor and cumulative hazard functions

Syntax

sts [graph] [*if*] [*in*] [, ...]

sts list [*if*] [*in*] [, ...]

sts test *varlist* [*if*] [*in*] [, ...]

sts generate *newvar* = ... [*if*] [*in*] [, ...]

You must stset your data before using sts; see [ST] **stset**.

fweights, iweights, and pweights may be specified using stset; see [ST] **stset**.

See [ST] **sts graph**, [ST] **sts list**, [ST] **sts test**, and [ST] **sts generate** for details of syntax.

Description

sts reports and creates variables containing the estimated survivor and related functions, such as the Nelson–Aalen cumulative hazard function. For the survivor function, sts tests and produces Kaplan–Meier estimates or, via Cox regression, adjusted estimates.

sts graph is equivalent to typing sts by itself—it graphs the survivor function.

sts list lists the estimated survivor and related functions.

sts test tests the equality of the survivor function across groups.

sts generate creates new variables containing the estimated survivor function, the Nelson–Aalen cumulative hazard function, or related functions.

sts can be used with single- or multiple-record or single- or multiple-failure st data.

▷ Example 1

```
. use http://www.stata-press.com/data/r10/drugtr
```

Graph the Kaplan–Meier survivor function
```
. sts graph
. sts graph, by(drug)
```

Graph the Nelson–Aalen cumulative hazard function
```
. sts graph, cumhaz
. sts graph, cumhaz by(drug)
```

Graph the estimated hazard function
```
. sts graph, hazard
. sts graph, hazard by(drug)
```

List the Kaplan–Meier survivor function
```
. sts list
. sts list, by(drug) compare
```

List the Nelson–Aalen cumulative hazard function
```
. sts list, cumhaz
. sts list, cumhaz by(drug) compare
```

Generate variable containing the Kaplan–Meier survivor function	. sts gen surv = s
	. sts gen surv_by_drug = s, by(drug)
Generate variable containing the Nelson–Aalen cumulative hazard function	. sts gen haz = na
	. sts gen haz_by_drug = na, by(drug)
Test equality of survivor functions	. sts test drug
	. gen agecat = autocode(age,4,47,67)
	. sts test drug, strata(agecat)

◁

Remarks

Remarks are presented under the following headings:

> Listing, graphing, and generating variables
> Comparing survivor or cumulative hazard functions
> Testing equality of survivor functions
> Adjusted estimates
> Counting the number lost due to censoring

sts concerns the survivor function $S(t)$, the probability of surviving to t or beyond, the cumulative hazard function $H(t)$, and the hazard function $h(t)$. Its subcommands can list and generate variables containing $\widehat{S}(t)$ and $\widehat{H}(t)$ and test the equality of $S(t)$ over groups. Also:

1. All subcommands share a common syntax.

2. All subcommands deal with either the Kaplan–Meier product-limit or the Nelson–Aalen estimates unless you request adjusted survival estimates.

3. If you request an adjustment, all subcommands perform the adjustment in the same way, which is described below.

The full details of each subcommand are found in the entries following this one, but each subcommand provides so many options to control exactly how the listing looks, how the graph appears, the form of the test to be performed, or what exactly is to be generated, that the simplicity of sts can be easily overlooked.

So, without getting burdened by the details of syntax, let us demonstrate the sts commands by using the Stanford heart transplant data introduced in [ST] **stset**.

Listing, graphing, and generating variables

You can list the overall survivor function by typing sts list, and you can graph it by typing sts graph or sts. sts assumes that you mean graph when you do not type a subcommand.

Or, you can list the Nelson–Aalen cumulative hazard function by typing sts list, cumhaz, and you can graph it by typing sts graph, cumhaz.

When you type sts list, you are shown all the details:

```
. use http://www.stata-press.com/data/r10/stan3
(Heart transplant data)
. stset, noshow
```

```
. sts list
```

Time	Beg. Total	Fail	Net Lost	Survivor Function	Std. Error	[95% Conf. Int.]	
1	103	1	0	0.9903	0.0097	0.9331	0.9986
2	102	3	0	0.9612	0.0190	0.8998	0.9852
3	99	3	0	0.9320	0.0248	0.8627	0.9670
5	96	1	0	0.9223	0.0264	0.8507	0.9604
(output omitted)							
1586	2	0	1	0.1519	0.0493	0.0713	0.2606
1799	1	0	1	0.1519	0.0493	0.0713	0.2606

When you type `sts graph` or just `sts`, you are shown a graph of the same result detailed by `list`:

```
. sts graph
```

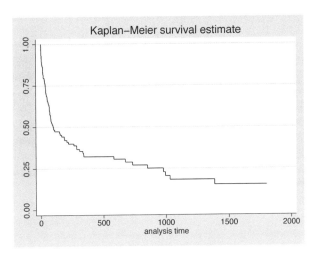

sts generate is a rarely used command. Typing `sts generate survf = s` creates a new variable `survf` containing the same survivor function that `list` just listed and `graph` just graphed:

```
. sts gen survf = s
. sort t1
. list t1 survf in 1/10
```

	t1	survf
1.	1	.99029126
2.	1	.99029126
3.	1	.99029126
4.	1	.99029126
5.	2	.96116505
6.	2	.96116505
7.	2	.96116505
8.	2	.96116505
9.	2	.96116505
10.	2	.96116505

sts generate is provided if you want to make a calculation, listing, or graph that sts cannot already do for you.

Comparing survivor or cumulative hazard functions

sts allows you to compare survivor or cumulative hazard functions. sts graph and sts graph, cumhaz are probably most successful at this. For example, survivor functions can be plotted using

. sts graph, by(posttran)

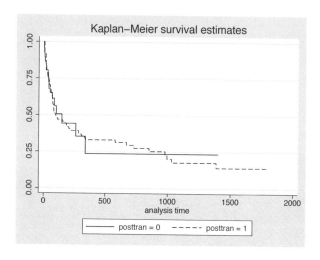

and Nelson–Aalen cumulative hazard functions can be plotted using

. sts graph, cumhaz by(posttran)

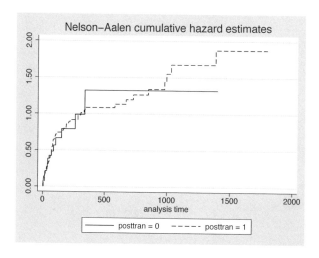

To compare survivor functions, we typed sts graph, just as before, and then we added by(posttran) to see the survivor functions for the groups designated by posttran. Here there are two groups, but as far as the sts command is concerned, there could have been more. cumhaz was also added to compare cumulative hazard functions.

You can also plot and compare estimated hazard functions by using sts graph, hazard. The hazard is estimated as a kernel smooth of the increments that sum to form the estimated cumulative hazard. The increments themselves do not estimate the hazard, but the smooth is weighted so that it estimates the hazard; see [ST] **sts graph**.

Just as you can compare survivor functions graphically by typing sts graph, by(posttran) and cumulative hazard functions by typing sts graph, cumhaz by(posttran), you can obtain detailed listings by typing sts list, by(posttran) and sts list, cumhaz by(posttran), respectively. Below we list the survivor function and specify enter, which adds a number-who-enter column:

```
. sts list, by(posttran) enter
```

Time	Beg. Total	Fail	Lost	Enter	Survivor Function	Std. Error	[95% Conf. Int.]	
posttran=0								
0	0	0	0	103	1.0000	.	.	.
1	103	1	3	0	0.9903	0.0097	0.9331	0.9986
2	99	3	3	0	0.9603	0.0195	0.8976	0.9849
(output omitted)								
427	2	0	1	0	0.2359	0.1217	0.0545	0.4882
1400	1	0	1	0	0.2359	0.1217	0.0545	0.4882
posttran=1								
1	0	0	0	3	1.0000	.	.	.
2	3	0	0	3	1.0000	.	.	.
3	6	0	0	3	1.0000	.	.	.
4	9	0	0	2	1.0000	.	.	.
5	11	0	0	3	1.0000	.	.	.
5.1	14	1	0	0	0.9286	0.0688	0.5908	0.9896
6	13	0	0	1	0.9286	0.0688	0.5908	0.9896
8	14	0	0	2	0.9286	0.0688	0.5908	0.9896
10	16	0	0	2	0.9286	0.0688	0.5908	0.9896
(output omitted)								
1586	2	0	1	0	0.1420	0.0546	0.0566	0.2653
1799	1	0	1	0	0.1420	0.0546	0.0566	0.2653

sts list's compare option allows you to compare survivor or cumulative hazard functions by listing the groups side by side.

```
. sts list, by(posttran) compare
```

posttran	Survivor Function 0	1
time 1	0.9903	1.0000
225	0.4422	0.3934
449	0.2359	0.3304
673	0.2359	0.3139
897	0.2359	0.2535
1121	0.2359	0.1774
1345	0.2359	0.1774
1569	.	0.1420
1793	.	0.1420
2017	.	.

If we include the `cumhaz` option, the cumulative hazard functions are listed:

```
. sts list, cumhaz by(posttran) compare
                Nelson-Aalen Cum. Haz.
    posttran              0           1

    time       1      0.0097      0.0000
             225      0.7896      0.9145
             449      1.3229      1.0850
             673      1.3229      1.1350
             897      1.3229      1.3411
            1121      1.3229      1.6772
            1345      1.3229      1.6772
            1569           .      1.8772
            1793           .      1.8772
            2017           .           .
```

When you specify `compare`, the same detailed survivor or cumulative hazard function is calculated, but it is then evaluated at 10 or so given times, and those evaluations are listed. Above we left it to `sts list` to choose the comparison times, but we can specify them ourselves with the `at()` option:

```
. sts list, by(posttran) compare at(0 100 to 1700)
                  Survivor Function
    posttran            0           1

    time       0     1.0000      1.0000
             100     0.5616      0.4814
             200     0.4422      0.4184
             300     0.3538      0.3680
             400     0.2359      0.3304
             500     0.2359      0.3304
             600     0.2359      0.3139
             700     0.2359      0.2942
             800     0.2359      0.2746
             900     0.2359      0.2535
            1000     0.2359      0.2028
            1100     0.2359      0.1774
            1200     0.2359      0.1774
            1300     0.2359      0.1774
            1400     0.2359      0.1420
            1500          .      0.1420
            1600          .      0.1420
            1700          .      0.1420
```

Testing equality of survivor functions

`sts test` tests equality of survivor functions:

```
. sts test posttran
```

Log-rank test for equality of survivor functions

posttran	Events observed	Events expected
0	30	31.20
1	45	43.80
Total	75	75.00

```
                chi2(1)  =      0.13
                Pr>chi2  =    0.7225
```

When you do not specify otherwise, `sts test` performs the log-rank test, but it can also perform the Wilcoxon test:

```
. sts test posttran, wilcoxon
```

Wilcoxon (Breslow) test for equality of survivor functions

posttran	Events observed	Events expected	Sum of ranks
0	30	31.20	-85
1	45	43.80	85
Total	75	75.00	0

```
          chi2(1) =     0.14
          Pr>chi2 =   0.7083
```

`sts test` also performs stratified tests; see [ST] **sts test**.

Adjusted estimates

All the estimates of the survivor function we have seen so far are the Kaplan–Meier product-limit estimates. `sts` can make adjusted estimates to the survivor function. We want to illustrate this and explain how it is done.

The heart transplant dataset is not the best for demonstrating this feature because we are starting with survivor functions that are similar already, so let us switch to data on a fictional drug trial:

```
. use http://www.stata-press.com/data/r10/drug2, clear
(Patient Survival in Drug Trial)
. stset, noshow
. stdescribe
```

Category	total	mean	min	median	max
			per subject		
no. of subjects	48				
no. of records	48	1	1	1	1
(first) entry time		0	0	0	0
(final) exit time		15.5	1	12.5	39
subjects with gap	0				
time on gap if gap	0				
time at risk	744	15.5	1	12.5	39
failures	31	.6458333	0	1	1

This dataset contains 48 subjects, all observed from time 0. The `st` command shows us how the dataset is currently declared:

```
. st
-> stset studytime, failure(died) noshow
       failure event:  died != 0 & died < .
  obs. time interval:  (0, studytime]
   exit on or before:  failure
```

The dataset contains variables `age` and `drug`:

```
. summarize age drug
```

Variable	Obs	Mean	Std. Dev.	Min	Max
age	48	47.125	9.492718	32	67
drug	48	.5833333	.4982238	0	1

We are comparing the outcomes of drug = 1 with that of the placebo, drug = 0. Here are the survivor curves for the two groups:

```
. sts graph, by(drug)
```

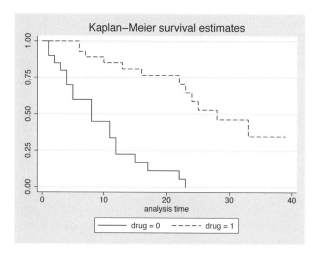

Here are the survivor curves adjusted for age (and scaled to age 50):

```
. generate age50 = age-50
. sts graph, by(drug) adjustfor(age50)
```

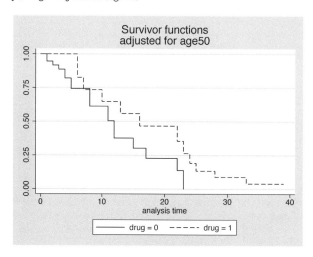

The age difference between the two samples accounts for much of the difference between the survivor functions.

When you type by(*group*) adjustfor(*vars*), sts fits a separate Cox proportional hazards model on *vars* (estimation via stcox) and retrieves the separately estimated baseline survivor functions. sts graph graphs the baseline survivor functions, sts list lists them, and sts generate saves them.

Thus `sts list` can list what `sts graph` plots:

```
. sts list, by(drug) adjustfor(age50) compare
          Adjusted Survivor Function
drug                    0          1

time        1      0.9463     1.0000
            5      0.7439     1.0000
            9      0.6135     0.7358
           13      0.3770     0.5588
           17      0.2282     0.4668
           21      0.2282     0.4668
           25         .       0.1342
           29         .       0.0872
           33         .       0.0388
           37         .       0.0388
           41         .          .

Survivor function adjusted for age50
```

In both the graph and the listing, we must adjust for variable $age50 = age - 50$ and not just age. Adjusted survivor functions are adjusted to the `adjustfor()` variables and scaled to correspond to the `adjustfor()` variables set to 0. Here is the result of adjusting for age, which is 0 at birth:

```
. sts list, by(drug) adjustfor(age) compare
          Adjusted Survivor Function
drug                    0          1

time        1      0.9994     1.0000
            5      0.9970     1.0000
            9      0.9951     0.9995
           13      0.9903     0.9990
           17      0.9853     0.9987
           21      0.9853     0.9987
           25         .       0.9965
           29         .       0.9958
           33         .       0.9944
           37         .       0.9944
           41         .          .

Survivor function adjusted for age
```

These are equivalent to what we obtained previously but not nearly so informative because of the scaling of the survivor function. Option `adjustfor(age)` scales the survivor function to correspond to $age = 0$. age is calendar age, so the survivor function is scaled to correspond to a newborn.

There is another way that `sts` will adjust the survivor function. Rather than specifying by(*group*) adjustfor(*vars*), we can specify strata(*group*) adjustfor(*vars*):

(Continued on next page)

```
. sts list, strata(drug) adjustfor(age50) compare
```

| | | Adjusted Survivor Function | |
drug		0	1
time	1	0.9526	1.0000
	5	0.7668	1.0000
	9	0.6417	0.7626
	13	0.4080	0.5995
	17	0.2541	0.5139
	21	0.2541	0.5139
	25	.	0.1800
	29	.	0.1247
	33	.	0.0614
	37	.	0.0614
	41	.	.

Survivor function adjusted for age50

When we specify `strata()` instead of `by()`, instead of fitting separate Cox models for each stratum, `sts list` fits one stratified Cox model and retrieves the stratified baseline survivor function. That is, `strata()` rather than `by()` constrains the effect of the `adjustfor()` variables to be the same across strata.

Counting the number lost due to censoring

`sts list`, in the detailed output, shows the number lost in the fourth column:

```
. sts list
```

Time	Beg. Total	Fail	Net Lost	Survivor Function	Std. Error	[95% Conf. Int.]	
1	48	2	0	0.9583	0.0288	0.8435	0.9894
2	46	1	0	0.9375	0.0349	0.8186	0.9794
3	45	1	0	0.9167	0.0399	0.7930	0.9679
(output omitted)							
8	36	3	1	0.7061	0.0661	0.5546	0.8143
9	32	0	1	0.7061	0.0661	0.5546	0.8143
10	31	1	1	0.6833	0.0678	0.5302	0.7957
(output omitted)							
39	1	0	1	0.1918	0.0791	0.0676	0.3634

`sts graph`, if you specify the `lost` option, will show that number, too:

```
. sts graph, lost
```

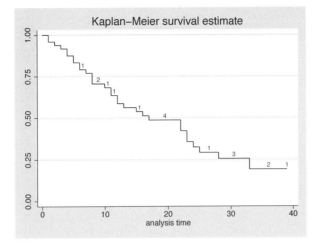

The number on the listing and on the graph is the number of net lost, defined as the number of censored minus the number who enter. With simple survival data—with 1 observation per subject—net lost corresponds to lost.

With more complicated survival data—meaning delayed entry or multiple records per subject—the number of net lost may surprise you. With complicated data, the vague term *lost* can mean many things. Sometimes subjects are lost, but mostly there are many censorings followed by reentries—a subject is censored at time 5 immediately to reenter the data with different covariates. This is called thrashing.

There are other possibilities: a subject can be lost, but only for a while, and so reenter the data with a gap; a subject can be censored out of one stratum to enter another. There are too many possibilities to dedicate a column in a table or a plotting symbol in a graph to each one. sts's solution is to define *lost* as *net lost*, meaning censored minus entered, and show that number. How we define *lost* does not affect the calculation of the survivor function; it merely affects a number that researchers often report.

Defining lost as censored minus entered results in exactly what is desired for simple survival data. Since everybody enters at time 0, calculating censored-minus-entered amounts to calculating censored − 0. The number of net lost is the number of censored.

In more complicated data, calculating censored-minus-entered results in the number really lost if there are no gaps and no delayed entry. Then the subtraction smooths the thrashing. In an interval, five might be censored and three reenter, so $5 - 3 = 2$ were lost.

In even more complicated data, calculating censored minus entered results in something reasonable once you understand how to interpret negative numbers and are cautious in interpreting positive ones. Five might be censored and three might enter (from the five? who can say?), resulting in two net lost; or three might be censored and five enter, resulting in -2 being lost.

sts, by default, reports the net lost but will, if you specify the enter option, report the pure number censored and the pure number who enter. Sometimes you will want to do that. Earlier in this entry, we used sts list to display the survivor functions in the Stanford heart transplant data for subjects pre- and posttransplantation, and we slipped in an enter option:

```
. use http://www.stata-press.com/data/r10/stan3, clear
(Heart transplant data)
```

```
. stset, noshow

. sts list, by(posttran) enter
```

	Beg.				Survivor	Std.		
Time	Total	Fail	Lost	Enter	Function	Error	[95% Conf. Int.]	
posttran=0								
0	0	0	0	103	1.0000	.	.	.
1	103	1	3	0	0.9903	0.0097	0.9331	0.9986
2	99	3	3	0	0.9603	0.0195	0.8976	0.9849
3	93	3	3	0	0.9293	0.0258	0.8574	0.9657
(output omitted)								
427	2	0	1	0	0.2359	0.1217	0.0545	0.4882
1400	1	0	1	0	0.2359	0.1217	0.0545	0.4882
posttran=1								
1	0	0	0	3	1.0000	.	.	.
2	3	0	0	3	1.0000	.	.	.
3	6	0	0	3	1.0000	.	.	.
4	9	0	0	2	1.0000	.	.	.
5	11	0	0	3	1.0000	.	.	.
5.1	14	1	0	0	0.9286	0.0688	0.5908	0.9896
6	13	0	0	1	0.9286	0.0688	0.5908	0.9896
8	14	0	0	2	0.9286	0.0688	0.5908	0.9896
(output omitted)								
1586	2	0	1	0	0.1420	0.0546	0.0566	0.2653
1799	1	0	1	0	0.1420	0.0546	0.0566	0.2653

We did that to keep you from being shocked at negative numbers for the net lost. In this complicated dataset, the value of posttran changes over time. All patients start with posttran = 0, and later some change to posttran = 1.

Thus at time 1 in the posttran = 0 group, three are lost—to the group but not to the experiment. Simultaneously, in the posttran = 1 group, we see that three enter. Had we not specified the enter option, you would not have seen that three enter, and you would have seen that −3 were, in net, lost:

```
. sts list, by(posttran)
```

	Beg.		Net	Survivor	Std.		
Time	Total	Fail	Lost	Function	Error	[95% Conf. Int.]	
posttran=0							
1	103	1	3	0.9903	0.0097	0.9331	0.9986
2	99	3	3	0.9603	0.0195	0.8976	0.9849
3	93	3	3	0.9293	0.0258	0.8574	0.9657
(output omitted)							
427	2	0	1	0.2359	0.1217	0.0545	0.4882
1400	1	0	1	0.2359	0.1217	0.0545	0.4882
posttran=1							
1	0	0	−3	1.0000	.	.	.
2	3	0	−3	1.0000	.	.	.
3	6	0	−3	1.0000	.	.	.
4	9	0	−2	1.0000	.	.	.
5	11	0	−3	1.0000	.	.	.
5.1	14	1	0	0.9286	0.0688	0.5908	0.9896
6	13	0	−1	0.9286	0.0688	0.5908	0.9896
8	14	0	−2	0.9286	0.0688	0.5908	0.9896
(output omitted)							
1586	2	0	1	0.1420	0.0546	0.0566	0.2653
1799	1	0	1	0.1420	0.0546	0.0566	0.2653

Here specifying `enter` makes the table easier to explain, but do not jump to the conclusion that specifying `enter` is always a good idea. In this same dataset, let's look at the overall survivor function, first with the `enter` option:

```
. sts list, enter
```

Time	Beg. Total	Fail	Lost	Enter	Survivor Function	Std. Error	[95% Conf. Int.]	
0	0	0	0	103	1.0000	.	.	.
1	103	1	3	3	0.9903	0.0097	0.9331	0.9986
2	102	3	3	3	0.9612	0.0190	0.8998	0.9852
3	99	3	3	3	0.9320	0.0248	0.8627	0.9670
(output omitted)								
1571	3	0	1	0	0.1519	0.0493	0.0713	0.2606
1586	2	0	1	0	0.1519	0.0493	0.0713	0.2606
1799	1	0	1	0	0.1519	0.0493	0.0713	0.2606

At time 1, three are lost and three enter. There is no delayed entry in this dataset, and there are no gaps; so, it is the same three that were lost and reentered, and no one was really lost. At time 1571, on the other hand, a patient really was lost. This is all more clearly revealed when we do not specify the `enter` option:

```
. sts list
```

Time	Beg. Total	Fail	Net Lost	Survivor Function	Std. Error	[95% Conf. Int.]	
1	103	1	0	0.9903	0.0097	0.9331	0.9986
2	102	3	0	0.9612	0.0190	0.8998	0.9852
3	99	3	0	0.9320	0.0248	0.8627	0.9670
(output omitted)							
1571	3	0	1	0.1519	0.0493	0.0713	0.2606
1586	2	0	1	0.1519	0.0493	0.0713	0.2606
1799	1	0	1	0.1519	0.0493	0.0713	0.2606

Thus to summarize:

1. The `sts list` and `graph` commands will show the number lost or censored. `sts list`, by default, shows this number on the detailed output. `sts graph` shows the number when you specify the `lost` option.

2. By default, the number lost is the net number lost, defined as censored minus entered.

3. Both commands allow you to specify the `enter` option and then show the number who actually entered, and the number lost becomes the actual number censored, not censored minus entered.

Saved Results

`sts test` saves the following in `r()`:

Scalars

`r(df)`	degrees of freedom	`r(chi2)`	χ^2

Methods and Formulas

sts is implemented as an ado-file.

Unless adjusted estimates are requested, sts estimates the survivor function by using the Kaplan–Meier product-limit method.

When the cumhaz option is specified, sts estimates the cumulative hazard function by using the Nelson–Aalen estimator.

For an introduction to the Kaplan–Meier product-limit method and the log-rank test, see Pagano and Gauvreau (2000, 495–499); for a detailed discussion, see Cox and Oakes (1984), Kalbfleisch and Prentice (2002), or Klein and Moeschberger (2003). For an introduction to survival analysis with examples using the sts commands, see Dupont (2002).

Let t_j, $j = 1, \ldots$, denote the times at which failure occurs. Let n_j be the number at risk of failure just before time t_j and d_j be the number of failures at time t_j. Then the nonparametric maximum likelihood estimate of the survivor function (Kaplan and Meier 1958) is

$$\widehat{S}(t) = \prod_{j|t_j \leq t} \left(\frac{n_j - d_j}{n_j} \right)$$

(Kalbfleisch and Prentice 2002, 15).

The failure function $\widehat{F}(t)$ is defined as $1 - \widehat{S}(t)$.

The standard error reported is given by Greenwood's (Greenwood 1926) formula

$$\widehat{\mathrm{Var}}\{\widehat{S}(t)\} = \widehat{S}^2(t) \sum_{j|t_j \leq t} \frac{d_j}{n_j(n_j - d_j)}$$

(Kalbfleisch and Prentice 2002, 17–18). These standard errors, however, are not used for confidence intervals. Instead, the asymptotic variance of $\ln[-\ln \widehat{S}(t)]$

$$\widehat{\sigma}^2(t) = \frac{\sum \frac{d_j}{n_j(n_j - d_j)}}{\left\{ \sum \ln\left(\frac{n_j - d_j}{n_j} \right) \right\}^2}$$

is used, where sums are calculated over $j|t_j \leq t$ (Kalbfleisch and Prentice 2002, 18). The confidence bounds are then $\widehat{S}(t)^{\exp(\pm z_{\alpha/2} \widehat{\sigma}(t))}$, where $z_{\alpha/2}$ is the $(1 - \alpha/2)$ quantile of the normal distribution. sts suppresses reporting the standard error and confidence bounds if the data are pweighted since these formulas are no longer appropriate.

When option adjustfor() is specified, the survivor function estimate $\widehat{S}(t)$ is the baseline survivor function estimate $\widehat{S}_0(t)$ of stcox; see [ST] **stcox**. If by() is specified, $\widehat{S}(t)$ is obtained from fitting separate Cox models on adjustfor() for each of the by() groups. If instead strata() is specified, a single Cox model on adjustfor(), stratified by strata(), is fitted.

The Nelson–Aalen estimator of the cumulative hazard rate function is derived from Nelson (1972) and Aalen (1978) and is defined up to the largest observed time as

$$\widehat{H}(t) = \sum_{j|t_j \leq t} \frac{d_j}{n_j}$$

Its variance (Aalen 1978) may be estimated by

$$\widehat{\text{Var}}\{\widehat{H}(t)\} = \sum_{j|t_j \leq t} \frac{d_j}{n_j{}^2}$$

Pointwise confidence intervals are calculated using the asymptotic variance of $\ln\widehat{H}(t)$

$$\widehat{\phi}^2(t) = \frac{\widehat{\text{Var}}\{\widehat{H}(t)\}}{\{\widehat{H}(t)\}^2}$$

The confidence bounds are then $\widehat{H}(t)\exp\{\pm z_{\alpha/2}\widehat{\phi}(t)\}$. If the data are `pweight`ed, these formulas are not appropriate and, then confidence intervals are not reported.

Major Greenwood (1880–1949) was born in London to a medical family. His given name "Major" was also that of his father and grandfather. Greenwood trained as a doctor but followed a career in medical research, learning statistics from Karl Pearson. He worked as a medical statistician and epidemiologist at the Lister Institute, the Ministry of Health, and the London School of Hygiene and Tropical Medicine. With interests ranging from clinical trials to historical subjects, Greenwood played a major role in developing biostatistics in the first half of the 20th century.

Edward Lynn Kaplan (1920–2006) was working at Bell Telephone Laboratories on the lifetimes of vacuum tubes when through John W. Tukey he became aware of the work of Paul Meier on essentially the same statistical problem. They had both previously been graduate students at Princeton. Their two separate papers were merged and the result was published after some years. Kaplan became a professor of mathematics at Oregon State University, where he wrote a book on mathematical programming and games.

Paul Meier (1924–) took degrees at Oberlin and Princeton and then served on the faculty at Johns Hopkins, Chicago, and Columbia. In addition to his key contribution with Kaplan, the most cited paper in statistical science, he worked as a biostatistician, making many theoretical and applied contributions in the area of clinical trials.

Wayne B. Nelson (1936–) was born in Chicago and received degrees in physics and statistics from Caltech and the University of Illinois. A longtime employee of General Electric, he now works as a consultant, specializing in reliability analysis and accelerated testing.

Odd Olai Aalen (1947–) was born in Oslo, Norway, and studied there and at Berkeley, where he was awarded a Ph.D. in 1975 for a thesis on counting processes. He is a professor of statistics at the University of Oslo and works on survival and event history analysis. Aalen was one of the prime movers in introducing martingale ideas to this branch of statistics.

Nelson and Aalen met for the first time at a conference at the University of South Carolina in 2003.

References

Aalen, O. O. 1978. Nonparametric inference for a family of counting processes. *Annals of Statistics* 6: 701–726.

Breslow, N. E. 1992. Introduction to Kaplan and Meier (1958) Nonparametric estimation from incomplete observations. In *Breakthroughs in Statistics. Volume II: Methodology and Distribution*, ed. S. Kotz and N. L. Johnson, 311–318. New York: Springer.

Cleves, M. A. 1999. stata53: censored option added to sts graph command. *Stata Technical Bulletin* 50: 34–36. Reprinted in *Stata Technical Bulletin Reprints*, vol. 9, pp. 4–7.

Cox, D. R., and D. Oakes. 1984. *Analysis of Survival Data*. London: Chapman & Hall/CRC.

Dupont, W. D. 2002. *Statistical Modeling for Biomedical Researchers: A Simple Introduction to the Analysis of Complex Data*. Cambridge: Cambridge University Press.

Greenwood, M. 1926. The natural duration of cancer. *Reports on Public Health and Medical Subjects* 33: 1–26.

Hogben, L. 1950. Major Greenwood. *Obituary Notices of Fellows of the Royal Society* 7: 139–154.

Kalbfleisch, J. D., and R. L. Prentice. 2002. *The Statistical Analysis of Failure Time Data*. 2nd ed. New York: Wiley.

Kaplan, E. L., and P. Meier. 1958. Nonparametric estimation from incomplete observations. *Journal of the American Statistical Association* 53: 457–481.

Klein, J. P., and M. L. Moeschberger. 2003. *Survival Analysis: Techniques for Censored and Truncated Data*. 2nd ed. New York: Springer.

Linhart, J. M., J. S. Pitblado, and J. Hassell. 2004. From the help desk: Kaplan–Meier plots with stsatrisk. *Stata Journal* 4: 56–65.

Nelson, W. 1972. Theory and applications of hazard plotting for censored failure data. *Technometrics* 14: 945–965.

Newman, S. C. 2001. *Biostatistical Methods in Epidemiology*. New York: Wiley.

Pagano, M., and K. Gauvreau. 2000. *Principles of Biostatistics*. 2nd ed. Belmont, CA: Duxbury.

Smythe, B. 2006. Obituary: Edward Kaplan 1920–2006. *IMS Bulletin* 35: 7.

Wilkinson, L. 1998. Greenwood, Major. In *Encyclopedia of Biostatistics*, vol. 2, ed. P. Armitage and T. Colton, 1778–1780. Chichester, UK: Wiley.

Also See

[ST] **stci** — Confidence intervals for means and percentiles of survival time

[ST] **stcox** — Fit Cox proportional hazards model

[ST] **sts generate** — Create variables containing survivor and related functions

[ST] **sts graph** — Graph the survivor and cumulative hazard functions

[ST] **sts list** — List the survivor or cumulative hazard function

[ST] **sts test** — Test equality of survivor functions

[ST] **stset** — Declare data to be survival-time data

[ST] **st** — Survival-time data

[ST] **survival analysis** — Introduction to survival analysis & epidemiological tables commands

Title

> **sts generate** — Create variables containing survivor and related functions

Syntax

sts <u>gen</u>erate *newvar* =

$\left\{ \text{s} \,|\, \text{se(s)} \,|\, \text{h} \,|\, \text{se(lls)} \,|\, \text{lb(s)} \,|\, \text{ub(s)} \,|\, \text{na} \,|\, \text{se(na)} \,|\, \text{lb(na)} \,|\, \text{ub(na)} \,|\, \text{n} \,|\, \text{d} \right\}$

$\left[\textit{newvar} = \left\{ \ldots \right\} \ldots \right]$ $\left[\textit{if} \right]$ $\left[\textit{in} \right]$ $\left[\text{, } \textit{options} \right]$

options	description
Options	
by(*varlist*)	calculate separately on different groups of *varlist*
<u>adj</u>ustfor(*varlist*)	adjust the estimates to zero values of *varlist*
<u>str</u>ata(*varlist*)	stratify on different groups of *varlist*
<u>l</u>evel(#)	set confidence level; default is level(95)

You must stset your data before using sts generate; see [ST] **stset**.

Description

sts generate creates new variables containing the estimated survivor (failure) function, the Nelson–Aalen cumulative hazard (integrated hazard) function, and related functions. See [ST] **sts** for an introduction to this command.

sts generate can be used with single- or multiple-record or single- or multiple-failure st data.

Functions

> Main

s produces the Kaplan–Meier product-limit estimate of the survivor function $\widehat{S}(t)$ or, if adjustfor() is specified, the baseline survivor function from a Cox regression model on the adjustfor() variables.

se(s) produces the Greenwood, pointwise standard error $\widehat{\text{se}}\{\widehat{S}(t)\}$. This option may not be used with adjustfor().

h produces the estimated hazard component $\Delta H_j = H(t_j) - H(t_{j-1})$, where t_j is the current failure time and t_{j-1} is the previous one. This is mainly a utility function used to calculate the estimated cumulative hazard $H(t_j)$, yet you can estimate the hazard via a kernel smooth of the ΔH_j; see [ST] **sts graph**. It is recorded at all the points at which a failure occurs and is computed as d_j/n_j, where d_j is the number of failures occurring at time t_j and n_j is the number at risk at t_j before the occurrence of the failures.

se(lls) produces $\widehat{\sigma}(t)$, the standard error of $\ln\{-\ln \widehat{S}(t)\}$. This option may not be used with adjustfor().

lb(s) produces the lower bound of the confidence interval for $\widehat{S}(t)$ based on $\ln\{-\ln\widehat{S}(t)\}$: $\widehat{S}(t)^{\exp(-z_{\alpha/2}\widehat{\sigma}(t))}$, where $z_{\alpha/2}$ is the $(1-\alpha/2)$ quantile of the standard normal distribution. This option may not be used with adjustfor().

ub(s) produces the upper bound of the confidence interval for $\widehat{S}(t)$ based on $\ln\{-\ln\widehat{S}(t)\}$: $\widehat{S}(t)^{\exp(z_{\alpha/2}\widehat{\sigma}(t))}$, where $z_{\alpha/2}$ is the $(1-\alpha/2)$ quantile of the standard normal distribution. This option may not be used with adjustfor().

na produces the Nelson–Aalen estimate of the cumulative hazard function. This option may not be used with adjustfor().

se(na) produces pointwise standard error for the Nelson–Aalen estimate of the cumulative hazard function, $\widehat{H}(t)$. This option may not be used with adjustfor().

lb(na) produces the lower bound of the confidence interval for $\widehat{H}(t)$ based on the log-transformed cumulative hazard function. This option may not be used with adjustfor().

ub(na) produces the corresponding upper bound. This option may not be used with adjustfor().

n produces n_j, the number at risk just before time t_j. This option may not be used with adjustfor().

d produces d_j, the number failing at time t_j. This option may not be used with adjustfor().

Options

┌─ Options ┐

by(*varlist*) produces separate survivor or cumulative hazard functions by making separate calculations for each group identified by equal values of the variables in *varlist*. by() may not be combined with strata().

adjustfor(*varlist*) adjusts the estimate of the survivor (failure) or hazard function to that for 0 values of the *varlist* specified. This option is available only with functions s or h. See [ST] **sts graph** for an example of how to adjust for values different from 0.

If you specify adjustfor() with by(), sts fits separate Cox regression models for each group using the adjustfor() variables as covariates. The separately calculated baseline survivor functions are then retrieved.

If you specify adjustfor() with strata(), sts fits a stratified-on-group Cox regression model using the adjustfor() variables as covariates. The stratified, baseline survivor function is then retrieved.

strata(*varlist*) requests estimates of the survivor (failure) or hazard functions stratified on variables in *varlist*. It requires specifying adjustfor() and may not be combined with by().

level(#) specifies the confidence level, as a percentage, for the lb(s), ub(s), lb(na) and ub(na) functions. The default is level(95) or as set by set level; see [U] **20.7 Specifying the width of confidence intervals**.

Remarks

sts generate is a seldom used command that gives you access to the calculations listed by sts list and graphed by sts graph.

Use of this command is demonstrated in [ST] **sts**.

Methods and Formulas

See [ST] **sts**.

References

See [ST] **sts**.

Also See

[ST] **sts** — Generate, graph, list, and test the survivor and cumulative hazard functions

[ST] **sts graph** — Graph the survivor and cumulative hazard functions

[ST] **sts list** — List the survivor or cumulative hazard function

[ST] **sts test** — Test equality of survivor functions

[ST] **stset** — Declare data to be survival-time data

Title

sts graph — Graph the survivor and cumulative hazard functions

Syntax

sts graph [*if*] [*in*] [, *options*]

options	description
Main	
survival	graph Kaplan–Meier survivor function; the default
failure	graph Kaplan–Meier failure function
cumhaz	graph Nelson–Aalen cumulative hazard function
hazard	graph smoothed hazard estimate
by(*varlist*)	calculate separately on different groups of *varlist*
adjustfor(*varlist*)	adjust the estimates to zero values of *varlist*
strata(*varlist*)	stratify on different groups of *varlist*
separate	show curves on separate graphs; default is to show curves one on top of another
ci	show pointwise confidence bands
At-risk table	
risktable	show table of number at risk beneath graph
risktable(*risk_spec*)	show customized table of number at risk beneath graph
Options	
level(#)	set confidence level; default is level(95)
per(#)	units to be used in reported rates
noshow	do not show st setting information
tmax(#)	show graph for $t \leq \#$
tmin(#)	show graph for $t \geq \#$
noorigin	begin survival (failure) curve at first exit time; default is to begin at $t = 0$
width(# [#...])	override default bandwidth(s)
kernel(*kernel*)	kernel function; use with hazard
noboundary	no boundary correction; use with hazard
lost	show number lost
enter	show number entered and number lost
atrisk	show numbers at risk at beginning of each interval
censored(single)	show one hash mark at each censoring time, no matter what number is censored
censored(number)	show one hash mark at each censoring time and number censored above hash mark
censored(multiple)	show multiple hash marks for multiple censoring at the same time
censopts(*hash_options*)	affect rendition of hash marks
lostopts(*marker_label_options*)	affect rendition of numbers lost
atriskopts(*marker_label_options*)	affect rendition of numbers at risk

Plot

<u>plot</u>opts(*cline_options*)	affect rendition of the plotted lines
<u>plot</u>#opts(*cline_options*)	affect rendition of the #th plotted line; may not be combined with separate

CI plot

<u>ci</u>opts(*area_options*)	affect rendition of the confidence bands
<u>ci</u>#opts(*area_options*)	affect rendition of the #th confidence band; may not be combined with separate

Add plots

<u>addplot</u>(*plot*)	add other plots to the generated graph

Y axis, X axis, Titles, Legend, Overall

twoway_options	any options documented in [G] ***twoway_options***
<u>byopts</u>(*byopts*)	how subgraphs are combined, labeled, etc.

See [R] **kdensity** for information on *kernel*, and see [G] ***marker_label_options***, [G] ***cline_options***, and [G] ***area_options***.

where *risk_spec* is

$\big[$ *numlist* $\big]$ $\big[$, *table_options* group(*group*) $\big]$

numlist specifies the points at which the number at risk is to be evaluated, *table_options* customizes the table of number at risk, and group(*group*) specifies a specific group/row for *table_options* to be applied.

table_options	description
Main	
axis_label_options	control table by using axis labeling options; seldom used
order(*order_spec*)	select which rows appear and their order
<u>righttitles</u>	place titles on right side of the table
<u>failevents</u>	show number failed in the at-risk table
text_options	affect rendition of table elements and titles
Row titles	
<u>rowtitle</u>($\big[$ *text* $\big]$ $\big[$, *rtext_options* $\big]$)	change title for a row
Title	
title($\big[$ *text* $\big]$ $\big[$, *ttext_options* $\big]$)	change overall table title

See [G] ***axis_label_options***.

where *order_spec* is

$\big[$ "*text*" $\big[$ "*text*" ... $\big]$ $\big]$ $\big[$ ... $\big]$

text_options	description
size(*textsizestyle*)	size of text
color(*colorstyle*)	color of text
justification(*justificationstyle*)	text left-justified, centered, or right-justified
format(%*fmt*)	format values per %*fmt*
topgap(*relativesize*)	margin above rows
bottomgap(*relativesize*)	margin beneath rows
†style(*textstyle*)	overall style of text

†style() does not appear in the dialog box.
See [G] *textsizestyle*, [G] *colorstyle*, [G] *justificationstyle*, [G] *relativesize*, and [G] *textstyle*.

rtext_options	description
size(*textsizestyle*)	size of text
color(*colorstyle*)	color of text
justification(*justificationstyle*)	text left-justified, centered, or right-justified
at(*#*)	override x position of titles
topgap(*relativesize*)	margin above rows
†style(*textstyle*)	overall style of text

†style() does not appear in the dialog box.
See [G] *textsizestyle*, [G] *colorstyle*, [G] *justificationstyle*, [G] *relativesize*, and [G] *textstyle*.

ttext_options	description
size(*textsizestyle*)	size of text
color(*colorstyle*)	color of text
justification(*justificationstyle*)	text left-justified, centered, or right-justified
at(*#*)	override x position of titles
topgap(*relativesize*)	margin above rows
bottomgap(*relativesize*)	margin beneath rows
†style(*textstyle*)	overall style of text

†style() does not appear in the dialog box.
See [G] *textsizestyle*, [G] *colorstyle*, [G] *justificationstyle*, [G] *relativesize*, and [G] *textstyle*.

group	description
#*rownum*	specify group by row number in table
value	specify group by value of group
label	specify group by text of value label associated with group

hash_options	description
line_options	change look of dropped lines
marker_label_options	add marker labels

See [G] *line_options* and [G] *marker_label_options*, except for mlabel().

risktable() may be repeated and is *merged-explicit*; see [G] **concept: repeated options**.

You must stset your data before using sts graph; see [ST] **stset**.

fweights, iweights, and pweights may be specified using stset; see [ST] **stset**.

Description

sts graph graphs the estimated survivor (failure) function, the Nelson–Aalen estimated cumulative (integrated) hazard function, or the estimated hazard function. See [ST] **sts** for an introduction to this command.

sts graph can be used with single- or multiple-record or single- or multiple-failure st data.

Options

<u>Main</u>

survival, failure, cumhaz, and hazard specify the function to graph.

survival specifies that the Kaplan–Meier survivor function be plotted. This option is the default if a function is not specified.

failure specifies that the Kaplan–Meier failure function $1 - S(t + 0)$ be plotted.

cumhaz specifies that the Nelson–Aalen estimate of the cumulative hazard function be plotted.

hazard specifies that an estimate of the hazard function be plotted. This estimate is calculated as a weighted kernel-density estimate using the estimated hazard contributions, $\Delta\widehat{H}(t_j) = \widehat{H}(t_j) - \widehat{H}(t_{j-1})$. These hazard contributions are the same as those obtained by sts generate *newvar* = h.

by(*varlist*) produces separate survivor, cumulative hazard, or hazard functions by making separate calculations for each group identified by equal values of the variables in *varlist* and plots all the groups on one graph. by() may not be combined with strata().

If you have more than one by() variable but need only one, use egen to create it; see [D] **egen**.

adjustfor(*varlist*) adjusts the estimate of the survivor or hazard functions to that for 0 values of the *varlist* specified. If you want to adjust the function to values different from 0, you need to center the variables around those values before issuing the command. Say that you want to plot the survivor function adjusted to age of patients and the ages in your sample are 40–60 years. Then

. sts graph, adjustfor(age)

will graph the survivor function adjusted to age 0. If you want to adjust the function to age 40, type

. gen age40 = age - 40

. sts graph, adjustfor(age40)

adjustfor() is not available with cumhaz or ci.

If you specify adjustfor() with by(), sts fits separate Cox regression models for each group using the adjustfor() variables as covariates. The separately calculated baseline survivor functions are then retrieved.

If you specify adjustfor() with strata(), sts fits a stratified-on-group Cox regression model using the adjustfor() variables as covariates. The stratified, baseline survivor function is then retrieved.

strata(*varlist*) produces estimates of the survivor (failure) or hazard functions stratified on variables in *varlist* and plots all the groups on one graph. It requires specifying adjustfor() and may not be combined with by().

If you have more than one strata() variable but need only one, use egen to create it; see [D] **egen**.

separate is meaningful only with by() or strata(); it requests that each group be placed on its own graph rather than one on top of the other. Sometimes curves have to be placed on separate graphs—such as when you specify ci—because, otherwise, it would be too confusing.

ci includes pointwise confidence bands. The default is not to produce these bands. ci is not allowed with adjustfor() or pweights.

⌐‾‾‾⌐ At-risk table ⌐‾‾‾

risktable[([*numlist*][, *table_options*])] displays a table showing the number at risk beneath the plot. risktable may not be used with separate or adjustfor().

risktable displays the table in the default format with number at risk shown for each time reported on the x axis.

risktable([*numlist*][, *table_options*]) specifies that the number at risk be evaluated at the points specified in *numlist* or that the rendition of the table be changed by *table_options*.

There are two ways to change the points at which the numbers at risk are evaluated.

1. The x axis of the graph may be altered. For example:

        . sts graph, xlabel(0(5)40) risktable

2. A *numlist* can be specified directly in the risktable() option, which affects only the at-risk table. For example:

        . sts graph, risktable(0(5)40)

The two examples produce the same at-risk table, but the first also changes the time labels on the graph's x axis.

table_options affect the rendition of the at-risk table and may be any of the following:

group(#*rownum* | *value* | *label*) specifies that all the suboptions specified in the risktable() apply only to the specified group. Because the risktable() option may be repeated, this option allows different rows of the at-risk table to be displayed with different colors, font sizes, etc.

When both a value and a value label are matched, the value label takes precedence.

risktable() may be specified with or without the group() suboption. When specified without group(), each suboption is applied to all available groups or rows. risktable() specified without group() is considered to be global and is itself merged-explicit. See [G] **concept: repeated options** for more information on how repeated options are merged.

Consider the following example:

        . sts graph, by(drug) risktable(, color(red) size(small))
        > risktable(, color(navy))

The example above would produce a table where all rows are colored navy with small text.

Combining global `risktable()` options with group-specific `risktable()` options can be useful. When global options are combined with group-specific options, group-specific options always take precedence.

Consider the following example:

```
. sts graph, by(drug) risktable(, color(navy))
> risktable(, color(red) group(#1))
```

The example above would produce a table with the first row colored red and all remaining rows colored navy.

◢ Main ◣

axis_label_options control the table by using axis labeling options. These options are seldom used. See [G] *axis_label_options*.

`order()` specifies which and in what order rows are to appear in the at-risk table. Optionally `order()` can be used to override the default text.

`order(# # # ...)` is the syntax used for identifying which rows to display and their order. `order(1 2 3)` would specify that row 1 is to appear first in the table, followed by row 2, followed by row 3. `order(1 2 3)` is the default if there are three groups. If there were four groups, `order(1 2 3 4)` would be the default, and so on. If there were four groups and you specified `order(1 2 3)`, the fourth row would not appear in the at-risk table. If you specified `order(2 1 3)`, row 2 would appear first, followed by row 1, followed by row 3.

`order(# "text" # "text" ...)` is the syntax used for specifying the row order and alternate row titles.

Consider the following at-risk table:

```
drug = 1    20    8     2
drug = 2    14    10    4    1
drug = 3    14    13    10   5
```

Specifying `order(1 "Placebo" 3 2)` would produce

```
Placebo     20    8     2
drug = 3    14    13    10   5
drug = 2    14    10    4    1
```

and specifying `order(1 "Placebo" 3 "Drug 2" 2 "Drug 1")` would produce

```
Placebo     20    8     2
Drug 2      14    13    10   5
Drug 1      14    10    4    1
```

`righttitles` specifies that row titles be placed to the right of the at-risk values. The default is to place row titles to the left of the at-risk values.

`failevents` specifies that the number of failure events be shown in parentheses, after the time in which the risk values were calculated.

text_options affect the rendition of both row titles and number at risk and may be any of the following:

size(*textsizestyle*) specifies the size of text.

color(*colorstyle*) specifies the color of text.

justification(*justificationstyle*) specifies how text elements are to be justified.

format(%*fmt*) specifies how numeric values are to be formatted.

topgap(*relativesize*) specifies how much space is to be placed above each row.

bottomgap(*relativesize*) specifies how much space is to be placed beneath each row.

style(*textstyle*) specifies the style of text. This option does not appear in the dialog box.

Row titles

rowtitle([*text*] [, *rtext_options*]) changes the default text or rendition of row titles. Specifying rowtitle(, color(navy)) would change the color of all row titles to navy.

rowtitle() is often combined with group() to change the text or rendition of a title. Specifying rowtitle(Placebo) group(#2) would change the title of the second row to Placebo. Specifying rowtitle(, color(red)) group(#3) would change the color of the row title for the third row to red.

Row titles may include more than one line. Lines are specified one after the other, each enclosed in double quotes. Specifying rowtitle("Experimental drug") group(#1) would produce a one-line row title, and specifying rowtitle("Experimental" "Drug") group(#1) would produce a multiple-line row title.

rtext_options affect the rendition of both row titles and number at risk and may be any of the following:

size(*textsizestyle*) specifies the size of text.

color(*colorstyle*) specifies the color of text.

justification(*justificationstyle*) specifies how text elements are to be justified.

at(#) allows you to reposition row titles or the overall table title to align with a specific location on the x axis.

topgap(*relativesize*) specifies how much space is to be placed above each row.

style(*textstyle*) specifies the style of text. This option does not appear on the dialog box.

Title

title([*title*] [, *ttext_options*]) may be used to override the default title for the at-risk table and affect the rendition of its text.

Titles may include one line of text or multiple lines. title("At-risk table") will produce a one-line title, and title("At-risk" "table") will produce a multiple-line title.

ttext_options affect the rendition of both row titles and number at risk and may be any of the following:

size(*textsizestyle*) specifies the size of text.

color(*colorstyle*) specifies the color of text.

justification(*justificationstyle*) specifies how text elements are to be justified.

at(*#*) allows you to reposition row titles or the overall table title to align with a specific location on the x axis.

at(rowtitles) places the overall table title at the default position calculated for the row titles. This option is sometimes useful for alignment when the default justification has not been used.

topgap(*relativesize*) specifies how much space is to be placed above each row.

bottomgap(*relativesize*) specifies how much space is to be placed beneath each row.

style(*textstyle*) specifies the style of text. This option does not appear on the dialog box.

Options

level(*#*) specifies the confidence level, as a percentage, for the pointwise confidence interval around the survivor, failure, or cumulative hazard function; see [U] **20.7 Specifying the width of confidence intervals**.

per(*#*) specifies the units used to report the survival or failure rates. For example, if the analysis time is in years, specifying per(100) results in rates per 100 person-years.

noshow prevents sts graph from showing the key st variables. This option is seldom used since most people type stset, show or stset, noshow to set whether they want to see these variables mentioned at the top of the output of every st command; see [ST] **stset**.

tmax(*#*) specifies that the plotted curve be graphed only for $t \leq \#$. This option does not affect the calculation of the function, rather the portion that is displayed.

tmin(*#*) specifies that the plotted curve be graphed only for $t \geq \#$. This option does not affect the calculation of the function, rather the portion that is displayed.

noorigin requests that the plot of the survival (failure) curve begin at the first exit time instead of beginning at $t = 0$ (the default). This option is ignored when cumhaz or hazard is specified.

width(*#* [*#* . . .]) is for use with hazard and specifies the bandwidth to be used in the kernel smooth used to plot the estimated hazard function. If width() is not specified, a default bandwidth is used as described in [R] **kdensity**. If it is used with by(), multiple bandwidths may be specified, one for each group. If there are more groups than the k bandwidths specified, the default bandwidth is used for the $k + 1, \ldots$ remaining groups. If any bandwidth is specified as . (dot), the default bandwidth is used for that group.

kernel(*kernel*) is for use with hazard and specifies the kernel function to be used in calculating the weighted kernel-density estimate required to produce a smoothed hazard-function estimator. The default kernel is Epanechnikov, yet *kernel* may be any of the kernels supported by kdensity; see [R] **kdensity**.

noboundary is for use with hazard. It specifies that no boundary-bias adjustments are to be made when calculating the smoothed hazard function estimator. By default, the smoothed hazards are adjusted near the boundaries. If the epan2, biweight, or rectangular kernel is used, the bias correction near the boundary is performed using boundary kernels. For other kernels, the plotted range of the smoothed hazard function is restricted to be within one bandwidth of each endpoint. For these other kernels, specifying noboundary merely removes this range restriction.

lost specifies that the numbers lost be shown on the plot. These numbers are shown as small numbers over the flat parts of the function.

If enter is not specified, the numbers displayed are the number censored minus the number who enter. If you do specify enter, the numbers displayed are the pure number censored. The underlying logic is described in [ST] **sts**.

lost may not be used with hazard.

enter specifies that the number who enter be shown on the graph, as well as the number lost. The number who enter are shown as small numbers beneath the flat parts of the plotted function.

enter may not be used with hazard.

atrisk specifies that the numbers at risk at the beginning of each interval be shown on the plot. The numbers at risk are shown as small numbers beneath the flat parts of the plotted function.

atrisk may not be used with hazard.

censored(single | number | multiple) specifies that hash marks be placed on the graph to indicate censored observations.

> censored(single) places one hash mark at each censoring time, regardless of the number of censorings at that time.

> censored(number) places one hash mark at each censoring time and displays the number of censorings about the hash mark.

> censored(multiple) places multiple hash marks for multiple censorings at the same time. For instance, if 3 observations are censored at time 5, three hash marks are placed at time 5. censored(multiple) is intended for use when there are few censored observations; if there are too many censored observations, the graph can look bad. In such cases, we recommend that censored(number) be used.

> censored() may not be used with hazard.

censopts(*hash_options*) specifies options that affect how the hash marks for censored observations are rendered; see [G] *line_options*. When combined with censored(number), censopts() also specifies how the count of censoring is rendered; see [G] *marker_label_options*, except mlabel() is not allowed.

lostopts(*marker_label_options*) specifies options that affect how the numbers lost are rendered; see [G] *marker_label_options*. This option implies the lost option.

atriskopts(*marker_label_options*) specifies options that affect how the numbers at risk are rendered; see [G] *marker_label_options*. This option implies the atrisk option.

Plot

plotopts(*cline_options*) affects the rendition of the plotted lines; see [G] *cline_options*. This option may not be combined with by(*varlist*) or strata(*varlist*), unless separate is also specified.

plot#opts(*cline_options*) affects the rendition of the #th plotted line; see [G] *cline_options*. This option may not be combined with separate.

CI plot

ciopts(*area_options*) affects the rendition of the confidence bands; see [G] *area_options*. This option may not be combined with by(*varlist*) or strata(*varlist*), unless separate is also specified.

ci#opts(*area_options*) affects the rendition of the #th confidence band; see [G] *area_options*. This option may not be combined with separate.

Add plots

addplot(*plot*) provides a way to add other plots to the generated graph; see [G] ***addplot_option***.

Y axis, X axis, Titles, Legend, Overall

twoway_options are any of the options documented in [G] ***twoway_options***. These include options for titling the graph (see [G] ***title_options***) and for saving the graph to disk (see [G] ***saving_option***).

byopts(*byopts*) affects the appearance of the combined graph when by() or adjustfor() is specified, including the overall graph title and the organization of subgraphs. byopts() may not be specified with separate. See [G] ***by_option***.

Remarks

Remarks are presented under the following headings:

> Including the number lost on the graph
> Graphing the Nelson–Aalen cumulative hazard function
> Graphing the hazard function
> Adding an at-risk table

If you have not read [ST] **sts**, please do so.

By default, sts graph displays the Kaplan–Meier product-limit estimate of the survivor (failure) function. Only one of sts graph's options, adjustfor(), modifies the calculation. All the other options merely determine how the results of the calculation are graphed.

We demonstrate many of sts graph's features in [ST] **sts**. This discussion picks up where that entry leaves off.

Including the number lost on the graph

In [ST] **sts**, we introduced a simple drug-trial dataset with 1 observation per subject. Here is a graph of the survivor functions, by drug, including the number lost because of censoring:

```
. use http://www.stata-press.com/data/r10/drug2
(Patient Survival in Drug Trial)
. sts graph, by(drug) lost
        failure _d:  died
   analysis time _t:  studytime
```

There is no late entry in these data, so we modify the data so that a few subjects entered late. Here is the same graph on the modified data:

```
. use http://www.stata-press.com/data/r10/drug2b
(Patient Survival in Drug Trial)
. sts graph, by(drug) lost
        failure _d:  died
  analysis time _t:  studytime
```

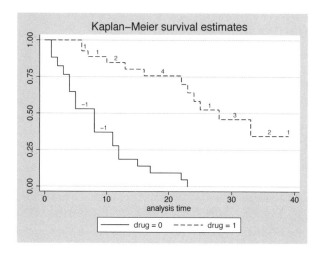

Note the negative numbers. These occur because, by default, lost means censored minus entered. Here −1 means that 1 entered, or 2 entered and 1 was lost, etc. If we specify the enter option, we will see the censored and entered separately:

```
. sts graph, by(drug) lost enter
        failure _d:  died
  analysis time _t:  studytime
```

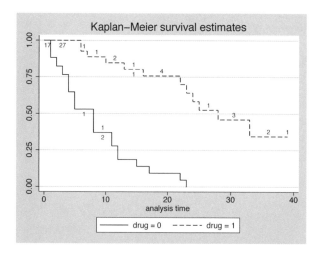

Although it might appear that specifying enter with lost is a good idea, that is not always true.

We have yet another version of the data—the correct data not adjusted to have late entry—but in this version we have multiple records per subject. The data are the same, but where there was one record in the first dataset, sometimes there are now two because we have a covariate that is changing over time. From this dataset, here is the graph with the number lost shown:

```
. use http://www.stata-press.com/data/r10/drug2c
(Patient Survival in Drug Trial)

. sts graph, by(drug) lost
        failure _d:  died
  analysis time _t:  studytime
               id:  id
```

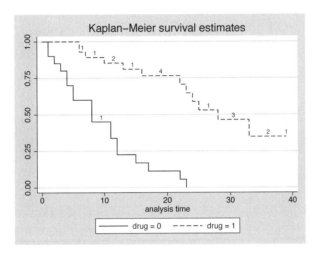

This looks just like the first graph we presented, as indeed it should. Again we emphasize that the data are logically, if not physically, equivalent. If, however, we graph the number lost and entered, we get a graph showing a lot of activity:

```
. sts graph, by(drug) lost enter
        failure _d:  died
  analysis time _t:  studytime
               id:  id
```

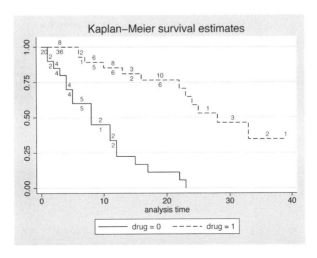

All that activity goes by the name *thrashing*—subjects are being censored to enter the data again, but with different covariates. This graph was better when we did not specify `enter` because the censored-minus-entered calculation smoothed out the thrashing.

Graphing the Nelson–Aalen cumulative hazard function

We can plot the Nelson–Aalen estimate of the cumulative (integrated) hazard function by specifying the `cumhaz` option. For example, from the 1-observation-per-subject drug-trial dataset, here is a graph of the cumulative hazard functions by drug:

```
. use http://www.stata-press.com/data/r10/drug2
(Patient Survival in Drug Trial)
. stset, noshow
. sts graph, cumhaz by(drug)
```

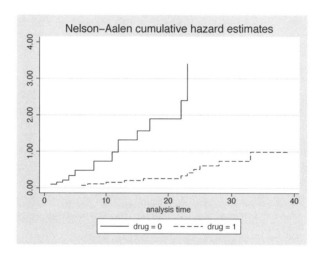

and here is a plot including the number lost because of censoring:

```
. sts graph, cumhaz by(drug) lost
```

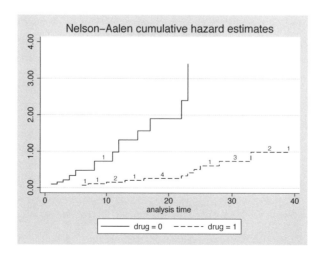

Graphing the hazard function

sts graph may also be used to plot an estimate of the hazard function. This graph is based on a weighted kernel smooth of the estimated hazard contributions, $\Delta\widehat{H}(t_j) = \widehat{H}(t_j) - \widehat{H}(t_{j-1})$, obtained by sts generate *newvar* = h. There are thus issues associated with selecting a kernel function and a bandwidth, although sts graph will use defaults if we do not want to worry about this.

```
. sts graph, hazard by(drug)
```

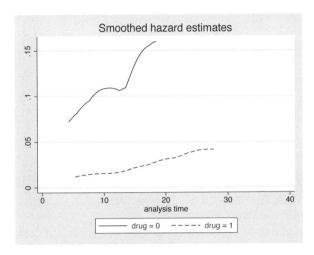

We can also adjust and customize the kernel smooth.

```
. sts graph, hazard by(drug) kernel(gauss) width(5 7)
> title(Comparison of hazard functions)
```

Adding an at-risk table

A table showing the number at risk may be added beneath a survivor, failure, or Nelson–Aalen cumulative hazard plot.

```
. sts graph, by(drug) risktable
```

By default, both the legend and the at-risk table share space at the bottom of the graph. Placing the legend in an empty area inside the plot may often be desirable.

```
. sts graph, by(drug) risktable legend(ring(0) position(2) rows(2))
```

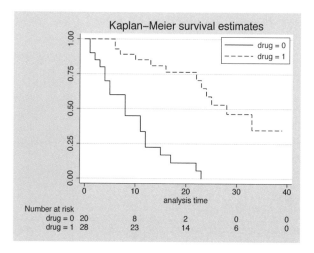

By default, row titles are placed on the left of the at-risk table and are right-justified. We can illustrate this by changing the text of the row titles to have an unequal length.

```
. sts graph, by(drug) risktable(, order(1 "Placebo" 2 "Test drug"))
```

If desired, the text of row titles can be left-justified.

```
. sts graph, by(drug) risktable(, order(1 "Placebo" 2 "Test drug")
> rowtitle(, justification(left)))
```

(Continued on next page)

In addition to left justification, the table title can be aligned with the row titles.

```
. sts graph, by(drug) risktable(, order(1 "Placebo" 2 "Test drug")
> rowtitle(, justification(left)) title(, at(rowtitle)))
```

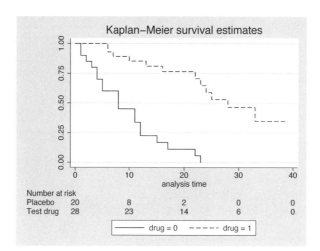

On boundary bias for smoothed hazards

sts graph uses the usual smoothing kernel technique to estimate the hazard function. Kernel estimators commonly encounter bias when estimating near the boundaries of the data range, and therefore estimates of the hazard function in the boundary regions are generally less reliable. To alleviate this problem, estimates that use the epan2, biweight, and rectangular kernels are adjusted at the boundaries with what are known as *boundary kernels* (e.g., Muller and Wang 1994). For estimates using other kernels, no boundary adjustment is made. Instead, the default graphing range is constrained to be the range $(h, \max + h)$, where max is the maximum analysis time at which failure occurred and h is the bandwidth.

Methods and Formulas

See [ST] **sts**.

The estimated hazard is calculated as a kernel smooth of the estimated hazard contributions, $\Delta \widehat{H}(t_j) = \widehat{H}(t_j) - \widehat{H}(t_{j-1})$, using

$$\widehat{h}(t) = b^{-1} \sum_{j=1}^{D} K\left(\frac{t - t_j}{b}\right) \Delta \widehat{H}(t_j)$$

where $K()$ is the kernel (Muller and Wang 1994) function, b is the bandwidth, and the summation is over the D times at which failure occurs (Klein and Moeschberger 2003, 167). If adjustfor() is specified, the $\Delta \widehat{H}(t_j)$ are instead obtained from stcox as the estimated baseline contributions from a Cox model; see [ST] **stcox** for details on how the $\Delta \widehat{H}(t_j)$ are calculated in this case.

Pointwise confidence bands for smoothed hazard functions are calculated using the method based on a log transformation,

$$\widehat{h}(t) \exp\left[\pm \frac{Z_{1-\alpha/2}\sigma\{\widehat{h}(t)\}}{\widehat{h}(t)} \right]$$

See Klein and Moeschberger (2003, 168) for details.

References

Müller, H. G., and J. L. Wang. 1994. Hazard rate estimation under random censoring with varying kernels and bandwidths. *Biometrics* 50: 61–76.

See [ST] **sts** for more references.

Also See

[ST] **sts** — Generate, graph, list, and test the survivor and cumulative hazard functions

[ST] **sts generate** — Create variables containing survivor and related functions

[ST] **sts list** — List the survivor or cumulative hazard function

[ST] **sts test** — Test equality of survivor functions

[ST] **stset** — Declare data to be survival-time data

[R] **kdensity** — Univariate kernel density estimation

Title

> **sts list** — List the survivor or cumulative hazard function

Syntax

sts <u>list</u> $\begin{bmatrix} if \end{bmatrix}$ $\begin{bmatrix} in \end{bmatrix}$ $\begin{bmatrix} , \ options \end{bmatrix}$

options	description
Main	
<u>s</u>urvival	report Kaplan–Meier survivor function; the default
<u>f</u>ailure	report Kaplan–Meier failure function
<u>c</u>umhaz	report Nelson–Aalen cumulative hazard function
by(*varlist*)	calculate separately on different groups of *varlist*
<u>adj</u>ustfor(*varlist*)	adjust the estimates to zero values of *varlist*
<u>str</u>ata(*varlist*)	stratify on different groups of *varlist*
Options	
<u>l</u>evel(#)	set confidence level; default is level(95)
at(# | *numlist*)	report estimated survivor/cumulative hazard function at specified times; default is to report at all unique time values
<u>e</u>nter	report number lost as pure censored instead of censored minus lost
<u>n</u>oshow	do not show st setting information
<u>c</u>ompare	report groups of survivor/cumulative hazard functions side by side

You must stset your data before using sts list; see [ST] **stset**.

fweights, iweights, and pweights may be specified using stset; see [ST] **stset**.

Description

sts list lists the estimated survivor (failure) or the Nelson–Aalen estimated cumulative (integrated) hazard function. See [ST] **sts** for an introduction to this command.

sts list can be used with single- or multiple-record or single- or multiple-failure st data.

Options

> **Main**

survival, failure, and cumhaz specify the function to report.

survival specifies that the Kaplan–Meier survivor function be listed. This option is the default if a function is not specified.

failure specifies that the Kaplan–Meier failure function $1 - S(t + 0)$ be listed.

cumhaz specifies that the Nelson–Aalen estimate of the cumulative hazard function be listed.

by(*varlist*) produces separate survivor or cumulative hazard functions by making separate calculations for each group identified by equal values of the variables in *varlist*. by() may not be combined with strata().

adjustfor(*varlist*) adjusts the estimate of the survivor (failure) function to that for 0 values of the *varlist* specified. This option is not available with the Nelson–Aalen function. See [ST] **sts graph** for an example of how to adjust for values different from 0.

If you specify adjustfor() with by(), sts fits separate Cox regression models for each group using the adjustfor() variables as covariates. The separately calculated baseline survivor functions are then retrieved.

If you specify adjustfor() with strata(), sts fits a stratified-on-group Cox regression model using the adjustfor() variables as covariates. The stratified, baseline survivor function is then retrieved.

strata(*varlist*) requests estimates of the survivor (failure) function stratified on variables in *varlist*. It requires specifying adjustfor() and may not be combined with by().

⌐ Options ⌐

level(*#*) specifies the confidence level, as a percentage, for the Greenwood pointwise confidence interval of the survivor (failure) or for the pointwise confidence interval of the Nelson–Aalen cumulative hazard function; see [U] **20.7 Specifying the width of confidence intervals**.

at(*# | numlist*) specifies the time values at which the estimated survivor (failure) or cumulative hazard function is to be listed.

The default is to list the function at all the unique time values in the data or, if functions are being compared, at about 10 times chosen over the observed interval. In any case, you can control the points chosen.

at(5 10 20 30 50 90) would display the function at the designated times.

at(10 20 to 100) would display the function at times 10, 20, 30, 40, ..., 100.

at(0 5 10 to 100 200) would display the function at times 0, 5, 10, 15, ..., 100, and 200.

at(20) would display the curve at (roughly) 20 equally spaced times over the interval observed in the data. We say roughly because Stata may choose to increase or decrease your number slightly if that would result in rounder values of the chosen times.

enter specifies that the table contain the number who enter, and, correspondingly, that the number lost be displayed as the pure number censored rather than censored minus entered. The logic underlying this is explained in [ST] **sts**.

noshow prevents sts list from showing the key st variables. This option is seldom used since most people type stset, show or stset, noshow to set whether they want to see these variables mentioned at the top of the output of every st command; see [ST] **stset**.

compare is specified only with by() or strata(). It compares the survivor (failure) or cumulative hazard functions and lists them side by side rather than first one and then the next.

Remarks

Only one of sts list's options—adjustfor()—modifies the calculation. All the other options merely determine how the results of the calculation are displayed.

If you do not specify adjustfor() or cumhaz, sts list displays the Kaplan–Meier product-limit estimate of the survivor (failure) function. Specify by() to perform the calculation separately on the different groups.

Specify adjustfor() to calculate an adjusted survival curve. Now if you specify by() or strata(), this further modifies how the adjustment is made.

sts list, cumhaz displays the Nelson–Aalen estimate of the cumulative hazard function.

We demonstrate many of sts list's features in [ST] **sts**. This discussion picks up where that entry leaves off.

By default, sts list will bury you in output. With the Stanford heart transplant data introduced in [ST] **stset**, the following commands produce 154 lines of output.

```
. use http://www.stata-press.com/data/r10/stan3
(Heart transplant data)

. stset, noshow

. sts list, by(posttran)
```

Time	Beg. Total	Fail	Net Lost	Survivor Function	Std. Error	[95% Conf. Int.]	
posttran=0							
1	103	1	3	0.9903	0.0097	0.9331	0.9986
2	99	3	3	0.9603	0.0195	0.8976	0.9849
3	93	3	3	0.9293	0.0258	0.8574	0.9657
(*output omitted*)							
1400	1	0	1	0.2359	0.1217	0.0545	0.4882
posttran=1							
1	0	0	-3	1.0000	.	.	.
2	3	0	-3	1.0000	.	.	.
(*output omitted*)							
5.1	14	1	0	0.9286	0.0688	0.5908	0.9896
6	13	0	-1	0.9286	0.0688	0.5908	0.9896
(*output omitted*)							
1799	1	0	1	0.1420	0.0546	0.0566	0.2653

at() and compare are the solutions. Here is another detailed, but more useful, view of the heart transplant data:

```
. sts list, at(10 40 to 170) by(posttran)
```

Time	Beg. Total	Fail	Survivor Function	Std. Error	[95% Conf. Int.]	
posttran=0						
10	74	12	0.8724	0.0346	0.7858	0.9256
40	31	11	0.6781	0.0601	0.5446	0.7801
70	17	2	0.6126	0.0704	0.4603	0.7339
100	11	1	0.5616	0.0810	0.3900	0.7022
130	10	1	0.5054	0.0903	0.3199	0.6646
160	7	1	0.4422	0.0986	0.2480	0.6204
posttran=1						
10	16	1	0.9286	0.0688	0.5908	0.9896
40	43	6	0.7391	0.0900	0.5140	0.8716
70	45	9	0.6002	0.0841	0.4172	0.7423
100	40	9	0.4814	0.0762	0.3271	0.6198
130	38	1	0.4687	0.0752	0.3174	0.6063
160	36	1	0.4561	0.0742	0.3076	0.5928

Note: survivor function is calculated over full data and evaluated at indicated times; it is not calculated from aggregates shown at left.

We specified at(10 40 to 170) when that is not strictly correct; at(10 40 to 160) would make sense and so would at(10 40 to 180), but sts list is not picky.

❏ Technical Note

When used with at(), sts list is designed only to give you a snapshot of the full Kaplan–Meier curve. That is, the Beg. Total information is that for the last observed failure time (before the failures occur).

When the at() option is used, the Beg. Total column in the output does not contain the number at risk at the time indicated in the Time column. It shows the number at risk at the time just before the previous failure.

❏

Similar output for the Nelson–Aalen estimated cumulative hazard can be produced by specifying the cumhaz option:

```
. sts list, cumhaz at(10 40 to 170) by(posttran)
```

Time	Beg. Total	Fail	Nelson-Aalen Cum. Haz.	Std. Error	[95% Conf. Int.]	
posttran=0						
10	74	12	0.1349	0.0391	0.0764	0.2382
40	31	11	0.3824	0.0871	0.2448	0.5976
70	17	2	0.4813	0.1124	0.3044	0.7608
100	11	1	0.5646	0.1400	0.3473	0.9178
130	10	1	0.6646	0.1720	0.4002	1.1037
160	7	1	0.7896	0.2126	0.4658	1.3385
posttran=1						
10	16	1	0.0714	0.0714	0.0101	0.5071
40	43	6	0.2929	0.1176	0.1334	0.6433
70	45	9	0.4981	0.1360	0.2916	0.8507
100	40	9	0.7155	0.1542	0.4691	1.0915
130	38	1	0.7418	0.1564	0.4908	1.1214
160	36	1	0.7689	0.1587	0.5130	1.1523

```
Note:  Nelson-Aalen function is calculated over full data and evaluated at
       indicated times; it is not calculated from aggregates shown at left.
```

Here is the result of the survivor functions with the compare option,

```
. sts list, at(10 40 to 170) by(posttran) compare
```

posttran	Survivor Function 0	1
time 10	0.8724	0.9286
40	0.6781	0.7391
70	0.6126	0.6002
100	0.5616	0.4814
130	0.5054	0.4687
160	0.4422	0.4561

(Continued on next page)

and of the cumulative hazard functions,

```
. sts list, cumhaz at(10 40 to 170) by(posttran) compare
                  Nelson-Aalen Cum. Haz.
      posttran              0            1

time        10         0.1349       0.0714
            40         0.3824       0.2929
            70         0.4813       0.4981
           100         0.5646       0.7155
           130         0.6646       0.7418
           160         0.7896       0.7689
```

Methods and Formulas

See [ST] **sts**.

References

See [ST] **sts**.

Also See

[ST] **sts** — Generate, graph, list, and test the survivor and cumulative hazard functions

[ST] **sts generate** — Create variables containing survivor and related functions

[ST] **sts graph** — Graph the survivor and cumulative hazard functions

[ST] **sts test** — Test equality of survivor functions

[ST] **stset** — Declare data to be survival-time data

Title

> **sts test** — Test equality of survivor functions

Syntax

> sts <u>test</u> *varlist* $\big[$ *if* $\big]$ $\big[$ *in* $\big]$ $\big[$, *options* $\big]$

options	description
Main	
<u>logrank</u>	perform log-rank test of equality; the default
<u>cox</u>	perform Cox test of equality
<u>wilcoxon</u>	perform Wilcoxon–Breslow–Gehan test of equality
<u>tware</u>	perform Tarone–Ware test of equality
<u>peto</u>	perform Peto–Peto–Prentice test of equality
<u>fh</u>(*p q*)	perform generalized Fleming–Harrington test of equality
<u>trend</u>	test trend of the survivor function across three or more ordered groups
<u>strata</u>(*varlist*)	perform stratified test on *varlist*, displaying overall test results
<u>detail</u>	display individual test results; modifies strata()
Options	
mat(*mname$_1$ mname$_2$*)	store vector **u** in *mname$_1$* and matrix **V** in *mname$_2$*
<u>noshow</u>	do not show st setting information
<u>noti</u>tle	suppress title

You must stset your data before using sts test; see [ST] **stset**.

Note that fweights, iweights, and pweights may be specified using stset; see [ST] **stset**.

Description

sts test tests the equality of survivor functions across two or more groups. The log-rank, Cox, Wilcoxon–Breslow–Gehan, Tarone–Ware, Peto–Peto–Prentice, and Fleming–Harrington tests are provided, in both unstratified and stratified forms.

sts test also provides a test for trend.

See [ST] **sts** for an introduction to this command.

sts test can be used with single- or multiple-record or single- or multiple-failure st data.

Options

> ⌐ Main ⌐

logrank, cox, wilcoxon, tware, peto, and fh(*p q*) specify the test of equality desired. logrank is the default, unless the data are pweighted, in which case cox is the default and is the only possibility.

wilcoxon specifies the Wilcoxon–Breslow–Gehan test, tware the Tarone–Ware test, peto the Peto–Peto–Prentice test, and fh() the generalized Fleming–Harrington test. The Fleming–Harrington test requires two arguments, p and q. When $p = 0$ and $q = 0$, the Fleming–Harrington test reduces to the log-rank test; when $p = 1$ and $q = 0$, the test reduces to the Mann–Whitney–Wilcoxon test.

trend specifies that a test for trend of the survivor function across three or more ordered groups be performed.

strata(*varlist*) requests that a stratified test be performed.

detail modifies strata(); it requests that, in addition to the overall stratified test, the tests for the individual strata be reported. detail is not allowed with cox.

_____ Options _____

mat(*mname₁ mname₂*) requests that the vector **u** be stored in *mname₁* and that matrix **V** be stored in *mname₂*. The other tests are rank tests of the form $\mathbf{u}'\mathbf{V}^{-1}\mathbf{u}$. This option may not be used with cox.

noshow prevents sts test from showing the key st variables. This option is seldom used since most people type stset, show or stset, noshow to set whether they want to see these variables mentioned at the top of the output of every st command; see [ST] **stset**.

notitle requests that the title printed above the test be suppressed.

Remarks

Remarks are presented under the following headings:

> The log-rank test
> The Wilcoxon (Breslow–Gehan) test
> The Tarone–Ware test
> The Peto–Peto–Prentice test
> The generalized Fleming–Harrington tests
> The "Cox" test
> The trend test

sts test tests the equality of the survivor function across groups. With the exception of the Cox test, these tests are members of a family of statistical tests that are extensions to censored data of traditional nonparametric rank tests for comparing two or more distributions. A technical description of these tests can be found in the *Methods and Formulas* section of this entry. Simply, at each distinct failure time in the data, the contribution to the test statistic is obtained as a weighted standardized sum of the difference between the observed and expected number of deaths in each of the k groups. The expected number of deaths is obtained under the null hypothesis of no differences between the survival experience of the k groups.

The weights or weight function used determines the test statistic. For example, when the weight is 1 at all failure times, the log-rank test is computed, and when the weight is the number of subjects at risk of failure at each distinct failure time, the Wilcoxon–Breslow–Gehan test is computed.

The following table summarizes the weights used for each statistical test.

Test	Weight at each distinct failure time (t_i)
Log-rank	1
Wilcoxon–Breslow–Gehan	n_i
Tarone–Ware	$\sqrt{n_i}$
Peto–Peto–Prentice	$\widetilde{S}(t_i)$
Fleming–Harrington	$\widehat{S}(t_{i-1})^p \left[1 - \widehat{S}(t_{i-1})\right]^q$

where $\widehat{S}(t_i)$ is the estimated Kaplan–Meier survivor function value for the combined sample at failure time t_i, $\widetilde{S}(t_i)$ is a modified estimate of the overall survivor function described in *Methods and Formulas*, and n_i is the number of subjects in the risk pool at failure time t_i.

These tests are appropriate for testing the equality of survivor functions across two or more groups. Up to 800 groups are allowed.

The "Cox" test is related to the log-rank test but is performed as a likelihood-ratio test (or, alternatively, as a Wald test) on the results from a Cox proportional hazards regression. The log-rank test should be preferable to what we have labeled the Cox test, but with `pweight`ed data the log-rank test is not appropriate. Whether you perform the log-rank or Cox test makes little substantive difference with most datasets.

`sts test, trend` can be used to test against the alternative hypothesis that the failure rate increases or decreases as the level of the k groups increases or decreases. This test is appropriate only when there is a natural ordering of the comparison groups, for example, when each group represents an increasing or decreasing level of a therapeutic agent.

`trend` is not valid when `cox` is specified.

The log-rank test

`sts test`, by default, performs the log-rank test, to be clear, is the exponential scores test (Savage 1956, Mantel and Haenszel 1959, Mantel 1963, Mantel 1966). This test is most appropriate when the hazard functions are thought to be proportional across the groups if they are not equal.

This test statistic is constructed by giving equal weights to the contribution of each failure time to the overall test statistic.

In [ST] **sts**, we demonstrated the use of this command with the heart transplant data, a multiple-record, single-failure st dataset.

(Continued on next page)

```
. use http://www.stata-press.com/data/r10/stan3
(Heart transplant data)

. sts test posttran

          failure _d:  died
    analysis time _t:  t1
                 id:  id
```

Log-rank test for equality of survivor functions

posttran	Events observed	Events expected
0	30	31.20
1	45	43.80
Total	75	75.00

```
                chi2(1) =      0.13
                Pr>chi2 =    0.7225
```

We cannot reject the hypothesis that the survivor functions are the same.

sts test, logrank can also perform the stratified log-rank test. Say that it is suggested that calendar year of acceptance also affects survival and that there are three important periods: 1967–69, 1970–72, and 1973–74. Therefore, a stratified test should be performed:

```
. stset, noshow

. generate group = 1 if year <= 69
(117 missing values generated)

. replace group=2 if year>=70 & year<=72
(78 real changes made)

. replace group=3 if year>=73
(39 real changes made)

. sts test posttran, strata(group)
```

Stratified log-rank test for equality of survivor functions

posttran	Events observed	Events expected(*)
0	30	31.51
1	45	43.49
Total	75	75.00

(*) sum over calculations within group

```
                chi2(1) =      0.20
                Pr>chi2 =    0.6547
```

Still finding nothing, we ask Stata to show the within-stratum tests:

```
. sts test posttran, strata(group) detail
```

Stratified log-rank test for equality of survivor functions

-> group = 1

posttran	Events observed	Events expected
0	14	13.59
1	17	17.41
Total	31	31.00

$$chi2(1) = \quad 0.03$$
$$Pr>chi2 = \quad 0.8558$$

-> group = 2

posttran	Events observed	Events expected
0	13	13.63
1	20	19.37
Total	33	33.00

$$chi2(1) = \quad 0.09$$
$$Pr>chi2 = \quad 0.7663$$

-> group = 3

posttran	Events observed	Events expected
0	3	4.29
1	8	6.71
Total	11	11.00

$$chi2(1) = \quad 0.91$$
$$Pr>chi2 = \quad 0.3410$$

-> Total

posttran	Events observed	Events expected(*)
0	30	31.51
1	45	43.49
Total	75	75.00

(*) sum over calculations within group

$$chi2(1) = \quad 0.20$$
$$Pr>chi2 = \quad 0.6547$$

The Wilcoxon (Breslow–Gehan) test

sts test, wilcoxon performs the generalized Wilcoxon test of Breslow (1970) and Gehan (1965). This test is appropriate when hazard functions are thought to vary in ways other than proportionally and when censoring patterns are similar across groups.

The Wilcoxon test statistic is constructed by weighting the contribution of each failure time to the overall test statistic by the number of subjects at risk. Thus it gives heavier weights to earlier failure times when the number at risk is higher. As a result, this test is susceptible to differences in the censoring pattern of the groups.

`sts test, wilcoxon` works the same way as `sts test, logrank`

```
. sts test posttran, wilcoxon
```

Wilcoxon (Breslow) test for equality of survivor functions

posttran	Events observed	Events expected	Sum of ranks
0	30	31.20	-85
1	45	43.80	85
Total	75	75.00	0

```
            chi2(1) =     0.14
            Pr>chi2 =   0.7083
```

and, with the `strata()` option, `sts test, wilcoxon` performs the stratified test:

```
. sts test posttran, wilcoxon strata(group)
```

Stratified Wilcoxon (Breslow) test for equality of survivor functions

posttran	Events observed	Events expected(*)	Sum of ranks(*)
0	30	31.51	-40
1	45	43.49	40
Total	75	75.00	0

(*) sum over calculations within group

```
            chi2(1) =     0.22
            Pr>chi2 =   0.6385
```

As with `sts test, logrank`, you can also specify the `detail` option to see the within-stratum tests.

The Tarone–Ware test

`sts test, tware` performs a test suggested by Tarone and Ware (1977), with weights equal to the square root of the number of subjects in the risk pool at time t_i.

Like Wilcoxon's test, this test is appropriate when hazard functions are thought to vary in ways other than proportionally and when censoring patterns are similar across groups. The test statistic is constructed by weighting the contribution of each failure time to the overall test statistic by the square root of the number of subjects at risk. Thus like the Wilcoxon test, it gives heavier weights, although not as large, to earlier failure times. Although less susceptible to the failure and censoring pattern in the data than Wilcoxon's test, this could remain a problem if large differences in these patterns exist between groups.

`sts test, tware` works the same way as `sts test, logrank`

```
. sts test posttran, tware
```

Tarone-Ware test for equality of survivor functions

posttran	Events observed	Events expected	Sum of ranks
0	30	31.20	-9.3375685
1	45	43.80	9.3375685
Total	75	75.00	0

```
            chi2(1) =     0.12
            Pr>chi2 =   0.7293
```

and, with the strata() option, sts test, tware performs the stratified test:

. sts test posttran, tware strata(group)

Stratified Tarone-Ware test for equality of survivor functions

posttran	Events observed	Events expected(*)	Sum of ranks(*)
0	30	31.51	-7.4679345
1	45	43.49	7.4679345
Total	75	75.00	0

(*) sum over calculations within group

$$chi2(1) = \quad 0.21$$
$$Pr>chi2 = \quad 0.6464$$

As with sts test, logrank, you can also specify the detail option to see the within-stratum tests.

The Peto–Peto–Prentice test

sts test, peto performs an alternative to the Wilcoxon test proposed by Peto and Peto (1972) and Prentice (1978). The test uses as the weight function an estimate of the overall survivor function, which is similar to that obtained using the Kaplan–Meier estimator. See *Methods and Formulas* for details.

This test is appropriate when hazard functions are thought to vary in ways other than proportionally, but unlike the Wilcoxon–Breslow–Gehan test, it is not affected by differences in censoring patterns across groups.

sts test, peto works the same way as sts test, logrank:

. sts test posttran, peto

Peto-Peto test for equality of survivor functions

posttran	Events observed	Events expected	Sum of ranks
0	30	31.20	-.86708453
1	45	43.80	.86708453
Total	75	75.00	0

$$chi2(1) = \quad 0.15$$
$$Pr>chi2 = \quad 0.6979$$

With the strata() option, sts test, peto performs the stratified test:

. sts test posttran, peto strata(group)

Stratified Peto-Peto test for equality of survivor functions

posttran	Events observed	Events expected(*)	Sum of ranks(*)
0	30	31.51	-.96898006
1	45	43.49	.96898006
Total	75	75.00	0

(*) sum over calculations within group

$$chi2(1) = \quad 0.19$$
$$Pr>chi2 = \quad 0.6618$$

As with the previous tests, you can also specify the detail option to see the within-stratum tests.

The generalized Fleming–Harrington tests

sts test, fh(p q) performs the Fleming and Harrington (1982) class of test statistics. The weight function at each distinct failure time t is the product of the Kaplan–Meier survivor estimate at time $t-1$ raised to the p power and $1 -$ the Kaplan–Meier survivor estimate at time $t-1$ raised to the q power. Thus, when specifying the Fleming and Harrington option, you must specify two nonnegative arguments, p and q.

When $p > q$, the test gives more weights to earlier failures than to later ones. When $p < q$, the opposite is true, and more weight is given to later failures than to earlier ones. When p and q are both zero, the weight is 1 at all failure times and the test reduces to the log-rank test.

sts test, fh(p q) works the same way as sts test, logrank. If we specify $p = 0$ and $q = 0$ we will get the same results as the log-rank test,

```
. sts test posttran, fh(0 0)
```

Fleming-Harrington test for equality of survivor functions

posttran	Events observed	Events expected	Sum of ranks
0	30	31.20	-1.1995511
1	45	43.80	1.1995511
Total	75	75.00	0

```
            chi2(1) =      0.13
            Pr>chi2 =    0.7225
```

which is what the log-rank test reported.

We could, for example, give more weight to later failures than to earlier ones.

```
. sts test posttran, fh(0 3)
```

Fleming-Harrington test for equality of survivor functions

posttran	Events observed	Events expected	Sum of ranks
0	30	31.20	-.09364975
1	45	43.80	.09364975
Total	75	75.00	0

```
            chi2(1) =      0.01
            Pr>chi2 =    0.9139
```

Similar to the previous tests, with the strata() option, sts test, fh() performs the stratified test:

```
. sts test posttran, fh(0 3) strata(group)
```

Stratified Fleming-Harrington test for equality of survivor functions

posttran	Events observed	Events expected(*)	Sum of ranks(*)
0	30	31.51	-.1623318
1	45	43.49	.1623318
Total	75	75.00	0

```
(*) sum over calculations within group
            chi2(1) =      0.05
            Pr>chi2 =    0.8266
```

As with the other tests, you can also specify the detail option to see the within-stratum tests.

The "Cox" test

The term *Cox test* is our own, and this test is a variation on the log-rank test using Cox regression.

One way of thinking about the log-rank test is as a Cox proportional hazards model on indicator variables for each of the groups. The log-rank test is a test that the coefficients are zero or, if you prefer, that the hazard ratios are one. The log-rank test is, in fact, a score test of that hypothesis performed on a slightly different (partial) likelihood function that handles ties more accurately.

Many researchers think that a (less precise) score test on the precise likelihood function is preferable to a (more precise) likelihood-ratio test on the approximate likelihood function used in Cox regression estimation. In our experience, it makes little difference:

```
. sts test posttran, cox
```

Cox regression-based test for equality of survival curves

posttran	Events observed	Events expected	Relative hazard
0	30	31.20	0.9401
1	45	43.80	1.0450
Total	75	75.00	1.0000

```
          LR chi2(1) =      0.13
          Pr>chi2 =      0.7222
```

By comparison, `sts test, logrank` also reported $\chi^2 = .13$, although the significance level was 0.7225, meaning that the χ^2 values differed in the fourth digit. As mentioned by Kalbfleisch and Prentice (2002, 20), a primary advantage of the log-rank test is the ease with which it can be explained to nonstatisticians, since the test statistic is the difference between the observed and expected number of failures within groups.

Our purpose in offering `sts test, cox` is not to promote its use instead of the log-rank test but to provide a test for researchers with sample-weighted data.

If you have sample weights (if you specified `pweights` when you `stset` the data), you cannot run the log-rank or Wilcoxon tests. The Cox regression model, however, has been generalized to sample-weighted data, and Stata's `stcox` can fit models with such data. In sample-weighted data, the likelihood-ratio statistic is no longer appropriate, but the Wald test based on the robust estimator of variance is.

Thus if we treated these data as sample-weighted data, we would obtain

```
. generate one = 1
. stset t1 [pw=one], id(id) time0(_t0) failure(died) noshow

                id:  id
     failure event:  died != 0 & died < .
obs. time interval:  (_t0, t1]
 exit on or before:  failure
            weight:  [pweight=one]

       172  total obs.
         0  exclusions

       172  obs. remaining, representing
       103  subjects
        75  failures in single failure-per-subject data
   31938.1  total analysis time at risk, at risk from t =         0
                              earliest observed entry t =         0
                                   last observed exit t =      1799
```

```
. sts test posttran, cox
```

Cox regression-based test for equality of survival curves

posttran	Events observed	Events expected	Relative hazard
0	30.00	31.20	0.9401
1	45.00	43.80	1.0450
Total	75.00	75.00	1.0000

```
              Wald chi2(1) =      0.13
                 Pr>chi2 =     0.7181
```

sts test, cox now reports the Wald statistic, which is, to two digits, 0.13 just like all the others.

The trend test

When the groups to be compared have a natural order, such as increasing or decreasing age groups or drug dosage, you may want to test the null hypothesis that there is no difference in failure rate among the groups versus the alternative hypothesis that the failure rate increases or decreases as you move from one group to the next.

We illustrate this test with a dataset from a carcinogenesis experiment reprinted in Marubini and Grazia (1995, 126). Twenty-nine experimental animals were exposed to three levels (0, 1.5, 2.0) of a carcinogenic agent. The time in days to tumor formation was recorded. Here are a few of the observations:

```
. use http://www.stata-press.com/data/r10/marubini, clear
. list time event group dose in 1/9
```

	time	event	group	dose
1.	67	1	2	1.5
2.	150	1	2	1.5
3.	47	1	3	2
4.	75	0	1	0
5.	58	1	3	2
6.	136	1	2	1.5
7.	58	1	3	2
8.	150	1	2	1.5
9.	43	0	2	1.5

In these data, there are two variables that indicate exposure level. The group variable is coded 1, 2, and 3, indicating a one-unit separation between exposures. The dose variable records the actual exposure dosage. To test the null hypothesis of no difference among the survival experience of the three groups versus the alternative hypothesis that the survival experience of at least one of the groups is different, it does not matter if we use group or dose.

```
. stset time, fail(event) noshow

    failure event:  event != 0 & event < .
obs. time interval:  (0, time]
 exit on or before:  failure
```

```
   29  total obs.
    0  exclusions
```

```
   29  obs. remaining, representing
   15  failures in single record/single failure data
 2564  total analysis time at risk, at risk from t =          0
                          earliest observed entry t =          0
                            last observed exit t =          246
```

```
. sts test group
```

Log-rank test for equality of survivor functions

group	Events observed	Events expected
1	4	6.41
2	6	6.80
3	5	1.79
Total	15	15.00

```
                chi2(2) =     8.05
                Pr>chi2 =   0.0179
```

```
. sts test dose
```

Log-rank test for equality of survivor functions

dose	Events observed	Events expected
0	4	6.41
1.5	6	6.80
2	5	1.79
Total	15	15.00

```
                chi2(2) =     8.05
                Pr>chi2 =   0.0179
```

For the trend test, however, the distance between the values is important, so using group or dose will produce different results.

(*Continued on next page*)

```
. sts test group, trend
```

Log-rank test for equality of survivor functions

group	Events observed	Events expected
1	4	6.41
2	6	6.80
3	5	1.79
Total	15	15.00

```
              chi2(2) =      8.05
              Pr>chi2 =    0.0179
```

Test for trend of survivor functions

```
              chi2(1) =      5.87
              Pr>chi2 =    0.0154
```

```
. sts test dose, trend
```

Log-rank test for equality of survivor functions

dose	Events observed	Events expected
0	4	6.41
1.5	6	6.80
2	5	1.79
Total	15	15.00

```
              chi2(2) =      8.05
              Pr>chi2 =    0.0179
```

Test for trend of survivor functions

```
              chi2(1) =      3.66
              Pr>chi2 =    0.0557
```

Although the above trend test was constructed using the log-rank test, any of the previously mentioned weight functions can be used. For example, a trend test on the data can be performed using the same weights as the Peto–Peto–Prentice test by specifying the option peto.

```
. sts test dose, trend peto
```

Peto-Peto test for equality of survivor functions

dose	Events observed	Events expected	Sum of ranks
0	4	6.41	-1.2792221
1.5	6	6.80	-1.3150418
2	5	1.79	2.5942639
Total	15	15.00	0

```
              chi2(2) =      8.39
              Pr>chi2 =    0.0150
```

Test for trend of survivor functions

```
              chi2(1) =      2.85
              Pr>chi2 =    0.0914
```

Saved Results

sts test saves the following in r():

Scalars

r(df)	degrees of freedom	r(chi2)	χ^2
r(df_tr)	degrees of freedom, trend test	r(chi2_tr)	χ^2, trend test

Methods and Formulas

sts test is implemented as an ado-file.

Let $t_1 < t_2 < \cdots < t_k$ denote the ordered failure times; let d_j be the number of failures at t_j and n_j be the population at risk just before t_j; and let d_{ij} and n_{ij} denote the same things for group i, $i = 1, \ldots, r$.

We are interested in testing the null hypothesis

$$H_o: \lambda_1(t) = \lambda_2(t) = \cdots = \lambda_r(t)$$

where $\lambda(t)$ is the hazard function at time t, against the alternative hypothesis that at least one of the $\lambda_i(t)$ is different for some t_j.

As described in Klein and Moeschberger (2003, 205–216), Kalbfleisch and Prentice (2002, 20–22), and Collett (2003, 48–49), if the null hypothesis is true, the expected number of failures in group i at time t_j is $e_{ij} = n_{ij}d_j/n_j$, and the test statistic

$$\mathbf{u}' = \sum_{j=1}^{k} W(t_j)(d_{1j} - e_{1j}, \ldots, d_{rj} - e_{rj})$$

is formed. $W(t_j)$ is a positive weight function defined as zero when n_{ij} is zero. The various test statistics are obtained by selecting different weight functions $W(t_j)$. See the table in the *Remarks* section of this entry for a list of these weight functions. For the Peto–Peto–Prentice test,

$$W(t_j) = \widetilde{S}(t_j) = \prod_{\ell:t_\ell \leq t_j} \left(1 - \frac{d_\ell}{n_\ell + 1}\right)$$

The variance matrix $\mathbf{V}$ for $\mathbf{u}$ has elements

$$V_{il} = \sum_{j=1}^{k} \frac{W(t_j)^2 n_{ij}d_j(n_j - d_j)}{n_j(n_j - 1)}\left(\delta_{il} - \frac{n_{ij}}{n_j}\right)$$

where $\delta_{il} = 1$ if $i = l$ and 0, otherwise.

For the unstratified test, statistic $\mathbf{u}'\mathbf{V}^{-1}\mathbf{u}$ is distributed as χ^2 with $r - 1$ degrees of freedom.

For the stratified test, let $\mathbf{u}_s$ and $\mathbf{V}_s$ be the results of performing the above calculation separately within stratum, and define $\mathbf{u} = \sum_s \mathbf{u}_s$ and $\mathbf{V} = \sum_s \mathbf{V}_s$. The χ^2 test is given by $\mathbf{u}'\mathbf{V}^{-1}\mathbf{u}$ redefined in this way.

The "Cox" test is performed by fitting a (possibly stratified) Cox regression using `stcox` on $r - 1$ indicator variables, one for each group with one of the indicators omitted. The χ^2 test reported is then the likelihood-ratio test (no `pweights`) or the Wald test (based on the robust estimate of variance); see [ST] **stcox**.

The reported relative hazards are the exponentiated coefficients from the Cox regression renormalized, and the renormalization plays no role calculating the test statistic. The renormalization is chosen so that the expected-number-of-failures-within-group weighted average of the regression coefficients is 0 (meaning that the hazard is 1). Let b_i, $i = 1, \dots, r - 1$ be the estimated coefficients, and define $b_r = 0$. The constant K is then calculated by

$$ K = \sum_{i=1}^{r} e_i b_i / d $$

where $e_i = \sum_j e_{ij}$ is the expected number of failures for group i, d is the total number of failures across all groups, and r is the number of groups. The reported relative hazards are $\exp(b_i - K)$.

The trend test assumes that there is natural ordering of the r groups, $r > 2$. Here we are interested in testing the null hypothesis

$$ H_o : \lambda_1(t) = \lambda_2(t) = \cdots = \lambda_r(t) $$

against the alternative hypothesis

$$ H_a : \lambda_1(t) \le \lambda_2(t) \le \cdots \le \lambda_r(t) $$

The test uses **u** as previously defined with any of the available weight functions. The test statistic is given by

$$ \frac{\left(\sum_{i=1}^{r} a_i u_i \right)^2}{\mathbf{a'Va}} $$

where $a_1 \le a_2 \le \cdots \le a_r$ are scores defining the relationship of interest. A score is assigned to each comparison group, equal to the value of the grouping variable for that group. **a** is the vector of these scores.

References

Breslow, N. E. 1970. A generalized Kruskal–Wallis test for comparing k samples subject to unequal patterns of censorship. *Biometrika* 57: 579–594.

Collett, D. 2003. *Modelling Survival Data in Medical Research*. 2nd ed. London: Chapman & Hall/CRC.

Gehan, E. A. 1965. A generalized Wilcoxon test for comparing arbitrarily singly censored data. *Biometrika* 52: 203–223.

Harrington, D. P., and T. R. Fleming. 1982. A class of rank test procedures for censored survival data. *Biometrika* 69: 553–566.

Kalbfleisch, J. D., and R. L. Prentice. 2002. *The Statistical Analysis of Failure Time Data*. 2nd ed. New York: Wiley.

Klein, J. P., and M. L. Moeschberger. 2003. *Survival Analysis: Techniques for Censored and Truncated Data*. 2nd ed. New York: Springer.

Mantel, N. 1963. Chi-squared tests with one degree of freedom: Extensions of the Mantel–Haenszel procedure. *Journal of the American Statistical Association* 58: 690–700.

——. 1966. Evaluation of survival data and two new rank-order statistics arising in its consideration. *Cancer Chemotherapy Reports* 50: 163–170.

Mantel, N., and W. Haenszel. 1959. Statistical aspects of the analysis of data from retrospective studies of disease. *Journal of the National Cancer Institute* 22: 719–748. Reprinted in *Evolution of Epidemiologic Ideas*, ed. S. Greenland, 112–141. Newton Lower Falls, MA: Epidemiology Resources.

Marubini, E., and M. Grazia-Valsecchi. 1995. *Analysing Survival Data from Clinical Trials and Observational Studies.* New York: Wiley.

Peto, R., and J. Peto. 1972. Asymptotically efficient rank invariant test procedures (with discussion). *Journal of the Royal Statistical Society* 135: 185–206.

Prentice, R. L. 1978. Linear rank tests with right-censored data. *Biometrika* 65: 167–179.

Savage, I. R. 1956. Contributions to the theory of rank-order statistics—the two-sample case. *Annals of Mathematical Statistics* 27: 590–615.

Tarone, R. E., and J. H. Ware. 1977. On distribution-free tests for equality of survival distributions. *Biometrika* 64: 156–160.

White, I. R., S. Walker, and A. Babiker. 2002. strbee: Randomization-based efficacy estimator. *Stata Journal* 2: 140–150.

Wilcoxon, F. 1945. Individual comparisons by ranking methods. *Biometrics* 1: 80–83.

Also See

[ST] **stcox** — Fit Cox proportional hazards model

[ST] **sts** — Generate, graph, list, and test the survivor and cumulative hazard functions

[ST] **sts generate** — Create variables containing survivor and related functions

[ST] **sts graph** — Graph the survivor and cumulative hazard functions

[ST] **sts list** — List the survivor or cumulative hazard function

[ST] **stset** — Declare data to be survival-time data

Title

> **stset** — Declare data to be survival-time data

Syntax

Single-record-per-subject survival data

> stset *timevar* [*if*] [*weight*] [, *single_options*]

> streset [*if*] [*weight*] [, *single_options*]

> st [, no**cmd** **not**able]

> stset, clear

Multiple-record-per-subject survival data

> stset *timevar* [*if*] [*weight*], id(*varname*) **f**ailure(*failvar*[==*numlist*])
>   [*multiple_options*]

> streset [*if*] [*weight*] [, *multiple_options*]

> streset, { **past** | **future** | **past** **future** }

> st [, no**cmd** **not**able]

> stset, clear

single_options	description
Main	
failure(*failvar*[==*numlist*])	failure event
noshow	prevent other st commands from showing st setting information
Options	
origin(**t**ime *exp*)	define when a subject becomes at risk
scale(*#*)	rescale time value
enter(**t**ime *exp*)	specify when subject first enters study
exit(**t**ime *exp*)	specify when subject exits study
Advanced	
if(*exp*)	select records for which *exp* is true; recommended rather than if *exp*
time0(*varname*)	mechanical aspect of interpretation about records in dataset; seldom used

multiple_options	description
Main	
* id(*varname*)	multiple-record ID variable
* <u>f</u>ailure(*failvar*[==*numlist*])	failure event
<u>nosh</u>ow	prevent other st commands from showing st setting information
Options	
<u>o</u>rigin([*varname*==*numlist*] <u>t</u>ime *exp*|min)	define when a subject becomes at risk
<u>sc</u>ale(#)	rescale time value
<u>en</u>ter([*varname*==*numlist*] <u>t</u>ime *exp*)	specify when subject first enters study
<u>ex</u>it(failure|[*varname*==*numlist*] <u>t</u>ime *exp*)	specify when subject exits study
Advanced	
if(*exp*)	select records for which *exp* is true; recommended rather than if *exp*
ever(*exp*)	select objects for which *exp* is ever true
never(*exp*)	select objects for which *exp* is never true
after(*exp*)	select records within subject on or after the first time *exp* is true
<u>befor</u>e(*exp*)	select records within subject before the first time *exp* is true
time0(*varname*)	mechanical aspect of interpretation about records in dataset; seldom used

  * id() and failure() are required with stset multiple-record-per-subject survival data.

fweights, iweights, and pweights are allowed; see [U] **11.1.6 weight**.

Examples

```
. stset ftime                              (Time measured from 0, all failed)
. stset ftime, failure(died)               (Time measured from 0, censoring)
. stset ftime, failure(died) id(id)        (Time measured from 0, censoring & ID)
. stset ftime, failure(died==2,3)          (Time measured from 0, failure codes)
. stset ftime, failure(died) origin(time dob)  (Time measured from dob, censoring)
```

You cannot harm your data by using stset, so feel free to experiment.

Description

st refers to survival-time data, which are fully described below.

stset declares the data in memory to be st data, informing Stata of key variables and their roles in a survival-time data analysis. When you stset your data, stset runs various data consistency checks to ensure that what you have declared makes sense. If the data are weighted, you specify the weights when you stset the data, not when you issue the individual st commands.

streset changes how the st dataset is declared. In multiple-record data, streset can also temporarily set the sample to include records from before the time at risk (called the past) and records after failure (called the future). Then typing streset without arguments resets the sample back to the analysis sample.

st displays how the dataset is currently declared.

Whenever you type stset or streset, Stata runs or reruns data consistency checks to ensure that what you are now declaring (or declared in the past) makes sense. Thus if you have made any changes to your data or simply wish to verify how things are, you can type streset with no options.

stset, clear is for use by programmers. It causes Stata to forget the st markers, making the data no longer st data to Stata. The data remain unchanged. It is not necessary to stset, clear before doing another stset.

Options for use with stset and streset

⌐ Main ⌐

id(*idvar*) specifies the subject-ID variable; observations with equal, nonmissing values of *idvar* are assumed to be the same subject. *idvar* may be string or numeric. Observations for which *idvar* is missing (. or "") are ignored.

When id() is not specified, each observation is assumed to represent a different subject and thus constitutes one-record-per-subject survival dataset.

When you specify id(), the data are said to be multiple-record data, even if it turns out that there is only one record per subject. Perhaps they would better be called potentially multiple-record data.

If you specify id(), stset requires that you specify failure().

Specifying id() never hurts; we recommend it because a few st commands, such as stsplit, require an ID variable to have been specified when the dataset was stset.

failure(*failvar*[==*numlist*]) specifies the failure event.

If failure() is not specified, all records are assumed to end in failure. This is allowed with single-record data only.

If failure(*failvar*) is specified, *failvar* is interpreted as an indicator variable; 0 and missing mean censored, and all other values are interpreted as representing failure.

If failure(*failvar*==*numlist*) is specified, records with *failvar* taking on any of the values in *numlist* are assumed to end in failure, and all other records are assumed to be censored.

noshow prevents other st commands from showing the key st variables at the top of their output.

⌐ Options ⌐

origin([*varname*==*numlist*] time *exp* | min) and scale(#) define analysis time; i.e., origin() defines when a subject becomes at risk. Subjects become at risk when time = origin(). All analyses are performed in terms of time since becoming at risk, called analysis time.

Let us use the terms *time* for how time is recorded in the data and t for analysis time. Analysis time t is defined

$$t = \frac{time - \texttt{origin()}}{\texttt{scale()}}$$

t is time from origin in units of scale.

By default, origin(time 0) and scale(1) are assumed, meaning that $t = time$. Then you must ensure that *time* in your data is measured as time since becoming at risk. Subjects are exposed at $t = time = 0$ and later fail. Observations with $t = time < 0$ are ignored because information before becoming at risk is irrelevant.

origin() determines when the clock starts ticking. scale() plays no substantive role, but it can be handy for making t units more readable (such as converting days to years).

origin(time *exp*) sets the origin to *exp*. For instance, if *time* were recorded as dates, such as 05jun1998, in your data and variable expdate recorded the date when subjects were exposed, you could specify origin(time expdate). If instead all subjects were exposed on 12nov1997, you could specify origin(time mdy(11,12,1997)).

origin(time *exp*) may be used with single- or multiple-record data.

origin(*varname*==*numlist*) is for use with multiple-record data; it specifies the origin indirectly. If *time* were recorded as dates in your data, variable obsdate recorded the (ending) date associated with each record, and subjects became at risk upon, say, having a certain operation— and that operation were indicated by code==217—then you could specify origin(code==217). origin(code==217) would mean, for each subject, that the origin time is the earliest time at which code==217 is observed. Records before that would be ignored (because $t < 0$). Subjects who never had code==217 would be ignored entirely.

origin(*varname*==*numlist* time *exp*) sets the origin to the later of the two times determined by *varname*==*numlist* and *exp*.

origin(min) sets origin to the earliest time observed, minus 1. This is an odd thing to do and is described in example 10.

origin() is an important concept; see *Key concepts*, *Two concepts of time*, and *The substantive meaning of analysis time*.

scale() makes results more readable. If you have *time* recorded in days (such as Stata dates, which are really days since 01jan1960), specifying scale(365.25) will cause results to be reported in years.

enter([*varname*==*numlist*] time *exp*) specifies when a subject first comes under observation, meaning that any failures, were they to occur, would be recorded in the data.

Do not confuse enter() and origin(). origin() specifies when a subject first becomes at risk. In many datasets, becoming at risk and coming under observation are coincident. Then it is sufficient to specify origin().

enter(time *exp*), enter(*varname*==*numlist*), and enter(*varname*==*numlist* time *exp*) follow the same syntax as origin(). In multiple-record data, both *varname*==*numlist* and time *exp* are interpreted as the earliest time implied, and if both are specified, the later of the two times is used.

exit(failure | [*varname*==*numlist*] time *exp*) specifies the latest time under which the subject is both under observation and at risk. The emphasis is on latest; obviously subjects also exit the risk pool when their data run out.

exit(failure) is the default. When the first failure event occurs, the subject is removed from the analysis risk pool, even if the subject has subsequent records in the data and even if some of those subsequent records document other failure events. Specify exit(time .) if you wish to keep all records for a subject after failure. You want to do this if you have multiple-failure data.

exit(*varname*==*numlist*), exit(time *exp*), and exit(*varname*==*numlist* time *exp*) follow the same syntax as origin() and enter(). In multiple-record data, both *varname*==*numlist* and time *exp* are interpreted as the earliest time implied. exit differs from origin() and enter() in that, if both are specified, the earlier of the two times is used.

if(*exp*), ever(*exp*), never(*exp*), after(*exp*), and before(*exp*) select relevant records.

if(*exp*) selects records for which *exp* is true. We strongly recommend specifying this if() option rather than if *exp* following stset or streset. They differ in that if *exp* removes the data from consideration before calculating beginning and ending times and other quantities. The if() option, on the other hand, sets the restriction after all derived variables are calculated. See *if() versus if exp*.

if() may be specified with single- or multiple-record data. The remaining selection options are for use with multiple-record data only.

ever(*exp*) selects only subjects for which *exp* is ever true.

never(*exp*) selects only subjects for which *exp* is never true.

after(*exp*) selects records within subject on or after the first time *exp* is true.

before(*exp*) selects records within subject before the first time *exp* is true.

time0(*varname*) is seldom specified because most datasets do not contain this information. time0() should be used exclusively with multiple-record data, and even then you should consider whether origin() or enter() would be more appropriate.

time0() specifies a mechanical aspect of interpretation about the records in the dataset, namely, the beginning of the period spanned by each record. See *Intermediate exit and reentry times (gaps)*.

Options unique to streset

past expands the stset sample to include the entire recorded past of the relevant subjects, meaning that it includes observations before becoming at risk and those excluded because of after(), etc.

future expands the stset sample to include the records on the relevant subjects after the last record that previously was included, if any, which typically means to include all observations after failure or censoring.

past future expands the stset sample to include all records on the relevant subjects.

Typing streset without arguments resets the sample to the analysis sample. See *Past and future records* for more information.

Options for st

nocmd suppresses displaying the last stset command.

notable suppresses displaying the table summarizing what has been stset.

Remarks

Remarks are presented under the following headings:

What are survival-time data?
Key concepts
Survival-time datasets
Using stset
Two concepts of time
The substantive meaning of analysis time
Setting the failure event
Setting multiple failures
First entry times
Final exit times
Intermediate exit and reentry times (gaps)
if( ) versus if exp
Past and future records
Using streset
Performance and multiple-record-per-subject datasets
Sequencing of events within t
Weights
Data warnings and errors flagged by stset
Using survival-time data in Stata

What are survival-time data?

Survival-time data—what we call st data—document spans of time ending in an event. For instance,

which indicates $x1 = 17$ and $x2 = 22$ over the time span 0 to 9, and $died = 1$. More formally: it means $x1 = 17$ and $x2 = 22$ for $0 < t \le 9$, which we often write as $(0, 9]$. However you wish to say it, this information might be recorded by the observation

id	end	x1	x2	died
101	9	17	22	1

and we call this single-record survival data.

The data can be more complicated. For instance, we might have

meaning

$$x1 = 17 \text{ and } x2 = 22 \text{ during } (0, 4]$$
$$x1 = 12 \text{ and } x2 = 22 \text{ during } (4, 9], \text{ and then } died = 1.$$

and this would be recorded by the data

id	begin	end	x1	x2	died
101	0	4	17	22	0
101	4	9	12	22	1

We call this multiple-record survival data.

These two formats allow you to record many different possibilities. The last observation on a person need not be failure,

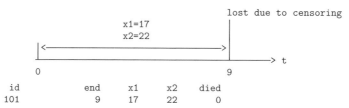

id	end	x1	x2	died
101	9	17	22	0

or

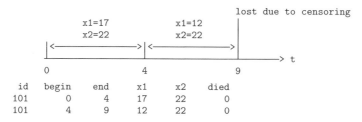

id	begin	end	x1	x2	died
101	0	4	17	22	0
101	4	9	12	22	0

Multiple-record data might have gaps,

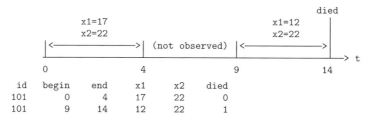

id	begin	end	x1	x2	died
101	0	4	17	22	0
101	9	14	12	22	1

or subjects might not be observed from the onset of risk,

begin	end	x1	x2	died
2	9	17	22	1

and

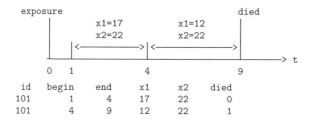

id	begin	end	x1	x2	died
101	1	4	17	22	0
101	4	9	12	22	1

The failure event might not be death but instead something that can be repeated:

id	begin	end	x1	x2	infarc
101	0	4	17	22	1
101	4	9	12	22	0
101	9	13	10	22	1

Our data may be in different time units; rather than t where $t = 0$ corresponds to the onset of risk, we might have time recorded as age,

id	age0	age1	x1	x2	died
101	20	29	17	22	1

or time recorded as calendar dates:

id	bdate	edate	x1	x2	died
101	01jan1998	02may1998	17	22	0
101	02may1998	15oct1998	12	22	1

Finally, we can mix these diagrams however we wish, so we might have time recorded according to the calendar, unobserved periods after the onset of risk, subsequent gaps, and multiple failure events.

The st commands analyze data like these, and the first step is to tell st about your data by using stset. You do not change your data to fit some predefined mold; you describe your data with stset, and the rest of the st commands just do the right thing.

Before we discuss using stset, let us describe one more style of recording time-to-event data because it is common and is inappropriate for use with st. It is inappropriate, but it is easy to convert to the survival-time form. It is called snapshot data, which are data for which you do not know spans of time but you have information recorded at various points in time:

id	t	x1	x2	died
101	0	17	22	0
101	4	12	22	0
101	9	.	.	1

In this snapshot dataset all we know are the values of x1 and x2 at $t = 0$ and $t = 4$, and we know that the subject died at $t = 9$. Snapshot data can be converted to survival-time data if we are willing to assume that x1 and x2 remained constant between times:

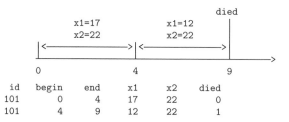

id	begin	end	x1	x2	died
101	0	4	17	22	0
101	4	9	12	22	1

The **snapspan** command makes this conversion. If you have snapshot data, first see [ST] **snapspan** to convert it to survival-time data and then use **stset** to tell st about the converted data; see example 10 first.

Key concepts

time, or better, *time units*, is how time is recorded in your data. It might be numbers (such as 0, 1, 2, ..., with *time* = 0 corresponding to some exposure event), a subject's age, or calendar time.

events are things that happen at an instant in time, such as being exposed to an environmental hazard, being diagnosed as myopic, becoming employed, being promoted, becoming unemployed, having a heart attack, and dying.

failure event is the *event* indicating failure as it is defined for analysis. This can be a single or compound event. The *failure* event might be when variable **dead** is 1, or it might be when variable **diag** is any of 115, 121, or 133.

at risk means the subject is at risk of the *failure event* occurring. For instance, if the *failure event* is becoming unemployed, a person must be employed. The subject is not *at risk* before being employed. Once employed, the subject becomes *at risk*; once again, the subject is no longer *at risk* once the *failure event* occurs. If subjects become *at risk* upon the occurrence of some *event*, it is called the exposure event. Gaining employment is the exposure event in our example.

origin is the *time* when the subject became at risk. If *time* is recorded as numbers such as 0, 1, 2, ..., with *time* = 0 corresponding to the exposure event, then *origin* = 0. Alternatively, *origin* might be the age of the subject when diagnosed or the date when the subject was exposed. Regardless, *origin* is expressed in *time units*.

scale is just a fixed number, typically 1, used in mapping *time* to analysis time t.

t, or *analysis time*, is $(time - origin)/scale$, meaning the time since onset of being at risk measured in *scale* units.

$t = 0$ corresponds to the onset of risk, and *scale* just provides a way to make the units of t more readable. You might have *time* recorded in days from 01jan1960 and want t recorded in years, in which case *scale* would be 365.25.

time is how time is recorded in your data, and t is how time is reported in the analysis.

under observation means that, should the *failure event* occur, it would be observed and recorded in the data. Sometimes subjects are *under observation* only after they are *at risk*. This would be the case, for instance, if subjects enrolled in a study after being diagnosed with cancer and if, to enroll in the study, subjects were required to be diagnosed with cancer.

Being *under observation* does not mean that the subject is necessarily *at risk*. A subject may come *under observation* before being *at risk*, and in fact, a subject *under observation* may never become *at risk*.

entry time and *exit time* mark when a subject is first and last *under observation*. The emphasis here is on the words *first* and *last; entry time* and *exit time* do not record observational gaps; there is only one *entry time* and one *exit time* per subject.

entry time and *exit time* might be expressed as *times* (recorded in *time units*), or they might correspond to the occurrence of some *event* (such as enrolling in the study).

Often the *entry time* corresponds to $t = 0$; i.e., since $t = (time - origin)/scale$, $time = origin$, meaning that *time* equals when the subject became at risk.

Often the *exit time* corresponds to when the *failure event* occurs or, failing that, the end of data for the subject.

delayed entry means that *entry time* corresponds to $t > 0$; the subject became at risk before coming under observation.

id refers to a subject identification variable; equal values of *id* indicate that the records are on the same subject. An *id* variable is required for multiple-record data and is optional, but recommended, with single-record data.

time0 refers to the beginning *time* (recorded in *time units*) of a record. Some datasets have this variable, but most do not. If the dataset does not contain the beginning time for each record, subsequent records are assumed to begin where previous records ended. A *time0* variable may be created for these datasets by using the snapspan command; see [ST] **snapspan**. Do not confuse *time0*—a mechanical aspect of datasets—with *entry time*—a substantive aspect of analysis.

gaps refer to gaps in observation between *entry time* and *exit time*. During a *gap* a subject is not *under observation*. *gaps* can arise only if the data contain a *time0* variable, because otherwise subsequent records beginning when previous records end would preclude there being *gaps* in the data. *gaps* are distinct from *delayed entry*.

past history is a term we use to mean information recorded in the data before the subject was both *at risk* and *under observation*. Complex datasets can contain such observations. Say that the dataset contains histories on subjects from birth to death. You might tell st that a subject becomes at risk once diagnosed with a particular kind of cancer. The *past history* on the subject would then refer to records before the subject was diagnosed.

The word *history* is often dropped, and the term simply becomes *past*. For instance, we might want to know whether the subject smoked in the *past*.

future history is a term meaning information recorded in the data after the subject is no longer *at risk*. Perhaps the failure event is not so serious as to preclude the possibility of data after failure.

The word *history* is often dropped, and the term simply becomes *future*. Perhaps the *failure event* is cardiac infarction, and you want to know whether the subject died soon in the *future* so that you can exclude the subject.

Survival-time datasets

In survival-time datasets, observations (records) document a span of time. The span might be explicitly indicated, such as

```
        begin   end    x1    x2
            3     9    17    22         <- spans (3,9]
```

or it might be implied that the record begins at 0,

```
         end    x1    x2
           9    17    22                 <- spans (0,9]
```

or it might be implied because there are multiple records per subject:

```
    id    end    x1    x2
     1      4    17    22                 <- spans (0,4]
     1      9    12    22                 <- spans (4,9]
```

Records may have an event indicator:

```
   begin    end    x1    x2    died
       3      9    17    22      1         <- spans (3,9], died at t=9


            end    x1    x2    died
              9    17    22      1         <- spans (0,9], died at t=9


    id      end    x1    x2    died
     1        4    17    22      0         <- spans (0,4],
     1        9    12    22      1         <- spans (4,9], died at t=9
```

The first two examples are called single-record survival-time data because there is one record per subject.

The final example is called multiple-record survival-time data. There are two records for subject with id = 1.

Either way, survival-time data document time spans. Characteristics are assumed to remain constant over the span, and the event is assumed to occur at the end of the span.

Using stset

Once you have stset your data, you can use the other st commands.

If you save your data after stsetting, you will not have to re-stset in the future; Stata will remember.

stset declares your data to be survival-time data. It does not change the data, although it does add a few variables to your dataset.

This means that you can re-stset your data as often as you wish. In fact, the streset command encourages this. Using complicated datasets often requires typing long stset commands, such as

```
. stset date, fail(event==27 28) origin(event==15) enter(event==22)
```

Later, you might want to try fail(event==27). You could retype the stset command, making the substitution, or you could type

```
. streset, fail(event==27)
```

streset takes what you type, merges it with what you have previously declared with stset, and performs the combined stset command.

▷ Example 1: Single-record data

Generators are run until they fail. Here is some of our dataset:

```
. use http://www.stata-press.com/data/r10/kva
(Generator experiment)

. list in 1/3
```

	failtime	load	bearings
1.	100	15	0
2.	140	15	1
3.	97	20	0

The stset command for this dataset is

```
. stset failtime

     failure event:  (assumed to fail at time=failtime)
obs. time interval:  (0, failtime]
 exit on or before:  failure

        12  total obs.
         0  exclusions

        12  obs. remaining, representing
        12  failures in single record/single failure data
       896  total analysis time at risk, at risk from t =         0
                            earliest observed entry t =         0
                                last observed exit t =       140
```

When you type stset *timevar*, *timevar* is assumed to be the time of failure. More generally, you will learn, *timevar* is the time of failure or censoring. Here *timevar* is failtime.

◁

▷ Example 2: Single-record data with censoring

Generators are run until they fail, but during the experiment, the room flooded, so some generators were run only until the flood. Here are some of our data:

```
. use http://www.stata-press.com/data/r10/kva2
(Generator experiment)

. list in 1/4
```

	failtime	load	bearings	failed
1.	100	15	0	1
2.	140	15	1	0
3.	97	20	0	1
4.	122	20	1	1

Here the second generator did not fail at time 140; the experiment was merely discontinued then. The stset command for this dataset is

```
. stset failtime, failure(failed)

     failure event:  failed != 0 & failed < .
obs. time interval:  (0, failtime]
 exit on or before:  failure
```

```
   12  total obs.
    0  exclusions
```

```
   12  obs. remaining, representing
   11  failures in single record/single failure data
  896  total analysis time at risk, at risk from t =          0
                          earliest observed entry t =          0
                                last observed exit t =        140
```

When you type stset *timevar*, failure(*failvar*), *timevar* is interpreted as the time of failure or censoring, which is determined by the value of *failvar*. *failvar* = 0 and *failvar* = . (missing) indicate censorings, and all other values indicate failure.

◁

▷ Example 3: Multiple-record data

Assume that we are analyzing survival time of patients with a particular kind of cancer. In this dataset, the characteristics of patients vary over time, perhaps because new readings were taken or because the drug therapy was changed. Some of the data are

```
. list, separator(0)
```

	patid	t	died	x1	x2
1.	90	100	0	1	0
2.	90	150	1	0	0
3.	91	50	1	1	1
4.	92	100	0	0	0
5.	92	150	0	0	1
6.	92	190	0	0	0
7.	93	100	0	0	0
		(output omitted)			

There are two records for patient 90 and that died is 0 in the first record but 1 in the second. The interpretation of these two records is

Interval (0,100]:	$x1 = 1$ and $x2 = 0$
Interval (100,150]:	$x1 = 0$ and $x2 = 0$
at $t = 150$:	the patient died

Similarly, here is how you interpret the other records:

Patient 91:

| Interval (0, 50]: | $x1 = 1$ and $x2 = 1$ |
| at $t = 50$: | the patient died |

Patient 92:

Interval (0,100]:	$x1 = 0$ and $x2 = 0$
Interval (100,150]:	$x1 = 0$ and $x2 = 1$
Interval (150,190]:	$x1 = 0$ and $x2 = 0$
at $t = 190$:	the patient was lost because of censoring

Look again at patient 92's data:

patid	t	died	x1	x2
92	100	0	0	0
92	150	0	0	1
92	190	0	0	0

died $= 0$ for the first event. Mechanically, this removes the subject from the data at $t = 100$—the patient is treated as censored. The next record, however, adds the patient back into the data (at $t = 100$) with new characteristics.

The stset command for this dataset is

```
. stset t, id(patid) failure(died)
                id:  patid
     failure event:  died != 0 & died < .
obs. time interval:  (t[_n-1], t]
 exit on or before:  failure
```

```
   126  total obs.
     0  exclusions

   126  obs. remaining, representing
    40  subjects
    26  failures in single failure-per-subject data
  2989  total analysis time at risk, at risk from t =         0
                          earliest observed entry t =         0
                            last observed exit t =          139
```

When you have multiple-record data, you specify stset's id(*idvar*) option. When you type 'stset *timevar*, id(*idvar*) failure(*failvar*)', *timevar* denotes the end of the period (just as it does in single-record data). The first record within *idvar* is assumed to begin at time 0, and later records are assumed to begin where the previous record left off. *failvar* should contain 0 on all but, possibly, the last record within *idvar* unless your data contain multiple failures (in which case you must specify the exit() option; see *Setting multiple failures* below).

◁

▷ Example 4: Multiple-record data with multiple events

We have the following data on hospital patients admitted to a particular ward:

patid	day	sex	x1	x2	code
101	5	1	10	10	177
101	13	1	20	8	286
101	21	1	16	11	208
101	24	1	11	17	401
102	8	0	20	19	204
102	18	0	19	1	401
103	*etc.*				

Variable code records various actions; code 401 indicates being discharged alive, and 402 indicates death. We stset this dataset by typing

```
. stset day, id(patid) fail(code==402)
                id:   patid
     failure event:   code == 402
obs. time interval:   (day[_n-1], day]
 exit on or before:   failure
```

```
     243   total obs.
       0   exclusions

     243   obs. remaining, representing
      40   subjects
      15   failures in single failure-per-subject data
    1486   total analysis time at risk, at risk from t =        0
                                earliest observed entry t =      0
                                  last observed exit t =        62
```

When you specify failure(*eventvar* == #), the failure event is as specified. You may include a list of numbers following the equal signs. If failure were codes 402 and 403, you could specify failure(code == 402 403). If failure were codes 402, 403, 404, 405, 406, 407, and 409, you could specify failure(code == 402/407 409).

◁

▷ Example 5: Multiple-record data recording time rather than t

More reasonably, the hospital data in the above example would not contain days since admission but would contain admission and current dates. In the dataset below, adday contains the day of admission, and curdate contains the ending date of the record, both recorded as number of days since the ward opened:

patid	adday	curday	sex	x1	x2	code
101	287	292	1	10	10	177
101	.	300	1	20	8	286
101	.	308	1	16	11	208
101	.	311	1	11	17	401
102	289	297	0	20	19	204
102	.	307	0	19	1	401
103	etc.					

This is the same dataset as shown in example 4. Previously the first record on patient 101 was recorded 5 days after admission. In this dataset, $292 - 287 = 5$. We would stset this dataset by typing

```
. stset curday, id(patid) fail(code==402) origin(time adday)
                id:   patid
     failure event:   code == 402
obs. time interval:   (curday[_n-1], curday]
 exit on or before:   failure
    t for analysis:   (time-origin)
            origin:   time adday
```

```
     243   total obs.
       0   exclusions

     243   obs. remaining, representing
      40   subjects
      15   failures in single failure-per-subject data
    1486   total analysis time at risk, at risk from t =        0
                                earliest observed entry t =      0
                                  last observed exit t =        62
```

origin() sets when a subject becomes at risk. It does this by defining *analysis time*.

When you specify stset *timevar*, ...origin(time *originvar*), analysis time is defined as $t = (timevar - originvar)/$scale(). In analysis time units, subjects become at risk at $t = 0$. See *Two concepts of time* and *The substantive meaning of analysis time* below.

◁

▷ Example 6: Multiple-record data with time recorded as a date

Even more reasonably, dates would not be recorded as integers 428, 433, and 453, meaning the number of days since the ward opened. The dates would be recorded as dates:

```
patid    addate    curdate   sex    x1    x2    code
  101  18aug1998  23aug1998    1     10    10    177
  101          .  31aug1998    1     20     8    286
  101          .  08sep1998    1     16    11    208
  101          .  11sep1998    1     11    17    401
  102  20aug1998  28aug1998    0     20    19    204
  102          .  07sep1998    0     19     1    401
  103      etc.
```

That, in fact, changes nothing. We still type what we previously typed:

```
. stset curdate, id(patid) fail(code==402) origin(time addate)
```

Stata dates are, in fact, integers—they are the number of days since 01jan1960—and it is merely Stata's %td display format that makes them display as dates.

◁

▷ Example 7: Multiple-record data with extraneous information

Perhaps we wish to study the outcome after a certain operation, said operation being indicated by code 286. Subjects become at risk when the operation is performed. Here we do not type

```
. stset curdate, id(patid) fail(code==402) origin(time addate)
```

We instead type

```
. stset curdate, id(patid) fail(code==402) origin(code==286)
```

The result of typing this would be to set analysis time t to

$$t = \text{curdate} - (\text{the value of curdate when code==286})$$

Let us work through this for the first patient:

```
patid    addate    curdate   sex    x1    x2    code
  101  18aug1998  23aug1998    1     10    10    177
  101          .  31aug1998    1     20     8    286
  101          .  08sep1998    1     16    11    208
  101          .  11sep1998    1     11    17    401
```

The event 286 occurred on 31aug1998, and thus the values of t for the four records are

$$t_1 = curdate_1 - 31\text{aug}1998 = 23\text{aug}1998 - 31\text{aug}1998 = -8$$
$$t_2 = curdate_2 - 31\text{aug}1998 = 31\text{aug}1998 - 31\text{aug}1998 = 0$$
$$t_3 = curdate_3 - 31\text{aug}1998 = 08\text{sep}1998 - 31\text{aug}1998 = 8$$
$$t_4 = curdate_4 - 31\text{aug}1998 = 11\text{sep}1998 - 31\text{aug}1998 = 11$$

Information prior to $t = 0$ is not relevant because the subject is not yet at risk. Thus the relevant data on this subject are

t in $(0, 8]$ sex $= 1$, x1 $= 16$, x2 $= 11$
t in $(8, 11]$ sex $= 1$, x1 $= 11$, x2 $= 17$, and the subject is censored (code $\neq 402$)

That is precisely the logic that stset went through. For your information, stset quietly creates the variables

_st	1 if the record is to be used, 0 if ignored
_t0	analysis time when record begins
_t	analysis time when record ends
_d	1 if failure, 0 if censored

You can examine these variables after issuing the stset command:

```
. list _st _t0 _t _d
```

	_st	_t0	_t	_d
1.	0	.	.	.
2.	0	.	.	.
203.	1	0	8	0
204.	1	8	11	0

Results are just as we anticipated. Do not let the observation numbers bother you; stset sorts the data in a way it finds convenient. Feel free to resort the data; if any of the st commands need the data in a different order, they will sort it themselves.

There are two ways of specifying origin():

origin(time *timevar*)   or   origin(time *exp*)
origin(*eventvar* == *numlist*)

In the first syntax—which is denoted by typing the word time—you directly specify when a subject becomes at risk. In the second syntax—which is denoted by typing a variable name and equal signs—you specify the same thing indirectly. The subject becomes at risk when the specified event occurs (which may be never).

Information prior to origin() is ignored. That information composes what we call the past history.

◁

▷ Example 8: Multiple-record data with delayed entry

In another analysis, we want to use the above data to analyze all patients, not just those undergoing a particular operation. In this analysis, subjects become at risk when they enter the ward. For this analysis, however, we need information from a particular test, and that information is available only if the test is administered to the patient. Even if the test is administered, some amount of time passes before that. Assume that when the test is administered, code==152 is inserted into the patient's hospital record.

To summarize, we want origin(time addate), but patients do not enter our sample until code==152. The way to stset these data is

```
. stset curdate, id(patid) fail(code==402) origin(time addate) enter(code==152)
```

Patient 107 has code 152:

patid	addate	curdate	sex	x1	x2	code
107	22aug1998	25aug1998	1	9	13	274
107	.	28aug1998	1	19	19	152
107	.	30aug1998	1	18	12	239
107	.	07sep1998	1	12	11	401

In analysis time, $t = 0$ corresponds to 22aug1998. The test was not administered, however, until 6 days later. The analysis times for these records are

$$t_1 = curdate_1 - 22\text{aug}1998 = 25\text{aug}1998 - 22\text{aug}1998 = 3$$

$$t_2 = curdate_2 - 22\text{aug}1998 = 28\text{aug}1998 - 22\text{aug}1998 = 6$$

$$t_3 = curdate_3 - 22\text{aug}1998 = 30\text{aug}1998 - 22\text{aug}1998 = 8$$

$$t_4 = curdate_4 - 22\text{aug}1998 = 07\text{sep}1998 - 22\text{aug}1998 = 16$$

and the data we want in our sample are

t in $(6, 8]$ sex $= 1$, x1 $= 18$, x2 $= 12$
t in $(8, 16]$ sex $= 1$, x1 $= 12$, x2 $= 11$, and patient was censored (code $\neq 402$)

The above `stset` command produced this:

```
. list _st _t0 _t _d
```

	_st	_t0	_t	_d
1.	0	.	.	.
2.	0	.	.	.
39.	1	6	8	0
40.	1	8	16	0

◁

▷ Example 9: Multiple-record data with extraneous information and delayed entry

Options `origin()` and `enter()` can be combined. For instance, we want to analyze patients receiving a particular operation (time at risk begins upon code == 286, but patients may not enter the sample before a test is administered, denoted by code == 152). We type

```
. stset curdate, id(patid) fail(code==402) origin(code==286) enter(code==152)
```

If we typed the above commands, it would not matter whether the test was performed before or after the operation.

A patient who had the test and then the operation would enter at analysis time $t = 0$.

A patient who had the operation and then the test would enter at analysis time $t > 0$, the analysis time being the time the test was performed.

If we wanted to require that the operation be performed after the test, we could type

```
. stset curdate, id(patid) fail(code==402) origin(code==286) after(code==152)
```

Admittedly this can be confusing. The way to proceed is to find a complicated case in your data and then list `_st _t0 _t _d` for that case after you `stset` the data.

◁

▷ Example 10: Real data

All of our hospital ward examples are artificial in one sense: it is unlikely the data would have come to us in survival-time form:

```
patid    addate    curdate    sex    x1    x2    code
  101  18aug1998  23aug1998     1     10    10     177
  101          .  31aug1998     1     20     8     286
  101          .  08sep1998     1     16    11     208
  101          .  11sep1998     1     11    17     401
  102  20aug1998  28aug1998     0     20    19     204
  102          .  07sep1998     0     19     1     401
  103      etc.
```

Rather, we would have received a snapshot dataset:

```
patid       date    sex    x1    x2    code
  101  18aug1998      1     10    10      22
  101  23aug1998      .     20     8     177
  101  31aug1998      .     16    11     286
  101  08sep1998      .     11    17     208
  101  11sep1998      .      .     .     401
  102  20aug1998      0     20    19      22
  102  28aug1998      .     19     1     204
  102  07sep1998      .      .     .     401
  103      etc.
```

In a snapshot dataset, we have a time (here, a date) and values of the variables as of that instant.

This dataset can be converted to the appropriate form by typing

```
. snapspan patid date code
```

The result would be as follows:

```
patid       date    sex    x1    x2    code
  101  18aug1998      .      .     .      22
  101  23aug1998      1     10    10     177
  101  31aug1998      .     20     8     286
  101  08sep1998      .     16    11     208
  101  11sep1998      .     11    17     401
  102  20aug1998      .      .     .      22
  102  28aug1998      0     20    19     204
  102  07sep1998      .     19     1     401
```

This is virtually the same dataset with which we have been working, but it differs in two ways:

1. The variable sex is not filled in for all the observations because it was not filled in on the original form. The hospital wrote down the sex on admission and then never bothered to document it again.

2. We have no admission date (addate) variable. Instead, we have an extra first record for each patient with code = 22 (22 is the code the hospital uses for admissions).

The first problem is easily fixed, and the second, it turns out, is not a problem because we can vary what we type when we stset the data.

First, let's fix the problem with variable sex. There are two ways to proceed. One would be simply to fill in the variable ourselves:

```
. by patid (date), sort: replace sex = sex[_n-1] if sex>=.
```

We could also perform a phony stset that is good enough to set all the data and then use stfill to fill in the variable for us. Let us begin with the phony stset:

```
. stset date, id(patid) origin(min) fail(code==-1)
                 id:  patid
      failure event:  code == -1
 obs. time interval:  (date[_n-1], date]
  exit on or before:  failure
     t for analysis:  (time-origin)
             origin:  min

      283  total obs.
        0  exclusions

      283  obs. remaining, representing
       40  subjects
        0  failures in single failure-per-subject data
     2224  total analysis time at risk, at risk from t =          0
                              earliest observed entry t =          0
                                 last observed exit t =         89
```

Typing stset date, id(patid) origin(min) fail(code == -1) does not produce anything we would want to use for analysis. This is a trick to get the dataset temporarily stset so that we can use some st data-management commands on it.

The first part of the trick is to specify origin(min). This defines the analysis time as $t = 0$, corresponding to the minimum observed value of the time variable minus 1. The time variable is date here. Why the minimum minus 1? Because st ignores observations for which analysis time $t < 0$. origin(min) provides a phony definition of t that ensures $t > 0$ for all observations.

The second part of the trick is to specify fail(code == -1), and you might have to vary what you type. We just wanted to choose an event that we know never happens, thus ensuring that no observations are ignored after failure.

Now that we have the dataset stset, we can use the other st commands. Do not use the st analysis commands unless you want ridiculous results, but one of the st data-management commands is just what we want:

```
. stfill sex, forward
          failure _d:  code == -1
    analysis time _t:  (date-origin)
              origin:  min
                  id:  patid
 replace missing values with previously observed values:
             sex:  203 real changes made
```

Problem one solved.

The second problem concerns the lack of an admission-date variable. That is not really a problem because we have a new first observation with code = 22 recording the date of admission, so every place we previously coded origin(time addate), we substitute origin(code == 22).

Problem two solved.

We also solved the big problem—converting a snapshot dataset into a survival-time dataset; see [ST] **snapspan**.

◁

Two concepts of time

The st system has two concepts of time. The first is *time* in italics, which corresponds to how time is recorded in your data. The second is analysis time, which we write as t. Substantively, analysis time is time at risk. stset defines analysis time in terms of *time* via

$$t = \frac{time - \mathtt{origin()}}{\mathtt{scale()}}$$

t and *time* can be the same thing, and by default they are because, by default, origin() is 0 and scale() is 1.

All the st analysis commands work with analysis time t.

By default, if you do not specify the origin() and scale() options, your time variables are expected to be the analysis time variables. This means that *time* = 0 corresponds to when subjects became at risk, and that means, among other things, that observations for which *time* < 0 are ignored because survival analysis concerns persons who are at risk, and no one is at risk before $t = 0$.

origin determines when the clock starts ticking. If you do not specify origin(), origin(time 0) is assumed, meaning that $t = time$ and that persons are at risk from $t = time = 0$.

time and t will often differ. *time* might be calendar time and t the length of time since some event, such as being born, being exposed to some risk factor, etc. origin() sets when $t = 0$. scale() merely sets a constant that makes t more readable.

The syntax for the origin() option makes it look more complicated than it really is:

$$\mathtt{origin(}\left[\mathit{varname} == \mathit{numlist}\right] \mathtt{time}\ \mathit{exp}\ |\ \mathtt{min)}$$

This says that there are four different ways to specify origin():

> origin(time *exp*)
> origin(*varname* == *numlist*)
> origin(*varname* == *numlist* time *exp*)
> origin(min)

The first syntax can be used with single- or multiple-record data. It states that the origin is given by *exp*, which can be a constant for all observations, a variable (and hence may vary subject by subject), or even an expression composed of variables and constants. Perhaps the origin is a fixed date or a date recorded in the data when the subject was exposed or when the subject turned 18.

The second and third syntaxes are for use with multiple-record data. The second states that the origin corresponds to the (earliest) time when the designated event occurred. Perhaps the origin is when an operation was performed. The third syntax calculates the origin both ways and then selects the later one.

The fourth syntax does something odd; it sets the origin to the minimum time observed minus 1. This is not useful for analysis but is sometimes useful for playing data-management tricks; see example 10 above.

Let's start with the first syntax. Say that you had the data

```
   faildate      x1      x2
   28dec1997     12      22
   12nov1997     15      22
   03feb1998     55      22
```

and that all the observations came at risk on the same date, 01nov1997. You could type

    . stset faildate, origin(time mdy(11,1,1997))

Remember that stset adds _t0 and _t to your dataset and that they contain the time span for each record, documented in analysis time units. After typing stset, you can list the results:

    . list faildate x1 x2 _t0 _t

	faildate	x1	x2	_t0	_t
1.	28dec1997	12	22	0	57
2.	12nov1997	15	22	0	11
3.	03feb1998	55	22	0	94

Record 1 reflects the period $(0, 57]$ in analysis time units, which are days here. stset calculated the 57 from $28\text{dec}1997 - 01\text{nov}1997 = 13{,}876 - 13{,}819 = 57$. (Dates such as 28dec1997 are really just integers containing the number of days from 01jan1960, and Stata's %td display format makes them display nicely. 28dec1997 is really the number 13,876.)

As another example, we might have data recording exposure and failure dates:

expdate	faildate	x1	x2
07may1998	22jun1998	12	22
02feb1998	11may1998	11	17

The way to stset this dataset is

    . stset faildate, origin(time expdate)

and the result, in analysis units, is

    . list expdate faildate x1 x2 _t0 _t

	expdate	faildate	x1	x2	_t0	_t
1.	07may1998	22jun1998	12	22	0	46
2.	02feb1998	11may1998	11	17	0	98

There is nothing magical about dates. Our original data could just as well have been

expdate	faildate	x1	x2
32	78	12	22
12	110	11	17

and the result would still be the same because $78 - 32 = 46$ and $110 - 12 = 98$.

Specifying an expression can sometimes be useful. Suppose that your dataset has the variable date recording the date of event and variable age recording the subject's age as of date. You want to make $t = 0$ correspond to when the subject turned 18. You could type $\text{origin}\big(\text{time}$ date-int$((\text{age-18})*365.25)\big)$.

origin(*varname* == *numlist*) is for use with multiple-record data. It states when each subject became at risk indirectly; the subject became at risk at the earliest time that *varname* takes on any of the enumerated values. Say that you had

```
patid       date      x1      x2    event
  101   12nov1997      15      22      127
  101   28dec1997      12      22      155
  101   03feb1998      55      22      133
  101   05mar1998      14      22      127
  101   09apr1998      12      22      133
  101   03jun1998      13      22      101
  102   22nov1997       .       .        .
```

and assume event $= 155$ represents the onset of exposure. You might stset this dataset by typing

```
. stset date, id(patid) origin(event==155) ...
```

If you did that, the information for patient 101 before 28dec1997 would be ignored in subsequent analysis. The prior information would not be removed from the dataset; it would just be ignored. Probably something similar would happen for patient 102, or if patient 102 has no record with event $= 155$, all the records on the patient would be ignored.

For analysis time, $t = 0$ would correspond to when event 155 occurred. Here are the results in analysis time units:

```
patid       date      x1      x2    event     _t0       _t
  101   12nov1997      15      22      127       .        .
  101   28dec1997      12      22      155       .        .
  101   03feb1998      55      22      133       0       37
  101   05mar1998      14      22      127      37       67
  101   09apr1998      12      22      133      67      102
  101   03jun1998      13      22      101     102      157
  102   22nov1997       .       .        .       .        .
```

Patient 101's second record is excluded from the analysis. That is not a mistake. Records document durations, date reflects the end of the period, and events occur at the end of periods. Thus event 155 occurred at the instant date $= 28$dec1997, and the relevant first record for the patient is $(28\text{dec}1997, 03\text{feb}1998]$ in time units, which is $(0, 37]$ in t units.

The substantive meaning of analysis time

In specifying origin(), you must ask yourself whether two subjects with identical characteristics face the same risk of failure. The answer is that they face the same risk when they have the same value of $t = (time - \text{origin}())/\text{scale}()$ or, equivalently, when the same amount of time has elapsed from origin().

Say that we have the following data on smokers who have died:

```
   ddate      x1      x2    reason
11mar1984      23      11        2
15may1994      21       9        1
22nov1993      22      13        2
etc.
```

We wish to analyze death due to reason==2. However, typing

```
. stset ddate, fail(reason==2)
```

would probably not be adequate. We would be saying that smokers were at risk of death from 01jan1960. Would it matter? It would if we planned on doing anything parametric because parametric hazard functions, except for the exponential, are functions of analysis time, and the location of 0 makes a difference.

Even if we were thinking of performing nonparametric analysis, there would probably be difficulties. We would be asserting that two "identical" persons (in terms of x1 and x2) face the same risk on the same calendar date. Does the risk of death due to smoking really change as the calendar changes?

It would be more reasonable to assume that the risk changes with how long a subject has been smoking and that our data would probably include that date. We would type

```
. stset ddate, fail(reason==2) origin(time smdate)
```

if smdate were the name of the date-started-smoking variable. We would now be saying that the risk is equal when the number of days smoked is the same. We might prefer to see t in years,

```
. stset ddate, fail(reason==2) origin(time smdate) scale(365.25)
```

but that would make no substantive difference.

Consider single-record data on firms that went bankrupt:

incorp	bankrupt	x1	x2	btype
22jan1983	11mar1984	23	11	2
17may1992	15may1994	21	9	1
03nov1991	22nov1993	22	13	2
etc.				

Say that we wish to examine the risk of a particular kind of bankruptcy, btype == 2, among firms that become bankrupt. Typing

```
. stset bankrupt, fail(btype==2)
```

would be more reasonable than it was in the smoking example. It would not be reasonable if we were thinking of performing any sort of parametric analysis, of course, because then location of $t = 0$ would matter, but it might be reasonable for semiparametric analysis. We would be asserting that two "identical" firms (with respect to the characteristics we model) have the same risk of bankruptcy when the calendar dates are the same. We would be asserting that the overall state of the economy matters.

It might be reasonable to instead measure time from the date of incorporation:

```
. stset bankrupt, fail(btype==2) origin(time incorp)
```

Understand that the choice of origin() is a substantive decision.

Setting the failure event

You set the failure event by using the failure() option.

In single-record data, if failure() is not specified, every record is assumed to end in a failure. For instance, with

	failtime	load	bearings
1.	100	15	0
2.	140	15	1
etc.			

you would type stset failtime, and the first observation would be assumed to fail at time = 100, the second at time = 140, and so on.

failure(*varname*) specifies that a failure occurs whenever *varname* is not zero and is not missing. For instance, with

	failtime	load	bearings	burnout
1.	100	15	0	1
2.	140	15	1	0
3.	97	20	0	1
4.	122	20	1	0
5.	84	25	0	1
6.	100	25	1	1
etc.				

you might type stset failtime, failure(burnout). Observations 1, 3, 5, and 6 would be assumed to fail at times 100, 97, 84, and 100, respectively; observations 2 and 4 would be assumed to be censored at times 140 and 122.

Similarly, if the data were

	failtime	load	bearings	burnout
1.	100	15	0	1
2.	140	15	1	0
3.	97	20	0	2
4.	122	20	1	.
5.	84	25	0	2
6.	100	25	1	3
etc.				

the result would be the same. Nonzero, nonmissing values of the failure variable are assumed to represent failures. (Perhaps burnout contains a code on how the burnout occurred.)

failure(*varname* == *numlist*) specifies that a failure occurs whenever *varname* takes on any of the values of *numlist*. In the above example, specifying

    . stset failtime, failure(burnout==1 2)

would treat observation 6 as censored.

    . stset failtime, failure(burnout==1 2 .)

would also treat observation 4 as a failure.

    . stset failtime, failure(burnout==1/3 6 .)

would treat burnout==1, burnout==2, burnout==3, burnout==6, and burnout==. as representing failures and all other values as representing censorings. (Perhaps we want to examine "failure due to meltdown", and these are the codes that represent the various kinds of meltdown.)

failure() is treated the same way in both single- and multiple-record data. Consider

	patno	t	x1	x2	died
1.	1	4	23	11	1
2.	2	5	21	9	0
3.	2	8	22	13	1
4.	3	7	20	5	0
5.	3	9	22	5	0
6.	3	11	21	5	0
7.	4	...			

Typing

    . stset t, id(patno) failure(died)

would treat

patno==1	as dying	at t==4
patno==2	as dying	at t==8
patno==3	as being censored	at t==11

Intervening records on the same subject are marked as "censored". Technically, they are not really censored if you think about it carefully; they are simply marked as not failing. Look at the data for subject 3:

patno	t	x1	x2	died
3	9	22	5	0
3	11	21	5	0

The subject is not censored at $t = 9$ because there are more data on the subject; it is merely the case that the subject did not die at that time. At $t = 9$, x1 changed from 22 to 21. The subject is really censored at $t = 11$ because the subject did not die and there are no more records on the subject.

Typing stset t, id(patno) failure(died) would mark the same persons as dying and the same persons as censored, as in the previous case. If died contained not 0 and 1, but 0 and nonzero, nonmissing codes for the reason for death would be

	patno	t	x1	x2	died
1.	1	4	23	11	103
2.	2	5	21	9	0
3.	2	8	22	13	207
4.	3	7	20	5	0
5.	3	9	22	5	0
6.	3	11	21	5	0
7.	4	...			

Typing

    . stset t, id(patno) failure(died)

or

    . stset t, id(patno) failure(died==103 207)

would yield the same results; subjects 1 and 2 would be treated as dying and subject 3 as censored.

Typing

    . stset t, id(patno) failure(died==207)

would treat subject 2 as dying and subjects 1 and 3 as censored. Thus when you specify the values for the code, the code variable need not ever contain 0. In

	patno	t	x1	x2	died
1.	1	4	23	11	103
2.	2	5	21	9	13
3.	2	8	22	13	207
4.	3	7	20	5	11
5.	3	9	22	5	12
6.	3	11	21	5	12
7.	4	...			

typing

    . stset t, id(patno) failure(died==207)

treats patient 2 as dying and 1 and 3 as censored. Typing

    . stset t, id(patno) failure(died==103 207)

treats patients 1 and 2 as dying and 3 as censored.

Setting multiple failures

In multiple-record data, records after the first failure event are ignored unless you specify the
exit() option. Consider the following data:

	patno	t	x1	x2	code
1.	1	4	21	7	14
2.	1	5	21	7	11
3.	1	7	20	7	17
4.	1	8	22	7	22
5.	1	9	22	7	22
6.	1	11	21	7	29
7.	2	...			

Perhaps code 22 represents the event of interest—say, the event "visited the doctor". Were you to
type stset t, id(patno) failure(code == 22), the result would be as if the data contained

	patno	t	x1	x2	code
1.	1	4	21	7	14
2.	1	5	21	7	11
3.	1	7	20	7	17
4.	1	8	22	7	22

Records after the first occurrence of the failure event are ignored. If you do not want this, you must
specify the exit() option. Probably you would want to specify exit(time .), here meaning that
subjects are not to exit the risk group until their data run out. Alternatively, perhaps code 142 means
"entered the nursing home" and, once that event happens, you no longer want them in the risk group.
Then you would code exit(code == 142); see *Final exit times* below.

First entry times

Do not confuse enter() with origin(). origin() specifies when a subject first becomes at
risk. enter() specifies when a subject first comes under observation. In most datasets, becoming at
risk and coming under observation are coincident. Then it is sufficient to specify origin() alone,
although you could specify both options.

Some persons enter the data after they have been at risk of failure. Say that we are studying deaths
due to exposure to substance X and we know the date at which a person was first exposed to the
substance. We are willing to assume that persons are at risk from the date of exposure forward. A
person arrives at our door who was exposed 15 years ago. Can we add this person to our data? The
statistical issue is labeled *left-truncation*, and the problem is that, had the person died before arriving
at our door, we would never have known about her. We can add her to our data, but we must be
careful to treat her subsequent survival time as conditional on having already survived 15 years.

Say that we are examining visits to the widget repair facility, "failure" being defined as a visit
(so failures can be repeated). The risk begins once a person buys a widget. We have a woman who
bought a widget 3 years ago, and she has no records on when she has visited the facility in the last
3 years. Can we add her to our data? Yes, as long as we are careful to treat her subsequent behavior
as already being 3 years after she first became at risk.

The jargon for this is "under observation". All this means is that any failures would be observed.
Before being under observation, failure would not be observed.

If enter() is not specified, we assume that subjects are under observation at the time they enter
the risk group as specified by origin(), 0 if origin() is not specified, or possibly time0(). To
be precise, subject i is assumed to first enter the analysis risk pool at

$$time_i = \max\left(\text{earliest time0() for } i, \text{enter()}, \text{origin()}\right)$$

Say that we have multiple-record data recording "came at risk" (`mycode == 1`), "enrolled in our study" (`mycode == 2`), and "failed due to risk" (`mycode == 3`). We `stset` this dataset by typing

```
. stset time, id(id) origin(mycode==1) enter(mycode==2) failure(mycode==3)
```

The above `stset` correctly handles the came at risk/came under observation problem regardless of the order of events 1, 2, and 3. For instance, if the subject comes under observation before he or she becomes at risk, the subject will be treated as entering the analysis risk pool at the time he or she came at risk.

Say that we have the same data in single-record format: variable `riskdate` documents becoming at risk and variable `enr_date` the date of enrollment in our study. We would `stset` this dataset by typing

```
. stset time, origin(time riskdate) enter(time enr_date) failure(mycode==3)
```

For a final example, let's return to the multiple-record way of recording our data and say that we started enrolling people in our study on 12jan1998 but that, up until 16feb1998, we do not trust that our records are complete (we had startup problems). We would `stset` that dataset by typing

```
. stset time, origin(mycode==1) enter(mycode==2 time mdy(2,16,1998))
> fail(mycode==3)
```

`enter(`*varname*`==`*numlist* `time` *exp*`)` is interpreted as

$$\max(\text{time of earliest event in } numlist, exp)$$

Thus, persons having `mycode == 2` occurring before 16feb1998 are assumed to be under observation from 16feb1998, and those having `mycode == 2` thereafter are assumed to be under observation from the time of `mycode == 2`.

Final exit times

`exit()` specifies the latest time under which the subject is both under observation and at risk of the failure event. The emphasis is on latest; obviously subjects also exit the data when their data run out.

When you type

```
. stset ..., ... failure(outcome==1/3 5) ...
```

the result is as if you had typed

```
. stset ..., ... failure(outcome==1/3 5) exit(failure) ...
```

which, in turn, is the same as

```
. stset ..., ... failure(outcome==1/3 5) exit(outcome==1/3 5) ...
```

When are people to be removed from the analysis risk pool? When their data end, of course, and when the event 1, 2, 3, or 5 first occurs. How are they to be removed? According to their status at that time. If the event is 1, 2, 3, or 5 at that instant, they exit as a failure. If the event is something else, they exit as censored.

Perhaps events 1, 2, 3, and 5 represent death due to heart disease, and that is what we are studying. Say that `outcome == 99` represents death for some other reason. Obviously, once the person dies, she is no longer at risk of dying from heart disease, so we would want to specify

```
. stset ..., ... failure(outcome==1/3 5) exit(outcome==1/3 5 99) ...
```

When we explicitly specify `exit()`, we must list all the reasons for which a person is to be removed other than simply running out of data. Here it would have been a mistake to specify just `exit(99)` because that would have left persons in the analysis risk pool who died for reasons 1, 2, 3, and 5. We would have treated those people as if they were still at risk of dying.

In fact, it probably would not have mattered had we specified `exit(99)` because, once a person is dead, he or she is unlikely to have any subsequent records, anyway. By that logic, we did not even have to specify `exit(99)` because death is death and there should be no records following it.

For other kinds of events, however, `exit()` becomes important. Let us assume that the failure event is to be diagnosed with heart disease. A person may surely have records following diagnosis, but even so,

        . stset ..., ... failure(outcome==22) ...

would be adequate because, by not specifying `exit()`, we are accepting the default that `exit()` is equivalent to `failure()`. Once outcome 22 occurs, subsequent records on the subject will be ignored—they constitute the future history of the subject.

Say, however, that we wish to treat as censored persons diagnosed with kidney disease. We would type

        . stset ..., ... failure(outcome==22) exit(outcome==22 29) ...

assuming that `outcome = 29` is "diagnosed with kidney disease". It is now of great importance that we specified `exit(outcome==22 29)` and not just `exit(outcome==29)` because, had we omitted code 22, persons would have remained in the analysis risk pool even after the failure event, i.e., being diagnosed with heart disease.

If, in addition, our data were untrustworthy after 22nov1998 (perhaps not all the data have been entered yet), we would type

        . stset ..., ... failure(outcome==22) exit(outcome==22 29 time
        > mdy(11,22,1998)) ...

If we type `exit(`*varname*`==`*numlist* `time` *exp*`)`, the exit time is taken to be

$$\min(\text{time of earliest event in } numlist, exp)$$

For some analyses, repeated failures are possible. If you have repeated failure data, you specify the `exit()` option and include whatever reasons, if any, that would cause the person to be removed. If there are no such reasons and you wish to retain all observations for the person, you type

        . stset ..., ... exit(time .) ...

`exit(time .)` specifies that the maximum time a person can be in the risk pool is infinite; thus, subjects will not be removed until their data run out.

Intermediate exit and reentry times (gaps)

Gaps arise when a subject is temporarily not under observation. The statistical importance of gaps is that, if failure is death and if the person died during such a gap, he would not have been around to be found again. The solution to this is to remove the person from the risk pool during the observational gap.

To determine that you have gaps, your data must provide starting and ending times for each record. Most datasets provide only ending times, making it impossible to know that you have gaps.

You use time0() to specify the beginning times of records. time0() specifies a mechanical aspect of interpreting the records in the dataset, namely, the beginning of the period spanned by each record. Do not confuse time0() with origin(), which specifies when a subject became at risk, or with enter(), which specifies when a subject first comes under observation.

time0() merely identifies the beginning of the time span covered by each record. Say that we had two records on a subject, the first covering the span (40,49] and the second (49,57]:

```
            |<—— record 1 ——>|<– record 2 –>|
 ————————————                              ————————————————> time
            40                49             57
```

A time0() variable would contain

40 in record 1

49 in record 2

and not, for instance, 40 and 40. A time0() variable varies record by record for a subject.

Most datasets merely provide an end-of-record time value, *timevar*, which you specify by typing stset *timevar*, ... When you have multiple records per subject and you do not specify a time0() variable, stset assumes that each record begins where the previous one left off.

if( ) versus if exp

Both the if *exp* and if(*exp*) options select records for which *exp* is true. We strongly recommend specifying the if() option in preference to if *exp*. They differ in that if *exp* removes data from consideration before calculating beginning and ending times, and other quantities as well. The if() option, on the other hand, sets the restriction after all derived variables are calculated. To appreciate this difference, consider the following multiple-record data:

```
patno     t     x1    x2    code
   3      7     20     5     14
   3      9     22     5     23
   3     11     21     5     29
```

Consider the difference in results between typing

```
. stset t if x1!=22, failure(code==14)
```

and

```
. stset t,  if(x1!=22) failure(code==14)
```

The first would remove record 2 from consideration at the outset. In constructing beginning and ending times, stset and streset would see

```
patno     t     x1    x2    code
   3      7     20     5     14
   3     11     21     5     29
```

and would construct the result:

```
            x1=20                 x1=21
            x2= 5                 x2= 5
     |<———————————————>|<———————————————>|
 ————                                   ————
     0                 7                 11
```

In the second case, the result would be

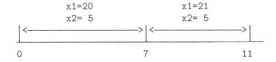

x2= 5   x2= 5

|<——————————————>| (gap) |<———>|

0   7   9   11

The latter result is correct and the former incorrect because $x1 = 21$ is not true in the interval $(7, 9)$.

The only reason to specify if *exp* is to ignore errors in the data—observations that would confuse stset and streset—without actually dropping the offending observations from the dataset.

You specify the if() option to ignore information in the data that are not themselves errors. Specifying if() yields the same result as specifying if *exp* on the subsequent st commands after the dataset has been stset.

Past and future records

Consider the hospital ward data that we have seen before:

```
patid    addate      curdate    sex    x1    x2    code
  101  18aug1998  23aug1998      1     10    10     177
  101          .  31aug1998      1     20     8     286
  101          .  08sep1998      1     16    11     208
  101          .  11sep1998      1     11    17     401
  etc.
```

Say that you stset this dataset such that you selected the middle two records. Perhaps you typed

```
. stset curdate, id(patid) origin(time addate) enter(code==286) failure(code==208)
```

The first record for the subject, since it was not selected, is called a *past history record*. Any earlier records that were not selected would also be called past history records.

The last record for the subject, since it was not selected, is called a *future history record*. Any later records that were not selected would also be called future history records.

If you typed

```
. streset, past
```

the first three records for this subject would be selected.

Typing

```
. streset, future
```

would select the last three records for this subject.

If you typed

```
. streset, past future
```

all four records for this subject would be selected.

If you then typed

```
. streset
```

the original two records would be selected, and things would be back just as they were before.

After typing `streset, past`; `streset, future`; or `streset, past future`, you would not want to use any analysis commands. `streset` did some strange things, especially with the analysis time variable, to include the extra records. It would be the wrong sample, anyway.

You might, however, want to use certain data-management commands on the data, especially those for creating new variables.

Typically, `streset, past` is of greater interest than the other commands. Past records—records prior to being at risk or excluded for other reasons—are not supposed to play a role in survival analysis. `stset` makes sure they do not. But it is sometimes reasonable to ask questions about them such as, was the subject ever on the drug cisplatin? Has the subject ever been married? Did the subject ever have a heart attack?

To answer questions like that, you sometimes want to dig into the past. Typing `streset, past` makes that easy, and once the past is set, the data can be used with `stgen` and `st_is` 2. You might well type the following:

```
. stset curdate, id(patid) origin(addate) enter(code==286) failure(code==208)
. streset, past
. stgen attack = ever(code==177)
. streset
. stcox attack ...
```

Do not be concerned about doing something inappropriate while having the past or future set; st will not let you:

```
. stset curdate, id(patid) origin(time addate) enter(code==286) failure(code==208)
  (output omitted )
. streset, past
  (output omitted )
. stcox x1
you last "streset, past"
you must type "streset" to restore the analysis sample
r(119);
```

Using streset

`streset` is a useful tool for gently modifying what you have previously `stset`. Rather than typing the whole `stset` command, you can type `streset` followed by just what has changed.

For instance, you might

```
. stset curdate, id(patid) origin(time addate) enter(code==286) failure(code==208)
```

and then later want to restrict the analysis to subjects who ever have x1>20. You could retype the whole `stset` command and add `ever(x1>20)`, but it would be easier to type

```
. streset, ever(x1>20)
```

If later you decide you want to remove the restriction, type

```
. streset, ever(.)
```

That is the general rule for resetting options to the default: type '.' as the option's argument.

Be careful using `streset` because you can make subtle mistakes. In another analysis with another dataset, consider the following:

```
. stset date, fail(code==2) origin(code==1107)
. ...
```

```
. streset date, fail(code==9) origin(code==1422) after(code==1423)
. ...
. streset, fail(code==2) origin(code==1107)
```

If, in the last step, you are trying to get back to the results of the first stset, you will fail. The last streset is equivalent to

```
. stset date, fail(code==9) origin(code==1107) after(code==1423)
```

streset() remembers the previously specified options and uses them if you do not override them. Both stset and streset display the current command line. Make sure that you verify that the command is what you intended.

Performance and multiple-record-per-subject datasets

stset and streset do not drop data; they simply mark data to be excluded from consideration. Some survival-time datasets can be large, although the relevant subsamples are small. In such cases, you can reduce memory requirements and speed execution by dropping the irrelevant observations.

stset and streset mark the relevant observations by creating a variable named _st (it is always named this) containing 1 and 0; _st = 1 marks the relevant observations and _st = 0 marks the irrelevant ones. If you type

```
. drop if _st==0
```

or equivalently

```
. keep if _st==1
```

or equivalently

```
. keep if _st
```

you will drop the irrelevant observations. All st commands produce the same results whether you do this or not. Be careful, however, if you are planning future stsets or stresets. Observations that are irrelevant right now might be relevant later.

One solution to this conundrum is to keep only those observations that are relevant after setting the entire history:

```
. stset date, fail(code==9) origin(code==1422) after(code==1423)
. streset, past future
. keep if _st
. streset
```

Final note: You may drop the irrelevant observations as marked by _st = 0, but do not drop the _st variable itself. The other st commands expect to find variable _st.

Sequencing of events within t

Consider the following bit of data:

etime	failtime	fail
0	5	1
0	5	0
5	7	1

Note all the different events happening at time 5: the first observation fails, the second is censored, and the third enters.

What does it mean for something to happen at time 5? In particular, is it at least potentially possible for the second observation to have failed at time 5; i.e., was it in the risk group when the first observation failed? How about the third observation? Was it in the risk group, and could it have potentially failed at time 5?

Stata sequences events within a time as follows:

first,   at time t the failures occur
then,   at time $t+0$ the censorings are removed from the risk group
finally, at time $t+0+0$ the new entries are added to the risk group

Thus, to answer the questions:

Could the second observation have potentially failed at time 5? Yes.

Could the third observation have potentially failed at time 5? No, because it was not yet in the risk group.

By this logic, the following makes no sense:

```
etime   failtime      fail
    5          5         1
```

because this would mark a subject as failing before being at risk. It would make no difference if fail were 0—the subject would then be marked as being censored too soon. Either way, stset would flag this as an error. If you had a subject who entered and immediately exited, you would code this as

```
etime   failtime      fail
 4.99          5         1
```

Weights

stset allows you to specify fweights, pweights, and iweights.

fweights are Stata's frequency or replication weights. Consider the data

```
failtime    load   bearings    count
     100      15          0        3
     140      15          1        2
      97      20          0        1
```

and the stset command

```
. stset failtime [fw=count]

     failure event:  (assumed to fail at time=failtime)
obs. time interval:  (0, failtime]
 exit on or before:  failure
            weight:  [fweight=count]

        3  total obs.
        0  exclusions

        3  physical obs. remaining, equal to
        6  weighted obs., representing
        6  failures in single record/single failure data
      677  total analysis time at risk, at risk from t =         0
                           earliest observed entry t =         0
                              last observed exit t =       140
```

This combination is equivalent to the expanded data

failtime	load	bearings
100	15	0
100	15	0
100	15	0
140	15	1
140	15	1
97	20	0

and

```
. stset failtime
```

pweights are Stata's sampling weights—the inverse of the probability that the subject was chosen from the population. pweights are typically integers, but they do not have to be. For instance, you might have

time0	time	died	sex	reps
0	300	1	0	1.50
0	250	0	1	4.50
30	147	1	0	2.25

Here reps is how many patients each observation represents in the underlying population—perhaps when multiplied by 10. The stset command for these data is

```
. stset time [pw=reps], origin(time time0) failure(died)
```

For variance calculations, the scale of the pweights does not matter. reps in the 3 observations shown could just as well be 3, 9, and 4.5. Nevertheless, the scale of the pweights is used when you ask for counts. For instance, stsum would report the person-time at risk as

$$(300 - 0)\,1.5 + (250 - 0)\,4.5 + (147 - 30)\,2.25 = 1{,}838.25$$

for the 3 observations shown. stsum would count that $1.5 + 2.25 = 3.75$ persons died, and so the incidence rate for these 3 observations would be $3.75/1{,}838.25 = .0020$. The incidence rate is thus unaffected by the scale of the weights. Similarly, the coefficients and confidence intervals reported by, for instance, streg, dist(exponential) would be unaffected. The 95% confidence interval for the incidence rate would be $[.0003, .0132]$, regardless of the scale of the weights.

If these 3 observations were examined unweighted, the incidence rate would be .0030 and the 95% confidence interval would be $[.0007, .0120]$.

Finally, stset allows you to set iweights, which are Stata's "importance" weights, but we recommend that you do not. iweights are provided for those who wish to create special effects by manipulating standard formulas. The st commands treat iweights just as they would fweights, although they do not require that the weights be integers, and push their way through conventional variance calculations. Thus results—counts, rates, and variances—depend on the scale of these weights.

Data warnings and errors flagged by stset

When you stset your data, stset runs various checks to verify that what you are setting makes sense. stset refuses to set the data only if, in multiple-record, weighted data, weights are not constant within ID. Otherwise, stset merely warns you about any inconsistencies that it identifies.

Although `stset` will set the data, it will mark out records that it cannot understand; for instance,

```
. stset curdate, origin(time addate) failure(code==402) id(patid)
                        id:  patid
            failure event:  code == 402
      obs. time interval:  (curdate[_n-1], curdate]
       exit on or before:  failure
          t for analysis:  (time-origin)
                   origin:  time addate
```

```
        243  total obs.
          1  event time missing (curdate>=.)              PROBABLE ERROR
          4  multiple records at same instant             PROBABLE ERROR
             (curdate[_n-1]==curdate)
```

```
        238  obs. remaining, representing
         40  subjects
         15  failures in single failure-per-subject data
       1478  total analysis time at risk, at risk from t =        0
                            earliest observed entry t =           0
                              last observed exit t =             62
```

You must ensure that the result, after exclusions, is correct.

The warnings `stset` might issue include

```
            ignored because patid missing
            event time missing                    PROBABLE ERROR
            entry time missing                    PROBABLE ERROR
            entry on or after exit (etime>t)      PROBABLE ERROR
            obs. end on or before enter()
            obs. end on or before origin()
            multiple records at same instant (t[_n-1]==t)  PROBABLE ERROR
            overlapping records (t[_n-1]>entry time)       PROBABLE ERROR
            weights invalid                       PROBABLE ERROR
```

`stset` sets $\_st = 0$ when observations are excluded for whatever reason. Thus, observations with any of the above problems can be found among the $\_st = 0$ observations.

Using survival-time data in Stata

In the examples above, we have shown you how Stata expects survival-time data to be recorded. To summarize:

1. Each subject's history is represented by 1 or more observations in the dataset.

2. Each observation documents a span of time. The observation must contain when the span ends (exit time) and may optionally contain when the span begins (entry time). If the entry time is not recorded, it is assumed to be 0 or, in multiple-record data, the exit time of the subject's previous observation, if there is one. By *previous* we mean that the data have already been temporally ordered on exit times within subject. The physical order of the observations in your dataset does not matter.

3. Each observation documents an outcome associated with the exit time. Unless otherwise specified with `failure()`, 0 and missing mean censored, and nonzero means failed.

4. Each observation contains other variables (called covariates) that are assumed to be constant over the span of time recorded by the observation.

Data rarely arrive in this neatly organized form. For instance, Kalbfleisch and Prentice (2002, 4–5) present heart transplant survival data from Stanford (Crowley and Hu 1977). These data can be converted into the correct st format in at least two ways. The first method is shown in example 11. A second, shorter, method using the st commands is described as an example in the `stsplit` entry.

▷ Example 11

Here we will describe the process that uses the standard Stata commands.

```
. use http://www.stata-press.com/data/r10/stan2
(Heart transplant data)

. describe

Contains data from http://www.stata-press.com/data/r10/stan2.dta
  obs:           103                          Heart transplant data
  vars:            5                          26 Mar 2007 17:48
  size:        1,442 (99.9% of memory free)
```

variable name	storage type	display format	value label	variable label
id	int	%8.0g		Patient Identifier
died	byte	%8.0g		Survival Status (1=dead)
stime	float	%8.0g		Survival Time (Days)
transplant	byte	%8.0g		Heart Transplant
wait	int	%8.0g		Waiting Time

```
Sorted by:
```

The data are from 103 patients selected as transplantation candidates. There is one record on each patient, and the important variables, from an st-command perspective, are

id	the patient's ID number
transplant	whether the patient received a transplant
wait	when (after acceptance) the patient received the transplant
stime	when (after acceptance) the patient died or was censored
died	the patient's status at `stime`

To better understand, let us examine two records from this dataset:

```
. list id transplant wait stime died if id==44 | id==16
```

	id	transp~t	wait	stime	died
33.	44	0	0	40	1
34.	16	1	20	43	1

Patient 44 never did receive a new heart; he or she died 40 days after acceptance while still on the waiting list. Patient 16 did receive a new heart—20 days after acceptance—yet died 43 days after acceptance.

Our goal is to turn this into st data that contain the histories of each of these patients. That is, we want records that appear as

id	t1	died	posttran
16	20	0	0
16	43	1	1
44	40	1	0

or, even more explicitly, as

```
id        t0        t1      died  posttran
16         0        20        0        0
16        20        43        1        1
44         0        40        1        0
```

The new variable posttran would be 0 before transplantation and 1 afterward.

Patient 44 would have one record in this new dataset recording that he or she died at time 40 and that posttran was 0 over the entire interval.

Patient 16, however, would have two records: one documenting the duration $(0, 20]$ during which posttran was 0, and one documenting the duration $(20, 43]$ during which posttran was 1.

Our goal is to take the first dataset and convert it into the second, which we can then stset. We make the transformation by using Stata's other data-management commands. One way we could do this is by typing

```
. expand 2 if transplant
(69 observations created)

. by id, sort: gen byte posttran = (_n==2)

. by id: gen t1 = stime if _n==_N
(69 missing values generated)

. by id: replace t1 = wait if _n==1 & transplant
(69 real changes made)

. by id: replace died=0 if _n==1 & transplant
(45 real changes made)
```

expand 2 if transplant duplicated the observations for patients who had transplant $\neq 0$. Considering our two sample patients, we would now have the following data:

```
id  transp~t     wait      stime     died
44         0        0         40        1
16         1       20         43        1
16         1       20         43        1
```

We would have 1 observation for patient 44 and 2 identical observations for patient 16.

We then by id, sort: gen posttran = (_n==2), resulting in

```
id  transp~t     wait      stime     died  posttran
16         1       20         43        1         0
16         1       20         43        1         1
44         0        0         40        1         0
```

This type of trickiness is discussed in [U] **13.7 Explicit subscripting**. Statements such as _n==2 produce values 1 (meaning true) and 0 (meaning false), so new variable posttran will contain 1 or 0 depending on whether _n is or is not 2. _n is the observation counter and, combined with by id:, becomes the observation-within-ID counter. Thus we set posttran to 1 on second records and to 0 on all first records.

Finally, we produce the exit-time variable. Final exit time is just stime, and that is handled by the command by id: gen t1 = stime if _n==_N. _n is the observation-within-ID counter, and _N is the total number of observations within id, so we just set the last observation on each patient to stime. Now we have

```
id  transp~t     wait      stime     died  posttran       t1
16         1       20         43        1         0        .
16         1       20         43        1         1       43
44         0        0         40        1         0       40
```

All that is left to do is to fill in t1 with the value from wait on the interim records, meaning replace t1=wait if it is an interim record.

There are many ways we could identify the interim records. In the output above, we did it by

. by id: replace t1 = wait if _n==1 & transplant

meaning that an interim record is a first record of a person who did receive a transplant. More easily, but with more trickery, we could have just said

. replace t1=wait if t1>=.

because the only values of t1 left to be filled in are the missing ones. Another alternative would be

. by id: replace t1 = wait if _n==1 & _N==2

which would identify the first record of two-record pairs. There are many alternatives, but they would all produce the same thing:

id	transp~t	wait	stime	died	posttran	t1
16	1	20	43	1	0	20
16	1	20	43	1	1	43
44	0	0	40	1	0	40

There is one more thing we must do, which is to reset died to contain 0 on the interim records:

. by id: replace died=0 if _n==1 & transplant

The result is

id	transp~t	wait	stime	died	posttran	t1
16	1	20	43	0	0	20
16	1	20	43	1	1	43
44	0	0	40	1	0	40

We now have the desired result and are ready to stset our data:

```
. stset t1, failure(died) id(id)
                  id:  id
       failure event:  died != 0 & died < .
  obs. time interval:  (t1[_n-1], t1]
  exit on or before:   failure
```

172	total obs.	
2	multiple records at same instant (t1[_n-1]==t1)	PROBABLE ERROR

170	obs. remaining, representing	
102	subjects	
74	failures in single failure-per-subject data	
31933	total analysis time at risk, at risk from t =	0
	earliest observed entry t =	0
	last observed exit t =	1799

Well, something went wrong. Two records were excluded. There are few enough data here that we could just list the dataset and look for the problem, but let's pretend otherwise. We want to find the records that, within patient, are marked as exiting at the same time:

. by id: gen problem = t1==t1[_n-1]
. sort id died

```
. list id if problem
```

	id
61.	38

```
. list id transplant wait stime died posttran t1 if id==38
```

	id	transp~t	wait	stime	died	posttran	t1
60.	38	1	5	5	0	0	5
61.	38	1	5	5	1	1	5

There is no typographical error in these data—we checked that variables `transplant`, `wait`, and `stime` contain what the original source published. Those variables indicate that patient 38 waited 5 days for a heart transplant, received one on the fifth day, and then died on the fifth day, too.

That makes perfect sense, but not to Stata, which orders events within t as failures, followed by censorings, followed by entries. Reading `t1`, Stata went for this literal interpretation: patient 38 was censored at time 5 with `posttran` $= 0$; then, at time 5, patient 38 died and then, at time 5, patient 38 reentered the data, but this time with `posttran` $= 1$. That made no sense to Stata.

Stata's sequencing of events may surprise you, but trust us, there are good reasons for it, and really, the ordering convention does not matter. To fix this problem, we just have to put a little time between the implied entry at time 5 and the subsequent death:

```
. replace t1 = 5.1 in 61
(1 real change made)
. list id transplant wait stime died posttran t1 if id==38
```

	id	transp~t	wait	stime	died	posttran	t1
60.	38	1	5	5	0	0	5
61.	38	1	5	5	1	1	5.1

Now the data make sense both to us and to Stata: until time 5, the patient had `posttran` $= 0$; then at time 5 the value of `posttran` changed to 1; and then at time 5.1, the patient died.

```
. stset t1, id(id) failure(died)
                id:  id
     failure event:  died != 0 & died < .
obs. time interval:  (t1[_n-1], t1]
 exit on or before:  failure
```

```
      172  total obs.
        0  exclusions

      172  obs. remaining, representing
      103  subjects
       75  failures in single failure-per-subject data
  31938.1  total analysis time at risk, at risk from t =            0
                               earliest observed entry t =          0
                                last observed exit t =           1799
```

This dataset is now ready for use with all the other st commands. Here is an illustration:

```
. use http://www.stata-press.com/data/r10/stan3, clear
(Heart transplant data)

. stset, noshow

. stsum, by(posttran)
```

posttran	time at risk	incidence rate	no. of subjects	25%	Survival time 50%	75%
0	5936	.0050539	103	36	149	340
1	26002.1	.0017306	69	39	96	979
total	31938.1	.0023483	103	36	100	979

```
. stcox age posttran surgery year

Iteration 0:   log likelihood = -298.31514
Iteration 1:   log likelihood =  -289.7344
Iteration 2:   log likelihood = -289.53498
Iteration 3:   log likelihood = -289.53378
Iteration 4:   log likelihood = -289.53378
Refining estimates:
Iteration 0:   log likelihood = -289.53378

Cox regression -- Breslow method for ties

No. of subjects =          103                  Number of obs   =        172
No. of failures =           75
Time at risk    =      31938.1
                                                LR chi2(4)      =      17.56
Log likelihood  =    -289.53378                 Prob > chi2     =     0.0015
```

_t	Haz. Ratio	Std. Err.	z	P>|z|	[95% Conf. Interval]	
age	1.030224	.0143201	2.14	0.032	1.002536	1.058677
posttran	.9787243	.3032597	-0.07	0.945	.5332291	1.796416
surgery	.3738278	.163204	-2.25	0.024	.1588759	.8796
year	.8873107	.059808	-1.77	0.076	.7775022	1.012628

◁

Methods and Formulas

stset is implemented as an ado-file.

References

Cleves, M. A. 1999. ssa13: Analysis of multiple failure-time data with Stata. *Stata Technical Bulletin* 49: 30–39. Reprinted in *Stata Technical Bulletin Reprints*, vol. 9, pp. 338–349.

Cleves, M. A., W. W. Gould, and R. G. Gutierrez. 2004. *An Introduction to Survival Analysis Using Stata*. Rev. ed. College Station, TX: Stata Press.

Crowley, J., and M. Hu. 1977. Covariance analysis of heart transplant data. *Journal of the American Statistical Association* 72: 27–36.

Hills, M., and B. L. De Stavola. 2006. *A Short Introduction to Stata for Biostatistics*. London: Timberlake.

Kalbfleisch, J. D., and R. L. Prentice. 2002. *The Statistical Analysis of Failure Time Data*. 2nd ed. New York: Wiley.

Also See

[ST] **snapspan** — Convert snapshot data to time-span data

[ST] **stdescribe** — Describe survival-time data

Title

| stsplit — Split and join time-span records |

Syntax

Split at designated times

> stsplit *newvar* $[$*if*$]$, $\{$at(*numlist*) | <u>ev</u>ery(#)$\}$ $[$*stsplitDT_options*$]$

Split at failure times

> stsplit $[$*if*$]$, at(<u>f</u>ailures) $[$*stsplitFT_options*$]$

Join episodes

> stjoin $[$, <u>c</u>ensored(*numlist*)$]$

stsplitDT_options	description
Main	
* at(*numlist*)	split records at specified analysis times
* <u>ev</u>ery(#)	split records when analysis time is a multiple of #
<u>af</u>ter(*spec*)	use time since *spec* for at() or every() rather than time since onset of risk; see *Options*
trim	exclude observations outside of range
† <u>nopreserve</u>	do not save original data; programmer's option

*Either at(*numlist*) or every(#) is required with stsplit at designated times.

stsplitFT_options	description
Main	
* at(<u>f</u>ailures)	split at observed failure times
<u>strata</u>(*varlist*)	restrict splitting to failures within stratum defined by *varlist*
<u>r</u>iskset(*newvar*)	create a risk-set ID variable named *newvar*
† <u>nopreserve</u>	do not save original data; programmer's option

*at(failures) is required with stsplit at failure times.

† nopreserve is not shown in the dialog box.

You must stset your dataset using the id() option before using stsplit and stjoin; see [ST] **stset**.

442

Description

stsplit with option at(*numlist*) or every(#) splits episodes into two or more episodes at the implied time points since being at risk or after a time point specified by after(). Each resulting record contains the follow-up on one subject through one time band. Expansion on multiple time scales may be obtained by repeatedly using stsplit. *newvar* specifies the name of the variable to be created containing the observation's category. The new variable records the interval to which each new observation belongs and is bottom coded.

stsplit, at(failures) performs episode splitting at the failure times (per stratum).

stjoin performs the reverse operation, namely, joining episodes back together when such can be done without losing information.

Options for stsplit

    Main

at(*numlist*) or every(#) is required in syntax one; at(failures) is required for syntax two. These options specify the analysis times at which the records are to be split.

at(5(5)20) splits records at $t = 5$, $t = 10$, $t = 15$, and $t = 20$.

If at([...] max) is specified, max is replaced by a suitably large value. For instance, to split records every five analysis time units from time zero to the largest follow-up time in our data, we could find out what the largest time value is by type summarize _t and then explicitly type it into the at() option, or we could just specify at(0(5)max).

every(#) is a shorthand for at(#(#)max); i.e., episodes are split at each positive multiple of #.

after(*spec*) specifies the reference time for at() or every(). Syntax one can be thought of as corresponding to after(*time of onset of risk*), although you cannot really type this. You could type, however, after(time=birthdate) or after(time=marrydate).

spec has syntax

$$\{\texttt{time} \,|\, \texttt{t} \,|\, \_\texttt{t}\} = \{exp \,|\, \min(exp) \,|\, \texttt{asis}(exp)\}$$

where

time specifies that the expression be evaluated in the same time units as *timevar* in stset timevar, ... This is the default.

t and _t specify that the expression be evaluated in units of analysis time. t and _t are synonyms; it makes no difference whether you specify one or the other.

exp specifies the reference time. For multiepisode data, *exp* should be constant within subject ID.

min(*exp*) specifies that for multiepisode data, the minimum of *exp* be taken within ID.

asis(*exp*) specifies that for multiepisode data, *exp* be allowed to vary within ID.

trim specifies that observations with values less than the minimum or greater than the maximum value listed in at() be excluded from subsequent analysis. Such observations are not dropped from the data; trim merely sets their value of variable _st to 0 so that they will not be used, yet they can still be retrieved the next time the dataset is stset.

strata(*varlist*) specifies up to five strata variables. Observations with equal values of the variables are assumed to be in the same stratum. strata() restricts episode splitting to failures that occur within the stratum, and memory requirements are reduced when strata are specified.

riskset(*newvar*) specifies the name for a new variable recording the unique risk set in which an episode occurs, and missing otherwise.

The following option is available with stsplit but is not shown in the dialog box:

nopreserve is intended for use by programmers. It speeds the transformation by not saving the original data, which can be restored should things go wrong or if you press *Break*. Programmers often specify this option when they have already preserved the original data. nopreserve does not affect the transformation.

Option for stjoin

censored(*numlist*) specifies values of the failure variable, *failvar*, from
stset..., failure(*failvar* =...) that indicate "no event" (censoring).

If you are using stjoin to rejoin records after stsplit, you do not need to specify censored().
Just do not forget to drop the variable created by stsplit before typing stjoin. See example 4
below.

Neither do you need to specify censored() if, when you stset your dataset, you specified
failure(*failvar*) and not failure(*failvar* =...). Then stjoin knows that *failvar* = 0 and
failvar = . (missing) correspond to no event. Two records can be joined if they are contiguous
and record the same data and the first record has *failvar* = 0 or *failvar* = ., meaning no event at
that time.

You may need to specify censored(), and you probably do if, when you stset the dataset, you
specified failure(*failvar* =...). If stjoin is to join records, it needs to know what events do
not count and can be discarded. If the only such event is *failvar* = ., you do not need to specify
censored().

Remarks

Remarks are presented under the following headings:

> *What stsplit does and why*
> *Using stsplit to split at designated times*
> *Time versus analysis time*
> *Splitting data on recorded ages*
> *Using stsplit to split at failure times*

What stsplit does and why

stsplit splits records into two or more records on the basis of analysis time or on a variable
that depends on analysis time, such as age. stsplit takes data like

id	_t0	_t	x1	x2	_d
1	0	18	12	11	1

and produces

id	_t0	_t	x1	x2	_d	tcat
1	0	5	12	11	0	0
1	5	10	12	11	0	5
1	10	18	12	11	1	10

or

id	_t0	_t	x1	x2	_d	agecat
1	0	7	12	11	0	30
1	7	17	12	11	0	40
1	17	18	12	11	1	50

The above alternatives record the same underlying data: subject 1 had $x1 = 12$ and $x2 = 11$ during $0 < t \leq 18$, and at $t = 18$, the subject failed.

The difference between the two alternatives is that the first breaks out the analysis times 0–5, 5–10, and 10–20 (although subject 1 failed before $t = 20$). The second breaks out age 30–40, 40–50, and 50–60. You cannot tell from what is presented above, but at $t = 0$, subject 1 was 33 years old.

In our example, that the subject started with one record is not important. The original data on the subject might have been

id	_t0	_t	x1	x2	_d
1	0	14	12	11	0
1	14	18	12	9	1

and then we would have obtained

id	_t0	_t	x1	x2	_d	tcat
1	0	5	12	11	0	0
1	5	10	12	11	0	5
1	10	14	12	11	0	10
1	14	18	12	9	1	10

or

id	_t0	_t	x1	x2	_d	agecat
1	0	7	12	11	0	30
1	7	14	12	11	0	40
1	14	17	12	9	0	40
1	17	18	12	9	1	50

Also, we could just as easily have produced records with analysis time or age recorded in single-year categories. That is, we could start with

id	_t0	_t	x1	x2	_d
1	0	14	12	11	0
1	14	18	12	9	1

and produce

id	_t0	_t	x1	x2	_d	tcat
1	0	1	12	11	0	0
1	1	2	12	11	0	1
1	2	3	12	11	0	2

. . .

or

id	_t0	_t	x1	x2	_d	agecat
1	0	1	12	11	0	30
1	1	2	12	11	0	31
1	2	3	12	11	0	32

. . .

Moreover, we can even do this splitting on more than one variable. Let's go back and start with

id	_t0	_t	x1	x2	_d
1	0	18	12	11	1

Let's split it into the analysis time intervals 0–5, 5–10, and 10–20, *and* let's split it into 10-year age intervals 30–40, 40–50, and 50–60. The result would be

```
id    _t0    _t    x1    x2    _d    tcat    agecat
 1      0     5    12    11     0       0        30
 1      5     7    12    11     0       5        30
 1      7    10    12    11     0       5        40
 1     10    17    12    11     0      10        40
 1     17    18    12    11     1      10        50
```

Why would we want to do any of this?

We might want to split on a time-dependent variable, such as age, if we want to estimate a Cox proportional hazards model and include current age among the regressors (although we could instead use stcox's tvc() option), or if we want to make tables by age groups (see [ST] **strate**).

Using stsplit to split at designated times

stsplit's syntax to split at designated times is, ignoring other options,

$$\text{stsplit } \textit{newvar } \big[\textit{if}\big], \text{ at}(\textit{numlist})$$

$$\text{stsplit } \textit{newvar } \big[\textit{if}\big], \text{ at}(\textit{numlist}) \text{ after}(\textit{spec})$$

at() specifies the analysis times at which records are to be split. Typing at(5 10 15) splits records at the indicated analysis times and separates records into the four intervals 0–5, 5–10, 10–15, and 15+.

In the first syntax, the splitting is done on analysis time t. In the second syntax, the splitting is done on 5, 10, and 15 analysis time units after the time given by after(*spec*).

In either case, stsplit also creates *newvar* containing the interval to which each observation belongs. Here *newvar* would contain 0, 5, 10, and 15; it would contain 0 if the observation occurred in the interval 0–5, 5 if the observation occurred in the interval 5–10, and so on. To be precise,

Category	Precise meaning	*newvar* value
0–5	$(-\infty, 5]$	0
5–10	$(5, 10]$	5
10–15	$(10, 15]$	10
15+	$(15, \infty)$	15

If any of the at() numbers are negative (which would be allowed only by specifying the after() option and would be unusual), the first category is labeled one less than the minimum value specified by at().

Consider the data

```
id    yr0    yr1    yrborn    x1    event
 1   1990   1995      1960     5       52
 2   1993   1997      1964     3       47
```

In these data, subjects became at risk in yr0. The failure event of interest is event = 47, so we stset our dataset by typing

```
. stset yr1, id(id) origin(time yr0) failure(event==47)
(output omitted)
```

and that results in

id	_t0	_t	yr0	yr1	yrborn	x1	event	_d
1	0	5	1990	1995	1960	5	52	0
2	0	4	1993	1997	1964	3	47	1

In the jargon of st, variables _t0 and _t record the span of each record in analysis time (t) units. Variables yr0 and yr1 also record the time span, but in time units. Variable _d records 1 for failure and 0 otherwise.

Typing stsplit cat, at(2 4 6 8) would split the records on the basis of analysis time:

```
. stsplit cat, at(2 4 6 8)
(3 observations (episodes) created)
. order id _t0 _t yr0 yr1 yrborn x1 event _d cat
. list id-cat
```

	id	_t0	_t	yr0	yr1	yrborn	x1	event	_d	cat
1.	1	0	2	1990	1992	1960	5	.	0	0
2.	1	2	4	1990	1994	1960	5	.	0	2
3.	1	4	5	1990	1995	1960	5	52	0	4
4.	2	0	2	1993	1995	1964	3	.	0	0
5.	2	2	4	1993	1997	1964	3	47	1	2

The first record, which represented the analysis time span $(0, 5]$, was split into three records: $(0, 2]$, $(2, 4]$, and $(4, 5]$. The yrborn and x1 values from the single record were duplicated in $(0, 2]$, $(2, 4]$, and $(4, 5]$. The original event variable was changed to missing at $t = 2$ and $t = 4$ because we do not know the value of event; all we know is that event is 52 at $t = 5$. The _d variable was correspondingly set to 0 for $t = 2$ and $t = 4$ because we do know, at least, that the subject did not fail.

stsplit also keeps your original time variables up to date in case you want to streset or re-stset your dataset. yr1 was updated, too.

Now let's go back to our original dataset after we stset it but before we split it,

id	_t0	_t	yr0	yr1	yrborn	x1	event	_d
1	0	5	1990	1995	1960	5	52	0
2	0	4	1993	1997	1964	3	47	1

and consider splitting on age. In 1990, subject 1 is age $1990 - \text{yrborn} = 1990 - 1960 = 30$, and subject 2 is 29. If we type

```
. stsplit acat, at(30 32 34) after(time=yrborn)
```

we will split the data according to

```
         age <= 30   (called acat=0)
30 < age <= 32   (called acat=30)
32 < age <= 34   (called acat=32)
34 < age         (called acat=34)
```

(Continued on next page)

The result will be

id	_t0	_t	yr0	yr1	yrborn	x1	event	_d	acat
1	0	2	1990	1992	1960	5	.	0	30
1	2	4	1990	1994	1960	5	.	0	32
1	4	5	1990	1995	1960	5	52	0	34
2	0	1	1993	1994	1964	3	.	0	0
2	1	3	1993	1996	1964	3	.	0	30
2	3	4	1993	1997	1964	3	47	1	32

The original record on subject 1 corresponding to $(0,5]$ was split into $(0,2]$, $(2,4]$, and $(4,5]$ because those are the t values at which age becomes 32 and 34.

You can stsplit the data more than once. Now having these data, if we typed

. stsplit cat, at(2 4 6 8)

the result would be

id	_t0	_t	yr0	yr1	yrborn	x1	event	_d	acat	cat
1	0	2	1990	1992	1960	5	.	0	30	0
1	2	4	1990	1994	1960	5	.	0	32	2
1	4	5	1990	1995	1960	5	52	0	34	4
2	0	1	1993	1994	1964	3	.	0	0	0
2	1	2	1993	1995	1964	3	.	0	30	0
2	2	3	1993	1996	1964	3	.	0	30	2
2	3	4	1993	1997	1964	3	47	1	32	2

Whether we typed

. stsplit acat, at(30 32 34) after(time=yrborn)
. stsplit cat, at(2 4 6 8)

or

. stsplit cat, at(2 4 6 8)
. stsplit acat, at(30 32 34) after(time=yrborn)

would make no difference.

Time versus analysis time

Be careful using the after() option if, when you stset your dataset, you specified stset's scale() option. We say be careful, but actually we mean be appreciative, because stsplit will do just what you would expect if you did not think too hard.

When you split a record on a time-dependent variable, at() is still specified in analysis time units, meaning the units of time/scale().

For instance, if your original data recorded time as Stata dates, i.e., number of days since 1960,

id	date0	date1	birthdate	x1	event
1	14apr1993	27mar1995	12jul1959	5	52
...					

and you previously stset your dataset by typing

. stset date1, id(id) origin(time date0) scale(365.25) ...

and you now wanted to split on the age implied by birthdate, you would specify the split points in *years* since birth:

. stsplit agecat, at(20(5)60) after(time=birth)

at(20(5)60) means to split the records at the ages, measured in years, of 20, 25, ..., 60.

When you `stset` your dataset, you basically told st how you recorded times (you recorded them as dates) and how to map such times (dates) into analysis time. That was implied by what you typed, and all of st remembers that. Typing

```
. stsplit agecat, at(20(5)60) after(time=birth)
```

tells `stsplit` to split the data on 20, 25, ..., 60 *analysis time units* after `birthdate` for each subject.

Splitting data on recorded ages

Recorded ages can sometimes be tricky. Consider the data

```
id     yr0    yr1    age    x1   event
 1    1980   1996     30     5      52
...
```

When was `age` = 30 recorded—1980 or 1996? Put aside that question because things are about to get worse. Say that you `stset` this dataset so that `yr0` is the `origin()`

```
id   _t0   _t    yr0    yr1    age   x1   event
 1     0   16   1980   1996     30    5      52
...
```

and then split on analysis time by typing `stsplit cat, at(5(5)20)`. The result would be

```
id   _t0   _t    yr0    yr1    age   x1   event
 1     0    5   1980   1985     30    5       .
 1     5   10   1980   1990     30    5       .
 1    10   15   1980   1995     30    5       .
 1    15   16   1980   1996     30    5      52
```

Regardless of the answer to the question on when age was measured, `age` is most certainly not 30 in the newly created records, although you might argue that age at baseline was 30 and that is what you wanted, anyway.

The only truly safe way to deal with ages is to convert them back to birthdates at the outset. Here we would, early on, type

```
. gen bdate = yr1 - age
```
(if age was measured at yr1)

or

```
. gen bdate = yr0 - age
```
(if age was measured at yr0)

In fact, `stsplit` tries to protect you from making age errors. Suppose that you did not do as we just recommended. Say that age was measured at `yr1`, and you typed, knowing that `stsplit` wants a date,

```
. stsplit acat, at(20(5)50) after(time= yr1-age)
```

on these already `stsplit` data. `stsplit` will issue the error message "after() should be constant within id". To use the earliest date, you need to type

```
. stsplit acat, at(20(5)50) after(time= min(yr1-age))
```

Nevertheless, be aware that when you `stsplit` data, if you have recorded ages in your data, and if the records were not already split to control for the range of those ages, then age values, just like all the other variables, are carried forward and no longer reflect the age of the newly created record.

▷ Example 1: Splitting on age

Consider the data from a heart disease and diet survey. The data arose from a study described more fully in Morris, Marr, and Clayton (1977) and analyzed in Clayton and Hills (1993). (Their results differ slightly from ours because the dataset has been updated.)

```
. use http://www.stata-press.com/data/r10/diet
(Diet data with dates)

. describe

Contains data from http://www.stata-press.com/data/r10/diet.dta
  obs:           337                          Diet data with dates
 vars:            11                          1 May 2007 19:01
 size:        17,861  (99.8% of memory free)

              storage  display     value
variable name   type   format      label      variable label

id              float  %9.0g                   Subject identity number
fail            int    %8.0g                   Outcome (CHD = 1 3 13)
job             int    %8.0g                   Occupation
month           byte   %8.0g                   month of survey
energy          float  %9.0g                   Total energy (1000kcals/day)
height          float  %9.0g                   Height (cm)
weight          float  %9.0g                   Weight (kg)
hienergy        float  %9.0g                   Indicator for high energy
doe             double %td                     Date of entry
dox             double %td                     Date of exit
dob             double %td                     Date of birth

Sorted by:  id
```

In this dataset, the outcome variable, `fail`, has been coded as 0, 1, 3, 5, 12, 13, 14, and 15. Codes 1, 3, and 13 indicated coronary heart disease (CHD), other nonzero values code other events such as cancer, and 0 is used to mean "no event" at the end of the study.

The variable `hienergy` is coded 1 if the total energy consumption is more than 2.75 Mcal and 0, otherwise.

We would like to expand the data, using age as the time scale with 10-year age bands. We do this by first `stset`ting the dataset, specifying the date of birth as the origin.

```
. stset dox, failure(fail) origin(time dob) enter(time doe) scale(365.25) id(id)

               id:  id
    failure event:  fail != 0 & fail < .
obs. time interval:  (dox[_n-1], dox]
 enter on or after:  time doe
 exit on or before:  failure
     t for analysis:  (time-origin)/365.25
           origin:  time dob

      337  total obs.
        0  exclusions

      337  obs. remaining, representing
      337  subjects
       80  failures in single failure-per-subject data
 4603.669  total analysis time at risk, at risk from t =          0
                             earliest observed entry t =   30.07529
                              last observed exit t =   69.99863
```

The origin is set to date of birth, making time-since-birth analysis time, and the scale is set to 365.25, so that time since birth is measured in years.

Let's list a few records and verify that the analysis time variables _t0 and _t are indeed recorded as we expect:

```
. list id dob doe dox fail _t0 _t if id==1 | id==34
```

	id	dob	doe	dox	fail	_t0	_t
1.	1	04jan1915	16aug1964	01dec1976	0	49.615332	61.908282
34.	34	12jun1899	16apr1959	31dec1966	3	59.841205	67.550992

We see that patient 1 was 49.6 years old at time of entry into our study and left at age 61.9. Patient 34 entered the study at age 59.8 and exited the study with CHD at age 67.6.

Now we can split the data by age:

```
. stsplit ageband, at(40(10)70)
(418 observations (episodes) created)
```

stsplit added 418 observations to the dataset in memory and generated a new variable, ageband, which identifies each observation's age group.

```
. list id _t0 _t ageband fail height if id==1 | id==34
```

	id	_t0	_t	ageband	fail	height
1.	1	49.615332	50	40	.	175.387
2.	1	50	60	50	.	175.387
3.	1	60	61.908282	60	0	175.387
61.	34	59.841205	60	50	.	177.8
62.	34	60	67.550992	60	3	177.8

The single record for the subject with id = 1 has expanded to three records. The first refers to the age band 40–49, coded 40, and the subject spends $\_t - \_t0 = .384668$ years in this band. The second refers to the age band 50–59, coded 50, and the subject spends 10 years in this band, and so on. The follow-up in each of the three bands is censored (fail = .). The single record for the subject with id = 34 is expanded to two age bands; the follow-up for the first band was censored (fail = .), and the follow-up for the second band ended in CHD (fail = 3).

The values for variables that do not change with time, such as height, are simply repeated in the new records. This can lead to much larger datasets after expansion. Dropping unneeded variables before using split may be necessary.

◁

▷ Example 2: Splitting on age and time in study

To use stsplit to expand the records on two time scales simultaneously, such as age and time in study, we can first expand on the age scale as described in example 1, and then on the time-in-study scale with the command

(Continued on next page)

```
. stsplit timeband, at(0(5)25) after(time=doe)
(767 observations (episodes) created)

. list id _t0 _t ageband fail if id==1 | id==34
```

	id	_t0	_t	ageband	fail
1.	1	49.615332	50	40	.
2.	1	50	54.615332	50	.
3.	1	54.615332	59.615332	50	.
4.	1	59.615332	60	50	.
5.	1	60	61.908282	60	0
111.	34	59.841205	60	50	.
112.	34	60	64.841205	60	.
113.	34	64.841205	67.550992	60	3

By splitting the data by using two time scales, we partitioned the data into time cells corresponding to a *Lexis diagram* as described, for example, in Clayton and Hills (1993). Also see Keiding (1998) for an overview of Lexis diagrams. Each new observation created by splitting the data records the time that the individual spent in a Lexis cell. We can obtain the time spent in the cell by calculating the difference $\_t - \_t0$. For example, the subject with id = 1 spent .384668 years $(50 - 49.615332)$ in the cell corresponding to age 40–49 and study time 0–5, and 4.615332 years $(54.615332 - 50)$ in the cell for age 50–59 and study time 0–5.

We can also do these expansions in reverse order, that is, split first on study time and then on age.

◁

▷ Example 3: Explanatory variables that change with time

In the previous examples, time, in the form of age or time in study, is the explanatory variable to be studied or controlled for, but in some studies other explanatory variables also vary with time. The stsplit command can sometimes be used to expand the records so that in each new record such an explanatory variable is constant over time. For example, in the Stanford heart data (see [ST] **stset**), we would like to split the data and generate the explanatory variable posttran, which takes the value 0 before transplantation and 1 thereafter. The follow-up must therefore be divided into time before transplantation and time after.

We first generate for each observation an entry time and an exit time that preserve the correct follow-up time in such a way that the time of transplants is the same for all individuals. By summarizing wait, the time to transplant, we obtain its maximum value of 310. By selecting a value greater than this maximum, say 320, we now generate two new variables:

```
. use http://www.stata-press.com/data/r10/stanford, clear
(Heart transplant data)

. generate enter = 320 - wait

. generate exit = 320 + stime
```

We have created a new artificial time scale where all transplants are coded as being performed at time 320. By defining enter and exit in this manner, we maintain the correct total follow-up time for each patient. We now stset and stsplit the data:

```
. stset exit, enter(time enter) failure(died) id(id)
                    id:  id
        failure event:  died != 0 & died < .
   obs. time interval:  (exit[_n-1], exit]
    enter on or after:  time enter
    exit on or before:  failure

        103  total obs.
          0  exclusions

        103  obs. remaining, representing
        103  subjects
         75  failures in single failure-per-subject data
    34589.1  total analysis time at risk, at risk from t =          0
                                 earliest observed entry t =         10
                                   last observed exit t =          2119
. stsplit posttran, at(0,320)
(69 observations (episodes) created)

. replace posttran=0 if transplant==0
(34 real changes made)

. replace posttran=1 if posttran==320
(69 real changes made)
```

We replaced posttran in the last command so that it is now a 0/1 indicator variable. We can now generate our follow-up time, t1, as the difference between our analysis time variables, list the data, and stset the dataset.

```
. generate  t1 =_t - _t0

. list id enter exit _t0 _t posttran if id==16 | id==44
```

	id	enter	exit	_t0	_t	posttran
41.	44	320	360	320	360	0
42.	16	300	320	300	320	0
43.	16	300	363	320	363	1

```
. stset t1, failure(died) id(id)
                    id:  id
        failure event:  died != 0 & died < .
   obs. time interval:  (t1[_n-1], t1]
    exit on or before:  failure

        172  total obs.
          0  exclusions

        172  obs. remaining, representing
        103  subjects
         75  failures in single failure-per-subject data
    31938.1  total analysis time at risk, at risk from t =          0
                                 earliest observed entry t =          0
                                   last observed exit t =          1799
```

Using stsplit to split at failure times

To split data at failure times, you would use `stsplit` with the following syntax, ignoring other options,

$$\text{stsplit } [\textit{if}] , \text{at(failures)}$$

This form of episode splitting is useful for Cox regression with time-varying covariates. Splitting at the failure times is useful because of a property of the maximum partial-likelihood estimator for a Cox regression model: the likelihood is evaluated only at the times at which failures occur in the data, and the computation depends only on the risk pools at those failure times. Changes in covariates between failure times do not affect estimates for a Cox regression model. Thus, to fit a model with time-varying covariates, all you have to do is define the values of these time-varying covariates at all failure times at which a subject was at risk (Collett 2003, chap. 8). After splitting at failure times, you define time-varying covariates by referring to the system variable _t (analysis time) or the *timevar* variable used to `stset` the data.

After splitting at failure times, all st commands still work fine and produce the same results as before splitting. To fit parametric models with time-varying covariates, it does not suffice to specify covariates at failure times. Stata can fit "piecewise constant" models by manipulating data using `stsplit, {at() | every()}`.

◁

▷ Example 4: Splitting on failure times to test the proportional-hazards assumption

Collett (2003, 187–190) presents data on 26 ovarian cancer patients who underwent two different chemotherapy protocols after a surgical intervention. Here are few of the observations:

```
. use http://www.stata-press.com/data/r10/ocancer, clear
. list patient time cens treat age rdisea in 1/6, separator(0)
```

	patient	time	cens	treat	age	rdisea
1.	1	156	1	1	66	2
2.	2	1040	0	1	38	2
3.	3	59	1	1	72	2
4.	4	421	0	2	53	2
5.	5	329	1	1	43	2
6.	6	769	0	2	59	2

The variable `treat` indicates the chemotherapy protocol administered, `age` records the age of the patient at the beginning of the treatment, and `rdisea` records each patient's residual disease after surgery. After `stset`ting this dataset, we fitted a Cox proportional-hazards regression model on `age` and `treat` to ascertain the effect of treatment, controlling for age.

```
. stset time, failure(cens) id(patient)

                id:  patient
     failure event:  cens != 0 & cens < .
obs. time interval:  (time[_n-1], time]
 exit on or before:  failure


        26  total obs.
         0  exclusions

        26  obs. remaining, representing
        26  subjects
        12  failures in single failure-per-subject data
     15588  total analysis time at risk, at risk from t =          0
                             earliest observed entry t =          0
                               last observed exit t =       1227

. stcox age treat, nolog nohr

         failure _d:  cens
   analysis time _t:  time
                id:  patient

Cox regression -- no ties

No. of subjects =           26                    Number of obs   =          26
No. of failures =           12
Time at risk    =        15588
                                                  LR chi2(2)      =       15.82
Log likelihood  =    -27.073767                   Prob > chi2     =      0.0004
```

_t	Coef.	Std. Err.	z	P>|z|	[95% Conf. Interval]
age	.1465698	.0458537	3.20	0.001	.0566982 .2364415
treat	-.7959324	.6329411	-1.26	0.209	-2.036474 .4446094

One way to test the proportional-hazards assumption is to include in the model a term for the interaction between age and time at risk, which is a continuously varying covariate. This can be easily done by first splitting the data at the failure times and then generating the interaction term.

```
. stsplit, at(failures)
(12 failure times)
(218 observations (episodes) created)

. generate tage = age * _t

. stcox age treat tage, nolog nohr

         failure _d:  cens
   analysis time _t:  time
                id:  patient

Cox regression -- no ties

No. of subjects =           26                    Number of obs   =         244
No. of failures =           12
Time at risk    =        15588
                                                  LR chi2(3)      =       16.36
Log likelihood  =    -26.806607                   Prob > chi2     =      0.0010
```

_t	Coef.	Std. Err.	z	P>|z|	[95% Conf. Interval]
age	.2156499	.1126093	1.92	0.055	-.0050602 .43636
treat	-.6635945	.6695492	-0.99	0.322	-1.975887 .6486978
tage	-.0002031	.0002832	-0.72	0.473	-.0007582 .000352

Other time-varying interactions of age and time at risk could be generated. For instance,

```
. generate lntage = age * ln(_t)
. generate dage = age * (_t >= 12)
```

Although in most analyses in which we include interactions we also include main effects, if we include in a Cox regression a multiplicative interaction between analysis time (or any transformation) and some covariate, we should not include the analysis time as a covariate in stcox. The analysis time is constant within each risk set, and hence, its effect is not identified.

❑ Technical Note

If our interest really were just in performing this test of the proportional-hazards assumption, we would not have had to use stsplit at all. We could have just typed

```
. stcox age treat, tvc(age)
```

to have fitted a model including t*age, and if we wanted instead to include $\ln(t)$*age or age*$t \geq 12$, we could have typed

```
. stcox age treat, tvc(age) texp(ln(_t))
. cstoc age treat, tvc(age) texp(_t>=12)
```

Still, it is worth understanding how stsplit could be used to obtain the same results for instances when stcox's tvc() and texp() options are not rich enough to handle the desired specification.

❑

Assume that we want to control for rdisea as a stratification variable. If the data are already split at all failure times, we can proceed with

```
. stcox age treat tage, strata(rdisea)
```

If the data are not yet split, and memory is scarce, then we could just split the data at the failure times within the respective stratum. That is, with the original data in memory we could type

```
. stset time, failure(cens) id(patient)
. stsplit, at(failures) strata(rdisea)
. generate tage = age * _t
. stcox treat age tage, strata(rdisea)
```

This would save memory by reducing the size of the split dataset.

◁

❑ Technical Note

Of course, the above model could also be obtained by typing

```
. stcox age treat, tvc(age) strata(rdisea)
```

without splitting the data.

❑

▷ Example 5: Cox regression versus conditional logistic regression

Cox regression with the "exact partial" method of handling ties is tightly related to conditional logistic regression. In fact, we can perform Cox regression via `clogit` as illustrated in the following example using Stata's cancer data. First, let's fit the Cox model.

```
. use http://www.stata-press.com/data/r10/cancer, clear
(Patient Survival in Drug Trial)
. generate id =_n
. stset studytime, failure(died) id(id)
               id:  id
    failure event:  died != 0 & died < .
obs. time interval:  (studytime[_n-1], studytime]
 exit on or before:  failure

        48  total obs.
         0  exclusions

        48  obs. remaining, representing
        48  subjects
        31  failures in single failure-per-subject data
       744  total analysis time at risk, at risk from t =          0
                            earliest observed entry t =          0
                                last observed exit t =          39
. stcox age drug, nolog nohr exactp
        failure _d:  died
   analysis time _t:  studytime
               id:  id
Cox regression -- exact partial likelihood

No. of subjects =          48                  Number of obs   =          48
No. of failures =          31
Time at risk    =         744
                                               LR chi2(2)      =       38.13
Log likelihood  =    -73.10556                 Prob > chi2     =      0.0000
```

_t _d	Coef.	Std. Err.	z	P>|z|	[95% Conf. Interval]
age	.1169906	.0374955	3.12	0.002	.0435008 .1904805
drug	-1.664873	.3437487	-4.84	0.000	-2.338608 -.9911376

We will now perform the same analysis by using `clogit`. To do this, we first split the data at failure times, specifying the `riskset()` option so that a risk set identifier is added to each observation. We then fit the conditional logistic regression, using _d as the outcome variable and the risk set identifier as the grouping variable.

(Continued on next page)

```
. stsplit, at(failures) riskset(RS)
(21 failure times)
(534 observations (episodes) created)

. clogit _d age drug, group(RS) nolog
note: multiple positive outcomes within groups encountered.
```

Conditional (fixed-effects) logistic regression	Number of obs	=	573
	LR chi2(2)	=	38.13
	Prob > chi2	=	0.0000
Log likelihood = -73.10556	Pseudo R2	=	0.2069

_d	Coef.	Std. Err.	z	P>|z|	[95% Conf. Interval]
age	.1169906	.0374955	3.12	0.002	.0435008	.1904805
drug	-1.664873	.3437487	-4.84	0.000	-2.338608	-.9911376

◁

▷ Example 6: Joining data that have been split with stsplit

Let's return to the first example. There we split the diet data into age bands, using the following commands:

```
. use http://www.stata-press.com/data/r10/diet, clear
(Diet data with dates)

. stset dox, failure(fail) origin(time dob) enter(time doe) scale(365.25) id(id)
  (output omitted)

. stsplit ageband, at(40(10)70)
(418 observations (episodes) created)
```

We can rejoin the data by typing stjoin:

```
. stjoin
(option censored(0) assumed)
(0 obs. eliminated)
```

Nothing happened! stjoin will combine records that are contiguous and record the same data. Here, when we split the data, stsplit created the new variable ageband, and that variable takes on different values across the split observations. Remember to drop the variable that stsplit creates:

```
. drop ageband

. stjoin
(option censored(0) assumed)
(418 obs. eliminated)
```

◁

Methods and Formulas

stsplit and stjoin are implemented as ado-files.

Wilhelm Lexis (1837–1914) was born near Aachen in Germany. He studied law, mathematics, and science at the University of Bonn and developed interests in the social sciences during a period in Paris. Lexis held posts at universities in Strassburg (now Strasbourg, in France), Dorpat (now Tartu, in Estonia), Freiburg, Breslau (now Wroclaw, in Poland), and Göttingen. During this peripatetic career he carried out original work in statistics on the analysis of dispersion, foreshadowing the later development of chi-squared and analysis of variance.

Acknowledgments

stsplit and stjoin are extensions of lexis by David Clayton, Cambridge Institute for Medical Research, and Michael Hills, London School of Hygiene and Tropical Medicine (retired) (Clayton and Hills 1995). The original stsplit and stjoin commands were written by Jeroen Weesie, Utrecht University, The Netherlands (Weesie 1998a, 1998b), as well as the revised stsplit command in this release.

References

Clayton, D. G., and M. Hills. 1993. *Statistical Models in Epidemiology*. Oxford: Oxford University Press.

——. 1995. ssa7: Analysis of follow-up studies. *Stata Technical Bulletin* 27: 19–26. Reprinted in *Stata Technical Bulletin Reprints*, vol. 5, pp. 219–227.

Cleves, M. A., W. W. Gould, and R. G. Gutierrez. 2004. *An Introduction to Survival Analysis Using Stata*. Rev. ed. College Station, TX: Stata Press.

Collett, D. 2003. *Modelling Survival Data in Medical Research*. 2nd ed. London: Chapman & Hall/CRC.

Hertz, S. 2001. Wilhelm Lexis. In *Statisticians of the Centuries*, ed. C. C. Heyde and E. Seneta, 204–207. New York: Springer.

Keiding, N. 1998. Lexis diagrams. In *Encyclopedia of Biostatistics*, ed. P. Armitage and T. Colton, 2844–2850. New York: Wiley.

Lexis, W. 1875. *Einleitung in die Theorie der Bevölkerungsstatistik*. Strassburg: Trübner.

Mander, A. 1998. gr31: Graphical representation of follow-up by time bands. *Stata Technical Bulletin* 45: 14–17. Reprinted in *Stata Technical Bulletin Reprints*, vol. 8, pp. 50–53.

Morris, J. N., J. W. Marr, and D. G. Clayton. 1977. Diet and heart: A postscript. *British Medical Journal* 19: 1307–1314.

Weesie, J. 1998a. ssa11: Survival analysis with time-varying covariates. *Stata Technical Bulletin* 41: 25–43. Reprinted in *Stata Technical Bulletin Reprints*, vol. 7, pp. 268–292.

——. 1998b. dm62: Joining episodes in multi-record survival-time data. *Stata Technical Bulletin* 45: 5–6. Reprinted in *Stata Technical Bulletin Reprints*, vol. 8, pp. 27–28.

Also See

[ST] **stset** — Declare data to be survival-time data

Title

stsum — Summarize survival-time data

Syntax

stsum [*if*] [*in*] [, by(*varlist*) <u>noshow</u>]

You must stset your data before using stsum; see [ST] **stset**.

by is allowed; see [D] **by**.

fweights, iweights, and pweights may be specified using stset; see [ST] **stset**.

Description

stsum presents summary statistics: time at risk, incidence rate, number of subjects, and the 25th, 50th, and 75th percentiles of survival time.

stsum can be used with single- or multiple-record or single- or multiple-failure st data.

Options

> Main

by(*varlist*) requests separate summaries for each group along with an overall total. Observations are in the same group if they have equal values of the variables in *varlist*. *varlist* may contain any number of string or numeric variables.

noshow prevents stsum from showing the key st variables. This option is seldom used since most people type stset, show or stset, noshow to set whether they want to see these variables mentioned at the top of the output of every st command; see [ST] **stset**.

Remarks

Single-failure data

Here is an example of stsum with single-record survival data:

```
. use http://www.stata-press.com/data/r10/page2
. stset, noshow
. stsum
```

	time at risk	incidence rate	no. of subjects	Survival time 25%	50%	75%
total	9118	.0039482	40	198	232	261

```
. stsum, by(group)
```

group	time at risk	incidence rate	no. of subjects	Survival time 25%	50%	75%
1	4095	.0041514	19	190	216	234
2	5023	.0037826	21	232	233	280
total	9118	.0039482	40	198	232	261

stsum works equally well with multiple-record survival data. Here is a summary of the multiple-record Stanford heart transplant data introduced in [ST] **stset**:

```
. use http://www.stata-press.com/data/r10/stan3
(Heart transplant data)
. stsum

        failure _d:  died
  analysis time _t:  t1
               id:  id
```

	time at risk	incidence rate	no. of subjects	—— Survival time ——		
				25%	50%	75%
total	31938.1	.0023483	103	36	100	979

stsum with the by() option may produce results with multiple-record data that, at first, you may think are in error.

```
. stsum, by(posttran) noshow
```

posttran	time at risk	incidence rate	no. of subjects	—— Survival time ——		
				25%	50%	75%
0	5936	.0050539	103	36	149	340
1	26002.1	.0017306	69	39	96	979
total	31938.1	.0023483	103	36	100	979

For the time at risk, $5{,}936 + 26{,}002.1 = 31{,}938.1$ but, for the number of subjects, $103 + 69 \neq 103$. Variable posttran is not constant for the subjects in this dataset:

```
. stset, noshow
. stvary posttran
```

	subjects for whom the variable is				
variable	constant	varying	never missing	always missing	sometimes missing
posttran	34	69	103	0	0

In this dataset, subjects have one or two records. All subjects were eligible for heart transplantation. They have one record if they die or are lost because of censoring before transplantation, and they have two records if the operation was performed. Then the first record records their survival up to transplantation and the second records their subsequent survival. posttran is 0 in the first record and 1 in the second.

Thus, all 103 subjects have records with posttran $= 0$, and when stsum reported results for this group, it summarized the pretransplantation survival. The incidence of death was .005, and median survival time was 149 days.

The posttran $= 1$ line of stsum's output summarizes the posttransplantation survival: 69 patients underwent transplantation, incidence of death was .002, and median survival time was 96 days. For these data, this is not 96 more days, but 96 days in total. That is, the clock was not reset at transplantation. Thus, without attributing cause, we can describe the differences between the groups as an increased hazard of death at early times followed by a decreased hazard later.

Multiple-failure data

If you simply type `stsum` with multiple-failure data, the reported survival time is the survival time to the first failure, assuming that the hazard function is not indexed by number of failures.

Here we have some multiple-failure data:

```
. use http://www.stata-press.com/data/r10/mfail2
. st
-> stset t, id(id) failure(d) time0(t0) exit(time .) noshow
              id:  id
    failure event:  d != 0 & d < .
  obs. time interval:  (t0, t]
   exit on or before:  time .
. stsum
```

	time at risk	incidence rate	no. of subjects	Survival time 25%	Survival time 50%	Survival time 75%
total	435444	.0018556	926	201	420	703

To understand this output, let's also obtain output for each failure separately:

```
. stgen nf = nfailures()
. stsum, by(nf)
```

nf	time at risk	incidence rate	no. of subjects	Survival time 25%	Survival time 50%	Survival time 75%
0	263746	.0020057	926	196	399	604
1	121890	.0018131	529	252	503	816
2	38807	.0014946	221	415	687	.
3	11001	0	58	.	.	.
total	435444	.0018556	926	201	420	703

The `stgen` command added, for each subject, a variable containing the number of previous failures. For a subject, up to and including the first failure, `nf` is 0. Then `nf` is 1 up to and including the second failure, and then it is 2, and so on; see [ST] **stgen**.

The first line of the output, corresponding to `nf` = 0, states that among those who had experienced no failures yet, the incidence rate for (first) failure is .0020. The distribution of the time to the first failure is as shown.

Similarly, the second line, corresponding to `nf` = 1, is for those who have already experienced one failure. The incidence rate for (second) failures is .0018, and the distribution of time of (second) failures is as shown.

When we simply typed `stsum`, we obtained the same information shown as the total line of the more detailed output. The total incidence rate is easy to interpret, but what is the "total" survival-time distribution? It is an estimate of the distribution of the time to the first failure assuming that the hazard function $h(t)$ is the same across failures—that the second failure is no different from the first failure. This is an odd definition of "same" because the clock t is not reset in $h(t)$. What is the hazard of a failure—any failure—at time t? The answer is $h(t)$.

Another definition of "same" would have it that the hazard of a failure is given by $h(\tau)$, where τ is the time since last failure—that the process repeats. These definitions are different unless $h()$ is a constant function of t (τ).

So let's examine these multiple-failure data under the process-replication idea. The key variables in these st data are `id`, `t0`, `t`, and `d`:

```
. st
-> stset t, id(id) failure(d) time0(t0) exit(time .) noshow
                id:  id
     failure event:  d != 0 & d < .
 obs. time interval:  (t0, t]
  exit on or before:  time .
```

Our goal is, for each subject, to reset t0 and t to 0 after every failure event. We are going to have to trick Stata, or at least trick stset, as it will not let us set data where the same subject has multiple records summarizing the overlapping periods. So, the trick is to create a new id variable that is different for every ID–nf combination (remember, nf is the variable we previously created that records the number of prior failures). Then all the "new" subjects can have their clocks start at time 0:

```
. egen newid = group(id nf)
. sort newid t
. by newid: replace t = t - t0[1]
(808 real changes made)
. by newid: gen newt0 = t0 - t0[1]
. stset t, failure(d) id(newid) time0(newt0)
                id:  newid
     failure event:  d != 0 & d < .
 obs. time interval:  (newt0, t]
  exit on or before:  failure

     1734  total obs.
        0  exclusions

     1734  obs. remaining, representing
     1734  subjects
      808  failures in single failure-per-subject data
   435444  total analysis time at risk, at risk from t =         0
                          earliest observed entry t =         0
                               last observed exit t =       797
```

stset no longer thinks that we have multiple-failure data. Whereas with id subjects had multiple failures, newid gives a unique identity to each ID–nf combination. Each "new" subject has at most one failure.

```
. stsum, by(nf)
          failure _d:  d
    analysis time _t:  t
                  id:  newid
```

nf	time at risk	incidence rate	no. of subjects	Survival time 25%	50%	75%
0	263746	.0020057	926	196	399	604
1	121890	.0018131	529	194	384	580
2	38807	.0014946	221	210	444	562
3	11001	0	58	.	.	.
total	435444	.0018556	1734	201	404	602

Compare this table with the one we previously obtained. The incidence rates are the same, but the survival times differ because now we measure the times from one failure to the next. Previously we measured the time from a fixed point. The time between events in these data appears to be independent of event number.

❏ Technical Note

The method shown for converting multiple-failure data to replicated-process single-event failure data is completely general. The generic outline of the conversion process is

```
. stgen nf = nfailures()
. egen newid = group(id nf)
. sort newid t
. by newid: replace t = t - t0[1]
. by newid: gen newt0 = t0 - t0[1]
. stset t, failure(d) id(newid) t0(newt0)
```

where *id*, *t*, *t0*, and *d* are the names of your key survival-time variables.

Once you have done this to your data, you need exercise only one caution. If, in fitting models with stcox, streg, etc., you wish to obtain robust estimates of variance, you should include the option vce(cluster *id*).

When you specify the vce(robust) option, stcox, streg, etc., assume that you mean vce(cluster *stset_id_variable*) which, here, will be vce(cluster newid). The data, however, are really more clustered than that. Two "subjects" with different newid values may, in fact, be the same real subject. vce(cluster *id*) is what is appropriate.

❏

Saved Results

stsum saves the following in r():

Scalars

r(p25)	25th percentile	r(risk)	time at risk
r(p50)	50th percentile	r(ir)	incidence rate
r(p75)	75th percentile	r(N_sub)	number of subjects

Methods and Formulas

stsum is implemented as an ado-file.

The 25th, 50th, and 75th percentiles of survival times are obtained from $S(t)$, the Kaplan–Meier product-limit estimate of the survivor function. The 25th percentile, for instance, is obtained as the minimum value of t such that $S(t) \le .75$.

Also See

[ST] **stdescribe** — Describe survival-time data

[ST] **stgen** — Generate variables reflecting entire histories

[ST] **stir** — Report incidence-rate comparison

[ST] **sts** — Generate, graph, list, and test the survivor and cumulative hazard functions

[ST] **stset** — Declare data to be survival-time data

[ST] **stvary** — Report whether variables vary over time

[ST] **stci** — Confidence intervals for means and percentiles of survival time

[ST] **stptime** — Calculate person-time, incidence rates, and SMR

Title

> **sttocc** — Convert survival-time data to case–control data

Syntax

> sttocc [*varlist*] [, *options*]

options	description
Main	
<u>match</u>(*matchvarlist*)	match cases and controls on analysis time and specified categorical variables; default is to match on analysis time only
<u>number</u>(#)	use # controls for each case; default is number(1)
<u>nodot</u>s	suppress displaying dots during calculation
Options	
<u>generate</u>(*case set time*)	new variable names; default is _case, _set, and _time

You must stset your data before using sttocc; see [ST] **stset**.

fweights, iweights, and pweights may be specified using stset; see [ST] **stset**.

Description

sttocc generates a nested case–control study dataset from a cohort-study dataset by sampling controls from the risk sets. For each case, the controls are chosen randomly from those members of the cohort who are at risk at the failure time of the case. That is, the resulting case–control sample is matched with respect to analysis time—the time scale used to compute risk sets. The following variables are added to the dataset:

_case	coded 0 for controls, 1 for cases
_set	case–control ID; matches cases and controls that belong together
_time	analysis time of the case's failure

The names of these three variables can be changed by specifying the generate() option. *varlist* defines variables that, in addition to those used in the creation of the case–control study, will be retained in the final dataset. If *varlist* is not specified, all variables are carried over into the resulting dataset.

When the resulting dataset is analyzed as a matched case–control study, odds ratios will estimate corresponding rate-ratio parameters in the proportional hazards model for the cohort study.

Randomness in the matching is obtained using Stata's uniform() function. To ensure that the sample truly is random, you should set the random-number seed; see [D] **generate**.

Options

―――――― Main ――

match(*matchvarlist*) specifies more categorical variables for matching controls to cases. When match() is not specified, cases and controls are matched with respect to time only. If match(*matchvarlist*) is specified, the cases will also be matched by *matchvarlist*.

number(#) specifies the number of controls to draw for each case. The default is 1, even though this is not a sensible choice.

nodots requests that dots not be placed on the screen at the beginning of each case–control group selection. By default, dots are displayed to show progress.

―――――― Options ―――

generate(*case set time*) specifies variable names for the three new variables, _case, _set, and _time.

Remarks

Nested case–control studies are an attractive alternative to full Cox regression analysis, particularly when time-varying explanatory variables are involved. They are also attractive when some explanatory variables involve laborious coding. For example, you can create a file with a subset of variables for all subjects in the cohort, generate a nested case–control study, and go on to code the remaining data only for those subjects selected.

In the same way as with Cox regression, the results of the analysis are critically dependent on the choice of analysis time (time scale). The choice of analysis time may be calendar time—so that controls would be chosen from subjects still being monitored on the date that the case fails—but other time scales, such as age or time in study, may be more appropriate in some studies. Remember that the analysis time set in selecting controls is implicitly included in the model in subsequent analysis.

match() requires that controls also be matched to the case with respect to other categorical variables, such as sex. This produces an analysis closely mirroring stratified Cox regression. If we wanted to match on calendar time and 5-year age bands, we could first type stsplit ageband ... to create the age bands and then specify match(ageband) on the sttocc command. Analyzing the resulting data as a matched case–control study would estimate rate ratios in the underlying cohort that are controlled for calendar time (very finely) and age (less finely). Such analysis could be carried out by Mantel–Haenszel (odds ratio) calculations, for example, using mhodds, or by conditional logistic regression using clogit.

When ties occur between entry times, censoring times, and failure times, the following convention is adopted:

$$\text{Entry time} < \text{Failure time} < \text{Censoring time}$$

Thus censored subjects and subjects entering at the failure time of the case are included in the risk set and are available for selection as controls. Tied failure times are broken at random. See Clayton and Hills (1997) for more information.

▷ Example 1: Creating a nested case–control study

Using the diet data introduced in [ST] **stsplit**, we will illustrate the use of sttocc, letting age be analysis time. Controls are chosen from subjects still being monitored at the age at which the case fails.

```
. use http://www.stata-press.com/data/r10/diet
(Diet data with dates)

. stset dox, failure(fail) enter(time doe) id(id) origin(time dob) scale(365.25)

                  id:  id
       failure event:  fail != 0 & fail < .
  obs. time interval:  (dox[_n-1], dox]
   enter on or after:  time doe
   exit on or before:  failure
       t for analysis:  (time-origin)/365.25
              origin:  time dob

       337  total obs.
         0  exclusions

       337  obs. remaining, representing
       337  subjects
        80  failures in single failure-per-subject data
  4603.669  total analysis time at risk, at risk from t =         0
                              earliest observed entry t =   30.07529
                                last observed exit t =   69.99863

. set seed 9123456

. sttocc, match(job) n(5) nodots
           failure _d:  fail
    analysis time _t:  (dox-origin)/365.25
              origin:  time dob
   enter on or after:  time doe
                  id:  id
         matching for:  job
There were 3 tied times involving failure(s)
  - failures assumed to precede censorings,
  - tied failure times split at random
There are 80 cases
Sampling 5 controls for each case
```

The above two commands create a new dataset in which there are five controls per case, matched on job, with the age of the subjects when the case failed recorded in the variable _time. The case indicator is given in _case and the matched set number in _set. Because we did not specify the optional *varlist*, all variables are carried over into the new dataset.

We can verify that the controls were correctly selected:

```
. gen ageentry=(doe-dob)/365.25

. gen ageexit=(dox-dob)/365.25

. sort _set _case id
```

(Continued on next page)

```
. list _set id _case _time ageentry ageexit job, sepby(_set)
```

	_set	id	_case	_time	ageentry	ageexit	job
1.	1	37	0	42.57358	35.2115	52.67351	0
2.	1	57	0	42.57358	40.04107	56.5859	0
3.	1	86	0	42.57358	38.14921	54.10815	0
4.	1	92	0	42.57358	36.67625	52.38877	0
5.	1	100	0	42.57358	36.15332	46.86653	0
6.	1	90	1	42.57358	31.4141	42.57358	0
7.	2	203	0	47.8987	41.26215	61.22108	2
8.	2	213	0	47.8987	47.23614	67.02532	2
9.	2	219	0	47.8987	41.86721	61.74127	2
10.	2	313	0	47.8987	41.50582	57.05133	2
11.	2	316	0	47.8987	40.68994	56.23545	2
12.	2	196	1	47.8987	45.46475	47.8987	2
13.	3	57	0	47.964408	40.04107	56.5859	0
14.	3	71	0	47.964408	47.52909	64.57221	0
				(output omitted)			
479.	80	136	0	68.596851	58.41205	69.99863	1
480.	80	108	1	68.596851	55.72074	68.59686	1

The controls do indeed belong to the appropriate risk set. The controls in each set enter at an age that is less than the age of the case at failure, and they exit at an age that is greater than the age of the case at failure. To estimate the effect of high energy, use clogit, just as you would for any matched case–control study:

```
. clogit _case hienergy, group(_set) or
Iteration 0:   log likelihood = -142.31278
Iteration 1:   log likelihood = -142.31276
Iteration 2:   log likelihood = -142.31276
Conditional (fixed-effects) logistic regression    Number of obs   =       480
                                                   LR chi2(1)      =      2.06
                                                   Prob > chi2     =    0.1516
Log likelihood = -142.31276                        Pseudo R2       =    0.0072
```

_case	Odds Ratio	Std. Err.	z	P>|z|	[95% Conf. Interval]	
hienergy	.7026801	.1734294	-1.43	0.153	.433183	1.13984

◁

Methods and Formulas

sttocc is implemented as an ado-file.

Acknowledgments

The original version of sttocc was written by David Clayton, Cambridge Institute for Medical Research, and Michael Hills, London School of Hygiene and Tropical Medicine (retired).

References

Clayton, D. G., and M. Hills. 1993. *Statistical Models in Epidemiology*. Oxford: Oxford University Press.

——. 1995. ssa7: Analysis of follow-up studies. *Stata Technical Bulletin* 27: 19–26. Reprinted in *Stata Technical Bulletin Reprints*, vol. 5, pp. 219–227.

——. 1997. ssa10: Analysis of follow-up studies with Stata 5.0. *Stata Technical Bulletin* 40: 27–39. Reprinted in *Stata Technical Bulletin Reprints*, vol. 7, pp. 253–268.

Coviello, V. 2001. sbe41: Ordinary case–cohort design and analysis. *Stata Technical Bulletin* 59: 12–18. Reprinted in *Stata Technical Bulletin Reprints*, vol. 10, pp. 121–129.

Langholz, B., and D. C. Thomas. 1990. Nested case–control and case–cohort methods of sampling from a cohort: A critical comparison. *American Journal of Epidemiology* 131: 169–176.

Also See

[ST] **stbase** — Form baseline dataset

[ST] **stdescribe** — Describe survival-time data

[ST] **stsplit** — Split and join time-span records

Title

---
sttoct — Convert survival-time data to count-time data

Syntax

> sttoct *newfailvar newcensvar* [*newentvar*] [, *options*]

options	description
by(*varlist*)	reflect counts by group, where groups are defined by observations with equal values of *varlist*
replace	proceed with transformation, even if current data are not saved
noshow	do not show st setting information

You must stset your data before using sttoct; see [ST] **stset**.

fweights, iweights, and pweights may be specified using stset; see [ST] **stset**.

There is no dialog-box interface for sttoct.

Description

sttoct converts survival-time (st) data to count-time (ct) data; see [ST] **ct**.

At present, there is absolutely no reason that you would want to do this.

Options

by(*varlist*) specifies that counts reflect counts by group where the groups are defined by observations with equal values of *varlist*.

replace specifies that it is okay to proceed with the transformation, even though the current dataset has not been saved on disk.

noshow prevents sttoct from showing the key st variables. This option is seldom used since most people type stset, show or stset, noshow to set whether they want to see these variables mentioned at the top of every st command; see [ST] **stset**.

Remarks

sttoct is a never-used command that is included only for completeness. The definition of ct data is found in [ST] **ct**. In the current version of Stata, all you can do with ct data is convert it to st data (which thus provides access to Stata's survival analysis capabilities to those with ct data), so there is little point in converting st data to ct data.

The converted dataset will contain

varlist	from by(*varlist*) if specified
t	the exit-time variable previously stset
newfailvar	number of failures at *t*
newcensvar	number of censored at *t* (after failures)
newentvar	if specified, number of entries at *t* (after censorings)

The resulting dataset will be ctset automatically.

There are two forms of the sttoct command:

1. sttoct *failvar censvar*, ...

2. sttoct *failvar censvar entvar*, ...

That is, specifying *entvar* makes a difference.

Case 1: entvar not specified

This is possible only if

a. the risk is not recurring;

b. the original st data is single-record data, or if it is multiple-record data, all subjects enter at time 0 and have no gaps thereafter; and

c. if by(*varlist*) is specified, subjects do not have changing values of the variables in *varlist* over their histories.

If you do not specify *entvar*, sttoct verifies that (a), (b), and (c) are true. If the assumptions are true, sttoct converts your data and counts each subject only once. That is, in multiple-record data, all thrashing (censoring followed by immediate reenter with different covariates) is removed.

Case 2: entvar specified

Any kind of survival-time data can be converted to count-data with an entry variable. You can convert your data in this way whether assumptions (a), (b), and (c) are true or not.

When you specify a third variable, thrashing is not removed, even if it could be—even if assumptions (a), (b), and (c) are true.

Methods and Formulas

sttoct is implemented as an ado-file.

Also See

[ST] **ct** — Count-time data

[ST] **st_is** — Survival analysis subroutines for programmers

[ST] **sttocc** — Convert survival-time data to case–control data

Title

> **stvary** — Report whether variables vary over time

Syntax

stvary $\big[$ *varlist* $\big]$ $\big[$ *if* $\big]$ $\big[$ *in* $\big]$ $\big[$, <u>nosh</u>ow $\big]$

You must stset your data before using stvary; see [ST] **stset**.

by is allowed; see [D] **by**.

fweights, iweights, and pweights may be specified using stset; see [ST] **stset**.

Description

stvary is for use with multiple-record datasets, for which id() has been stset. It reports whether values of variables within subject vary over time and reports their pattern of missing values. Although stvary is intended for use with multiple-record st data, it may be used with single-record data as well, but this produces little useful information.

stvary ignores weights, even if you have set them. stvary summarizes the variables in the computer or data sense of the word.

Option

Main

noshow prevents stvary from showing the key st variables. This option is seldom used since most people type stset, show or stset, noshow to set whether they want to see these variables mentioned at the top of the output of every st command; see [ST] **stset**.

Remarks

Consider a multiple-record dataset. A subject's sex, presumably, does not change, but his or her age might. stvary allows you to verify that values vary in the way that you expect:

```
. use http://www.stata-press.com/data/r10/stan3
(Heart transplant data)

. stvary

        failure _d:  died
   analysis time _t:  t1
                id:  id
```

		subjects for whom the variable is			
variable	constant	varying	never missing	always missing	sometimes missing
year	103	0	103	0	0
age	103	0	103	0	0
stime	103	0	103	0	0
surgery	103	0	103	0	0
transplant	103	0	103	0	0
wait	103	0	103	0	0
posttran	34	69	103	0	0

472

That 103 values for `year` are "constant" does not mean that `year` itself is a constant—it means merely that, for each subject, the value of `year` does not change across the records. Whether the values of `year` vary across subjects is still an open question.

Now look at the bottom of the table: `posttran` is constant over time for 34 subjects and varies for the remaining 69.

Below we have another dataset, and we will examine just two of the variables:

```
. use http://www.stata-press.com/data/r10/stvaryex
```

```
. stvary sex drug
```

| | subjects for whom the variable is | | | | |
	constant	varying	never missing	always missing	sometimes missing
variable					
sex	119	1	119	3	1
drug	121	2	123	0	0

Clearly, there are errors in the variable `sex`; for 119 of the subjects, `sex` does not change over time, but for one, it does. Also, we see that we do not know the sex of three of the patients, but for another, we sometimes know it and sometimes do not. The latter must be a simple data construction error. As for `drug`, we see that for two of our patients, the drug administered varied over time. Perhaps this is an error, or perhaps those two patients were treated differently from all the rest.

Saved Results

`stvary` saves the following in `r()`:

Scalars

`r(cons)`	number of subjects for whom variable is constant when not missing
`r(varies)`	number of subjects for whom nonmissing values vary
`r(never)`	number of subjects for whom variable is never missing
`r(always)`	number of subjects for whom variable is always missing
`r(miss)`	number of subjects for whom variable is sometimes missing

Methods and Formulas

`stvary` is implemented as an ado-file.

Reference

Cleves, M. A., W. W. Gould, and R. G. Gutierrez. 2004. *An Introduction to Survival Analysis Using Stata*. Rev. ed. College Station, TX: Stata Press.

Also See

[ST] **stdescribe** — Describe survival-time data

[ST] **stfill** — Fill in by carrying forward values of covariates

[ST] **stset** — Declare data to be survival-time data

Glossary

accelerated failure-time model. A model in which everyone has, in a sense, the same survival function $S(\tau)$ and an individual's τ_j is a function of his or her characteristics and of time, such as $\tau_j = t * \exp(\beta_0 + \beta_1 x_{1j} + \beta_2 x_{2j})$.

accrual period or **recruitment period** or **accrual**. The accrual period (or recruitment period) is the period during which subjects are being enrolled (recruited) into a study. Also see *follow-up period*.

administrative censoring. Administrative censoring is the right-censoring that occurs when the study observation period ends. All subjects complete the course of the study and are known to have experienced either of two outcomes at the end of the study: survival or failure. This type of censoring should not be confused with *withdrawal* and *loss to follow-up*. Also see *censoring*.

analysis time. Analysis time is like time, except that 0 has a special meaning: $t = 0$ is the time of onset of risk, the time when failure first became possible.

Analysis time is usually not what is recorded in a dataset. A dataset of patients might record calendar time. Calendar time must then be mapped to analysis time.

The letter t is reserved for time in analysis time units. The term *time* is used for time measured in other units.

The *origin* is the *time* corresponding to $t = 0$, which can vary subject to subject. Thus $t = time - origin$.

at risk. A subject is at risk from the instant the first failure event becomes possible and usually stays that way until failure, but a subject can have periods of being at risk and not at risk.

attributable fraction. An attributable fraction is the reduction in the risk of a disease or other condition of interest when a particular risk factor is removed.

baseline. In survival analysis, baseline is the state at which the covariates, usually denoted by the row vector **x**, are zero. For example, if the only measured covariate is systolic blood pressure, the baseline survival function would be the survival function for someone with zero systolic blood pressure. This may seem ridiculous, but covariates are usually centered so that the mathematical definition of baseline (covariate is zero) translates into something meaningful (mean systolic blood pressure).

case–control studies. In case–control studies, cases meeting a fixed criterion are matched to noncases ex post to study differences in possible covariates. Relative sample sizes are usually fixed at 1:1 or 1:2 but sometimes vary once the survey is complete. In any case, sample sizes do not reflect the distribution in the underlying population.

censored, **censoring**, **left-censoring**, and **right-censoring**. An observation is left-censored when the exact time of the onset of risk is not known; it is merely known that the onset of risk occurred before t_l.

An observation is right-censored when the time of failure is not known; it is merely known that the failure occurred after t_r.

In common usage, *censored* without a modifier means right-censoring.

Also see *truncation*.

cohort studies. In cohort studies, a group that is well defined is monitored over time to track the transition of noncases to cases. Cohort studies differ from incidence studies in that they can be retrospective as well as prospective.

competing risks. Competing risks models are survival-data models in which the failures are generated by more than one underlying process. For example, death may be caused by either heart attack or stroke. There are various methods for dealing with competing risks. One direct way is to duplicate failures for one competing risk as censored observations for the other risk, stratify on the risk type, and use clustering to account for the fact that both records (original and duplicate) come from the same subject.

confounding. In the analysis of epidemiological tables, factor or interaction effects are said to be confounded when the effect of one factor is combined with that of another. For example, the effect of alcohol consumption on esophageal cancer may be confounded with the effects of age and/or smoking. In the presence of confounding, it is often useful to stratify on the confounded factors that are not of primary interest, in the above example, age and smoking.

count-time data. See *ct data*.

covariates. Covariates are the explanatory variables that appear in a model. For instance, if survival time were to be explained by age, sex, and treatment, then those variables would be the covariates. Also see *time-varying covariates*.

cross-sectional or **prevalence studies**. Cross-sectional studies sample distributions of healthy and diseased subjects in the population at one point in time.

crude estimate. A crude estimate is an estimate that is chosen not for accuracy or precision but instead for ease of calculation.

ct data. ct stands for count time. ct data is an aggregate organized like a life table. Each observation records a time, the number known to fail at that time, the number censored, and the number of new entries. See [ST] **ctset**.

effect size. The effect size is the size of the clinically significant difference between the treatments being compared, often expressed as the hazard ratio (or the log of the hazard ratio) in survival analysis.

event. An event is something that happens at an instant in time, such as being exposed to an environmental hazard, being diagnosed as myopic, or becoming employed.

The failure event is of special interest in survival analysis, but there are other equally important events, such as the exposure event, from which analysis time is defined.

In st data, events occur at the end of the recorded time span.

exponential test. The exponential test is the parametric test comparing the hazard rates, λ_1 and λ_2, (or log hazards) from two independent exponential (constant only) regression models with the null hypothesis $H_0: \lambda_2 - \lambda_1 = 0$ (or $H_0: \ln(\lambda_2) - \ln(\lambda_1) = \ln(\lambda_2/\lambda_1) = 0$).

failure event. Survival analysis is really time-to-failure analysis, and the failure event is the event under analysis. The failure event can be death, heart attack, myopia, or finding employment. Many authors—including Stata—write as if the failure event can occur only once per subject, but when we do, we are being sloppy. Survival analysis encompasses repeated failures, and all Stata's survival analysis features can be used with repeated-failure data.

follow-up period or **follow-up**. The (minimum) follow-up period is the period after the last subject entered the study until the end of the study. The follow-up defines the phase of a study during which subjects are under observation and no new subjects enter the study. If T is the total duration of a study, and R is the accrual period of the study, then follow-up period f is equal to $T - R$. Also see *accrual period*.

frailty. In survival analysis, it is often assumed that subjects are alike—homogeneous—except for their observed differences. The probability that subject j fails at time t may be a function of j's covariates and random chance. Subjects j and k, if they have equal covariate values, are equally likely to fail.

Frailty relaxes that assumption. The probability that subject j fails at time t becomes a function of j's covariates and j's unobserved frailty value, ν_j. Frailty ν is assumed to be a random variable. Parametric survival models can be fitted even in the presence of such heterogeneity.

Shared frailty refers to the case in which groups of subjects share the same frailty value. For instance, subjects 1 and 2 may share frailty value ν because they are genetically related. Both parametric and semiparametric models can be fitted under the shared-frailty assumption.

future history. Future history is information recorded after a subject is no longer at risk. The word *history* is often dropped, and the term becomes simply *future*. Perhaps the failure event is cardiac infarction, and you want to know whether the subject died soon in the *future*, in which case you might exclude the subject from analysis.

Also see *past history*.

gaps. Gaps refers to gaps in observation between entry time and exit time; see *under observation*.

hazard, cumulative hazard, and **hazard ratio**. The hazard or hazard rate at time t, $h(t)$, is the instantaneous rate of failure at time t conditional on survival until time t. Hazard rates can exceed 1. Say that the hazard rate were 3. If an individual faced a constant hazard of 3 over a unit interval and if the failure event could be repeated, the individual would be expected to experience three failures during the time span.

The cumulative hazard $H(t)$ is the integral of the hazard function $h(t)$, from 0 (the onset of risk) to t. It is the total number of failures that would be expected to occur up until time t, if the failure event could be repeated. The relationship between the cumulative hazard function $H(t)$ and the survivor function $S(t)$ is

$$S(t) = \exp\{-H(t)\}$$

$$H(t) = -\ln\{S(t)\}$$

The hazard ratio is the ratio of the hazard function evaluated at two different values of the covariates: $h(t\,|\,\mathbf{x})/h(t\,|\,\mathbf{x}_0)$. The hazard ratio is often called the relative hazard, especially when $h(t\,|\,\mathbf{x}_0)$ is the baseline hazard function.

ID variable. An ID variable identifies groups; equal values of an ID variable indicate that the observations are for the same group. For instance, a stratification ID variable would indicate the strata to which each observation belongs.

When an ID variable is referred to without modification, it means subjects, and usually this occurs in multiple-record st data. In multiple-record data, each physical observation in the dataset represents a time span, and the ID variable ties the separate observations together:

idvar	t0	t
1	0	5
1	5	7

ID variables are usually numbered 1, 2, . . ., but that is not required. An ID variable might be numbered 1, 3, 7, 22, . . ., or -5, -4, . . ., or even 1, 1.1, 1.2, ...

incidence and **incidence rate**. Incidence is the number of new failures (e.g., number of new cases of a disease) that occur during a specified period in a population at risk (e.g., of the disease).

Incidence rate is incidence divided by the sum of the length of time each individual was exposed to the risk.

Do not confuse incidence with prevalence. Prevalence is the fraction of a population that has the disease. Incidence refers to the rate at which people contract a disease, whereas prevalence is the total number actually sick at a given time.

incidence studies, **longitudinal studies**, and **follow-up studies**. Whichever word is used, these studies monitor a population for a time to track the transition of noncases into cases. Incidence studies are prospective. Also see *cohort studies*.

Kaplan–Meier product-limit estimate. An estimate of the survivor function, which is the product of conditional survival to each time at which an event occurs. The simple form of the calculation, which requires tallying the number at risk and the number who die and at each time, makes accounting for censoring easy. The resulting estimate is a step function with jumps at the event times.

life table. Also known as a mortality table or actuarial table, a life table is a table that shows for each analysis time the fraction that survive to that time. In mortality tables, analysis time is often age.

loss to follow-up. Subjects are lost to follow-up if they do not complete the course of the study for reasons unrelated to the event of interest. For example, loss to follow-up occurs if subjects move to a different area or decide to no longer participate in a study. Loss to follow-up should not be confused with administrative censoring. If subjects are lost to follow-up, the information about the outcome these subjects would have experienced at the end of the study, had they completed the study, is unavailable. Also see *withdrawal*, *administrative censoring*, and *follow-up*.

matched case–control study. Also known as a retrospective study, a matched case–control study is a study in which persons with positive outcomes are each matched with one or more persons with negative outcomes but with similar characteristics.

multiarm trial. A multiarm trial is a trial comparing survivor functions of more than two groups.

odds and **odds ratio**. The odds in favor of an event are $o = p/(1 - p)$, where p is the probability of the event. Thus if $p = .2$, the odds are .25, and if $p = .8$, the odds are 4.

The log of the odds is $\ln(o) = \text{logit}(p) = \ln\{p/(1 - p)\}$, and logistic-regression models, for instance, fit $\ln(o)$ as a linear function of the covariates.

The odds ratio is a ratio of two odds: o_1/o_0. The individual odds that appear in the ratio are usually for an experimental group and a control group, or two different demographic groups.

offset variable and **exposure variable**. An offset variable is a variable that is to appear on the right-hand side of a model with coefficient one:

$$y_j = \text{offset}_j + b_0 + b_1 x_j + \cdots$$

In the above, b_0 and b_1 are to be estimated. The offset is not constant. Offset variables are often included to account for the amount of exposure. Consider a model where the number of events observed over a period is the length of the period multiplied by the number of events expected in a unit of time:

$$n_j = T_j e(X_j)$$

When we take logs, this becomes

$$\log(n_j) = \log(T_j) + \log\{e(X_j)\}$$

$\ln(T_j)$ is an offset variable in this model.

When the log of a variable is an offset variable, the variable is said to be an exposure variable. In the above, T_j is an exposure variable.

past history. Past history is information recorded about a subject before the subject was both *at risk* and *under observation*. Consider a dataset that contains information on subjects from birth to death and an analysis in which subjects became at risk once diagnosed with a particular kind of cancer. The past history on the subject would then refer to records before the subjects were diagnosed.

The word *history* is often dropped, and the term becomes simply *past*. For instance, we might want to know whether a subject smoked in the past.

Also see *future history*.

penalized log-likelihood function. A log-likelihood function that contains an added term, usually referred to as a roughness penalty, that reduces its value when the model overfits the data. In Cox models with frailty, such functions are used to prevent the variance of the frailty from growing too large, which would allow the individual frailty values to perfectly fit the data.

power. The power of a test is the probability of correctly rejecting the null hypothesis when it is false. It is often denoted as $1 - \beta$ in statistical literature, where β is the type II error probability. Commonly used values for power are 80% and 90%. Also see *type II error* and *type I error*.

prevented fraction. A prevented fraction is the reduction in the risk of a disease or other condition of interest caused by including a protective risk factor or public-health intervention.

proportional hazards model. A model in which, between individuals, the ratio of the instantaneous failure rates (the hazards) is constant over time.

prospective study. Also known as a prospective longitudinal study, a prospective study is a study based on observations over the same subjects for a given period.

risk factor. A variable associated with an increased or decreased risk of failure.

risk pool. At a particular point in time, the subjects at risk of failure.

risk ratio. In a log-linear model, the ratio of probability of survival associated with a one-unit increase in a risk factor relative to that calculated without such an increase, that is, $R(x + 1)/R(x)$. Given the exponential form of the model, $R(x + 1)/R(x)$ is constant and is given by the exponentiated coefficient.

semiparametric model. A model that is not fully parameterized. The Cox proportional hazards model is such a model:

$$h(t) = h_0(t) \exp(\beta_1 x_1 + \cdots + \beta_k x_k)$$

In the Cox model, $h_o(t)$ is left unparameterized and not even estimated. Meanwhile, the relative effects of covariates are parameterized as $\exp(\beta_1 x_1 + \cdots + \beta_k x_k)$.

singleton-group data. A singleton is a frailty group that contains only 1 observation. A dataset containing only singletons is known as singleton-group data.

SMR. SMR stands for standardized mortality (morbidity) ratio and is the observed number of deaths divided by the expected number of deaths. It is calculated using indirect standardization: you take the population of the group of interest—say, by age, sex, and other factors—and calculate the expected number of deaths in each cell (expected being defined as the number of deaths that would have been observed if those in the cell had the same mortality as some other population). You then take the ratio to compare the observed with the expected number of deaths. For instance,

Age	(1) Population of group	(2) Deaths per 100,000 in general pop.	(1)×(2) Expected # of deaths	(4) Observed deaths
25–34	95,965	105.2	100.9	92
34–44	78,280	203.6	159.4	180
44–54	52,393	428.9	224.7	242
55–64	28,914	964.6	278.9	312
Total			763.9	826

$$\text{SMR} = 826/763.9 = 1.08$$

snapshot data. Snapshot data are those in which each record contains the values of a set of variables for a subject at an instant in time. The name arises because each observation is like a snapshot of the subject.

In snapshot datasets, one usually has a group of observations (snapshots) for each subject.

Snapshot data must be converted to st data before they can be analyzed. This requires making assumptions about what happened between the snapshots. See [ST] **snapspan**.

spell data. Spell data are survival data in which each record represents a fixed period, consisting of a begin time, an end time, possibly a censoring/failure indicator, and other measurements (covariates) taken during that specific period.

st data. st stands for survival time. In survival-time data, each observation represents a span of survival, recorded in variables $t0$ and t. For instance, if in an observation $t0$ were 3 and t were 5, the span would be $(t0, t]$, meaning from just after $t0$ up to and including t.

Sometimes variable $t0$ is not recorded. $t0$ is then assumed to be 0. In such a dataset, an observation that had $t = 5$ would record the span $(0, 5]$.

Each observation also includes a variable d, called the failure variable, which contains 0 or nonzero (typically, 1). The failure variable records what happened at the end of the span: 0, the subject was still alive (had not yet failed) or 1, the subject died (failed).

Sometimes variable d is not recorded. d is then assumed to be 1. In such a dataset, all time-span observations would be assumed to end in failure.

Finally, each observation in an st dataset can record the entire history of a subject or each can record a part of the history. In the latter case, groups of observations record the full history. One observation might record the period $(0, 5]$ and the next, $(5, 8]$. In such cases, there is a variable ID that records the subject for which the observation records a time span. Such data are called multiple-record st data. When each observation records the entire history of a subject, the data are called single-record st data. In the single-record case, the ID variable is optional.

See [ST] **stset**.

survival-time data. See *st data*.

survivor function. Also known as the survivorship function and the survival function, the survivor function $S(t)$ is (1) the probability of surviving beyond time t, or equivalently, (2) the probability that there is no failure event prior to t, (3) the proportion of the population surviving to time t, or equivalently, (4) the reverse cumulative distribution function of T, the time to the failure event: $S(t) = \Pr(T > t)$. Also see *hazard*.

time-varying covariates. Time-varying covariates appear in a survival model whose values vary over time. The values of the covariates vary, not the effect. For instance, in a proportional hazards model, the log hazard at time t might be $b \times \text{age}_t + c \times \text{treatment}_t$. Variable age might be time varying, meaning that as the subject ages, the value of age changes, which correspondingly causes the hazard to change. The effect b, however, remains constant.

Time-varying variables are either continuously varying or discretely varying.

In the continuously varying case, the value of the variable x at time t is $x_t = x_o + f(t)$, where $f()$ is some function and often is the identity function, so that $x_t = x_o + t$.

In the discretely varying case, the value of x changes at certain times and often in no particular pattern:

idvar	t0	t	bp
1	0	5	150
1	5	7	130
1	7	9	135

In the above data, the value of bp is 150 over the period $(0,5]$, then 130 over $(5,7]$, and 135 over $(7,9]$.

truncation. In statistics, truncation refers to cases where subjects are unobserved (do not appear in the data). Censoring, on the other hand, refers to cases when subjects are known to fail within a certain time span, except that the exact failure time is unknown.

In survival analysis, truncation—sometimes called left-truncation—occurs when subjects are not observed before time t_c, only to appear in the study at time t_c. It is only because they didn't fail before t_c that we even knew about their existence. Left-truncation differs from left-censoring in that, in the censored case, we know that the subject failed before time t_c, but we just do not know exactly when.

Given these conventions, right-truncation is equivalent to right-censoring, since failure (at some point before time infinity) is inevitable.

type I error or **false-positive result**. The type I error of a test is the error of rejecting the null hypothesis when it is true. The probability of committing a type I error, significance level of a test, is often denoted as α in statistical literature. One traditionally used value for α is 5%. Also see *type II error* and *power*.

type II error or **false-negative result**. The type II error of a test is the error of not rejecting the null hypothesis when it is false. The probability of committing type II error is often denoted as β in statistical literature. Commonly used values for β are 20% or 10%. Also see *type I error* and *power*.

type I study. A type I study is a study in which all subjects fail (or experience an event) by the end of the study; that is, no censoring of subjects occurs.

type II study. A type II study is a study in which there are subjects who do not fail (or do not experience an event) by the end of the study. These subjects are known to be censored.

under observation. A subject is under observation when failure events, should they occur, would be observed (and so recorded in the dataset). Being under observation does not mean that a subject is necessarily at risk. Subjects usually come under observation before they are at risk. The statistical concern is with periods when subjects are at risk but not under observation, even when the subject is (later) known not to have failed during the hiatus.

In such cases, since failure events would not have been observed, the subject necessarily had to survive the observational hiatus, and that leads to bias in statistical results unless the hiatus is accounted for properly.

Entry time and exit time record when a subject first and last comes under observation, between which there may be observational gaps, but usually there are not. There is only one entry time and one exit time for each subject. Often, entry time corresponds to analysis time $t = 0$, or before, and exit time corresponds to the time of failure.

Delayed entry means that the entry time occurred after $t = 0$.

withdrawal. Withdrawal is the process under which subjects withdraw from a study for reasons unrelated to the event of interest. For example, withdrawal occurs if subjects move to a different area or decide to no longer participate in a study. Withdrawal should not be confused with administrative censoring. If subjects withdraw from the study, the information about the outcome those subjects would have experienced at the end of the study, had they completed the study, is unavailable. Also see *loss to follow-up* and *administrative censoring*.

Subject and author index

This is the subject and author index for the *Stata Survival Analysis and Epidemiological Tables Reference Manual*. Readers interested in topics other than survival analysis should see the combined subject index (and the combined author index) in the *Stata Quick Reference and Index*. The combined index indexes the *Getting Started* manuals, the *User's Guide*, and all the Reference manuals except the *Mata Reference Manual*.

Semicolons set off the most important entries from the rest. Sometimes no entry will be set off with semicolons, meaning that all entries are equally important.

A

Aalen–Nelson cumulative hazard, *see* Nelson–Aalen cumulative hazard
Aalen, O. O., [ST] **sts**
Abraira-García, L., [ST] **epitab**
Abramson, J. H., [ST] **epitab**
Abramson, Z. H., [ST] **epitab**
accelerated failure-time model, [ST] **glossary**, [ST] **streg**
accrual period, [ST] **glossary**, [ST] **stpower exponential**, [ST] **stpower logrank**
actuarial tables, *see* life table
adjusted Kaplan–Meier survivor function, [ST] **sts**
administrative censoring, [ST] **glossary**
AIC (Akaike information criterion), [ST] **streg**
Aisbett, C. W., [ST] **stcox**, [ST] **streg**
Akaike, H., [ST] **streg**
Allison, P. D., [ST] **discrete**
analysis time, [ST] **glossary**
association test, [ST] **epitab**
at risk, [ST] **glossary**
at-risk table, [ST] **sts graph**
attributable fraction, [ST] **epitab**, [ST] **glossary**
attributable proportion, [ST] **epitab**

B

Babiker, A., [ST] **epitab**, [ST] **stpower**, [ST] **stpower cox**, [ST] **sts test**
Barthel, F. M.-S., [ST] **stcox diagnostics**, [ST] **stpower**, [ST] **stpower cox**
baseline, [ST] **glossary**
baseline dataset, [ST] **stbase**
baseline hazard and survivor functions, [ST] **stcox**, [ST] **stcox diagnostics**
Boice, J. D., [ST] **epitab**
Box-Steffensmeier, J. M., [ST] **stcox**, [ST] **streg**
Breslow, N. E., [ST] **epitab**, [ST] **stcox**, [ST] **stcox diagnostics**, [ST] **sts**, [ST] **sts test**

C

Califf, R. M., [ST] **stcox postestimation**
Campbell, M., [ST] **stpower**, [ST] **stpower logrank**
Carlin, J., [ST] **epitab**
Carnes, B. A., [ST] **streg**
Carter, S. L., [ST] **stcox**, [ST] **streg**
case–cohort data, [ST] **sttocc**
case–control data, [ST] **epitab**, [ST] **sttocc**
case–control studies, [ST] **glossary**
categorical data, [ST] **epitab**
cc command, [ST] **epitab**
cci command, [ST] **epitab**
Chiang, C. L., [ST] **ltable**
chi-squared, test of independence, [ST] **epitab**
Chow, S.-C., [ST] **stpower**, [ST] **stpower exponential**
Clark, V. A., [ST] **ltable**
Clayton, D. G., [ST] **epitab**, [ST] **stptime**, [ST] **strate**, [ST] **stsplit**, [ST] **sttocc**
Cleves, M. A., [ST] **st**, [ST] **stcox**, [ST] **stcurve**, [ST] **stdescribe**, [ST] **streg**, [ST] **sts**, [ST] **stset**, [ST] **stsplit**, [ST] **stvary**, [ST] **survival analysis**
clinical trial, [ST] **stpower**
cluster estimator of variance,
    Cox proportional hazards model, [ST] **stcox**
    parametric survival models, [ST] **streg**
cohort studies, [ST] **glossary**
Collett, D., [ST] **stci**, [ST] **stpower**, [ST] **stpower logrank**, [ST] **streg postestimation**, [ST] **sts test**, [ST] **stsplit**
competing risks, [ST] **glossary**
concordance, estat subcommand, [ST] **stcox postestimation**
confidence intervals for odds and risk ratios, [ST] **epitab**, [ST] **stci**
confounding, [ST] **glossary**
constrained estimation, [ST] **estimation options**
    parametric survival models, [ST] **streg**
contingency tables, [ST] **epitab**
Cornfield confidence intervals, [ST] **epitab**
Cornfield, J., [ST] **epitab**
count-time data, [ST] **ct**, [ST] **glossary**; [ST] **ctset**, [ST] **cttost**, [ST] **sttoct**
covariates, [ST] **glossary**
Coviello, V., [ST] **sttocc**
Cox, D. R., [ST] **ltable**, [ST] **stcox**, [ST] **stcox diagnostics**, [ST] **stpower**, [ST] **stpower cox**, [ST] **streg**, [ST] **streg postestimation**, [ST] **sts**
Cox proportional hazards model, [ST] **stcox**
    power, [ST] **stpower cox**
    sample size, [ST] **stpower cox**
    test of assumption, [ST] **stcox**, [ST] **stcox diagnostics**, [ST] **stcox postestimation**, [ST] **stsplit**
    Wald test, power, [ST] **stpower cox**
Cox–Snell residual, [ST] **stcox**, [ST] **streg postestimation**
cox, stpower subcommand, [ST] **stpower cox**

cross-sectional studies, [ST] **glossary**
Crowder, M. J., [ST] **streg**
Crowley, J., [ST] **stcox**, [ST] **stset**
crude estimate, [ST] **epitab**, [ST] **glossary**
cs command, [ST] **epitab**
csi command, [ST] **epitab**
ct data, [ST] **glossary**, *also see* count-time data
ctset command, [ST] **ctset**
cttost command, [ST] **cttost**
Cui, J., [ST] **stcox**, [ST] **streg**
cumulative hazard function, [ST] **stcurve**, [ST] **sts**,
     [ST] **sts generate**, [ST] **sts graph**, [ST] **sts list**
cumulative hazard ratio, *see* hazard ratio
cumulative incidence data, [ST] **epitab**
Cutler, S. J., [ST] **ltable**

D

data,
     case–cohort, *see* case–cohort data
     case–control, *see* case–control data
     count-time, *see* count-time data
     discrete survival, *see* discrete survival data
     multiple-record st data, *see* multiple-record st data
     nested case–control, *see* nested case–control data
     time-span, *see* time-span data
Day, N. E., [ST] **epitab**
De Stavola, B. L., [ST] **stcox**, [ST] **stset**
Desu, M. M., [ST] **stpower**, [ST] **stpower exponential**
deviance residual, [ST] **stcox**, [ST] **streg**
discrete survival data, [ST] **discrete**
Dobbin, K., [ST] **stpower**
Dohoo, I., [ST] **epitab**
Doll, R., [ST] **epitab**
Drukker, D. M., [ST] **stcox**, [ST] **streg**
Dupont, W. D., [ST] **epitab**, [ST] **stcox**, [ST] **stir**,
     [ST] **sts**

E

Ederer, E., [ST] **ltable**
effect size, [ST] **glossary**, [ST] **stpower**, [ST] **stpower**
     cox, [ST] **stpower exponential**, [ST] **stpower**
     logrank
epidemiological tables, [ST] **epitab**
equality test, survivor functions, [ST] **sts test**
estat concordance command, [ST] **stcox**
     postestimation
estat phtest command, [ST] **stcox postestimation**
estimation options, [ST] **estimation options**
etiologic fraction, [ST] **epitab**
event, [ST] **glossary**, [ST] **stpower logrank**
excess fraction, [ST] **epitab**
exponential distribution, [ST] **streg**
exponential, stpower subcommand, [ST] **stpower**
     exponential

exponential survival
     power, [ST] **stpower exponential**
     regression, [ST] **streg**
     sample size, [ST] **stpower exponential**
exponential test,, [ST] **glossary**
     power, [ST] **stpower exponential**
     sample size, [ST] **stpower exponential**
exposure variable, [ST] **glossary**

F

failure event, [ST] **glossary**
failure tables, [ST] **ltable**
failure-time model, [ST] **stcox**, [ST] **stcox diagnostics**,
     [ST] **streg**
false-negative result, *see* type II error
false-positive result, *see* type I error
Fayers, P., [ST] **stpower**, [ST] **stpower logrank**
Feiveson, A. H., [ST] **stpower**
Feltbower, R., [ST] **epitab**
filling in values, [ST] **stfill**
Fisher, L. D., [ST] **epitab**
Fisher, R. A., [ST] **streg**
Fisher's exact test, [ST] **epitab**
Fleiss, J. L., [ST] **epitab**
Fleming, T. R., [ST] **stcox**, [ST] **sts test**
follow-up period, [ST] **glossary**
follow-up studies, *see* incidence studies
Foulkes, M. A., [ST] **intro**, [ST] **stpower**, [ST] **stpower**
     cox, [ST] **stpower exponential**
fourfold tables, [ST] **epitab**
frailty, [ST] **glossary**
frailty model, [ST] **streg**; [ST] **stcox**, [ST] **stcurve**
Freedman, L. S., [ST] **intro**, [ST] **stpower**,
     [ST] **stpower cox**, [ST] **stpower exponential**,
     [ST] **stpower logrank**
Freeman, J., [ST] **epitab**
future history, [ST] **glossary**, [ST] **stset**
Fyler, D. C., [ST] **epitab**

G

Gail, M. H., [ST] **intro**, [ST] **stpower**, [ST] **stpower**
     exponential, [ST] **strate**
gaps, [ST] **glossary**
Garrett, J. M., [ST] **stcox diagnostics**, [ST] **stcox**
     postestimation
Gauvreau, K., [ST] **ltable**, [ST] **sts**
Gehan, E. A., [ST] **sts test**
generalized gamma survival regression, [ST] **streg**
generate, sts subcommand, [ST] **sts generate**
generating variables, [ST] **stgen**, [ST] **sts generate**
George, S. L., [ST] **stpower**, [ST] **stpower exponential**
Gini, R., [ST] **epitab**
Glass, R. I., [ST] **epitab**
Gleason, J. R., [ST] **epitab**
Glidden, D. V., [ST] **stcox**

Gloeckler, L., [ST] **discrete**
Goldblatt, A., [ST] **epitab**
Gompertz survival regression, [ST] **streg**
Gould, W. W., [ST] **stcox**, [ST] **stdescribe**,
    [ST] **streg**, [ST] **stset**, [ST] **stsplit**, [ST] **stvary**,
    [ST] **survival analysis**
Grambsch, P. M., [ST] **stcox**, [ST] **stcox postestimation**
graph, sts subcommand, [ST] **sts graph**
graph,
    adjusted Kaplan–Meier survivor curves, [ST] **sts**
    baseline hazard and survivor, [ST] **stcox**, [ST] **sts**
    cumulative hazard function, [ST] **stcurve**, [ST] **sts graph**
    hazard function, [ST] **ltable**, [ST] **stcurve**, [ST] **sts graph**
    Kaplan–Meier survivor curves, [ST] **stcox diagnostics**, [ST] **sts**
    log-log curve, [ST] **stcox diagnostics**
    survivor function, [ST] **stcurve**, [ST] **sts graph**
Grazia-Valsecchi, M., [ST] **sts test**
Greenhouse, J. B., [ST] **epitab**
Greenhouse, S. W., [ST] **epitab**
Greenland, S., [ST] **epitab**
Greenwood confidence intervals, [ST] **sts**
Greenwood, M., [ST] **ltable**, [ST] **sts**
Gross, A. J., [ST] **ltable**
Gutierrez, R. G., [ST] **stcox**, [ST] **stdescribe**,
    [ST] **streg**, [ST] **stset**, [ST] **stsplit**, [ST] **stvary**,
    [ST] **survival analysis**

H

Haenszel, W., [ST] **epitab**, [ST] **sts test**
Haldane, J. B. S., [ST] **epitab**
Halley, E., [ST] **ltable**
Hankey, B., [ST] **strate**
Harley, J. B., [ST] **stpower cox**
Harrell, F. E., [ST] **stcox postestimation**
Harrell's C, [ST] **stcox postestimation**
Harrington, D. P., [ST] **stcox**, [ST] **sts test**
Hassell, J., [ST] **sts**
Hastorf, A. H., [ST] **epitab**
hazard function, [ST] **sts**, [ST] **sts generate**, [ST] **sts list**
    graph of, [ST] **ltable**, [ST] **stcurve**, [ST] **sts graph**
hazard ratio, [ST] **glossary**
    minimal detectable difference, [ST] **stpower**
    minimal effect size, [ST] **stpower**
hazard tables, [ST] **ltable**
Heagerty, P. J., [ST] **epitab**
Heinonen, O. P., [ST] **epitab**
Henry-Amar, M., [ST] **ltable**
Hertz, S., [ST] **stsplit**
Hess, K. R., [ST] **stcox diagnostics**
heterogeneity test, [ST] **epitab**
Hilgard, E. R., [ST] **epitab**
Hill, A. B., [ST] **epitab**
Hill, W. G., [ST] **epitab**

Hills, M., [ST] **epitab**, [ST] **stcox**, [ST] **stptime**,
    [ST] **strate**, [ST] **stset**, [ST] **stsplit**, [ST] **sttocc**
Hogben, L., [ST] **sts**
Holmgren, J., [ST] **epitab**
homogeneity test, [ST] **epitab**
Hooker, P. F., [ST] **streg**
Hosmer, D. W., Jr., [ST] **stcox**, [ST] **stpower**,
    [ST] **stpower cox**, [ST] **streg**
Hossain, K. M. B., [ST] **epitab**
Hougaard, P., [ST] **streg**
Hsieh, F. Y., [ST] **stpower**, [ST] **stpower cox**,
    [ST] **stpower logrank**
Hu, M., [ST] **stcox**, [ST] **stset**
Huq, M. I., [ST] **epitab**

I

ID variable, [ST] **glossary**
incidence, [ST] **glossary**
incidence studies, [ST] **glossary**
incidence-rate ratio, [ST] **epitab**, [ST] **stci**, [ST] **stir**,
    [ST] **stptime**, [ST] **stsum**
independence test, [ST] **epitab**
ir command, [ST] **epitab**
iri command, [ST] **epitab**

J

Jenkins, S. P., [ST] **discrete**, [ST] **stcox**
Jewell, N. P., [ST] **epitab**
Jick, H., [ST] **epitab**
joining time-span records, [ST] **stsplit**
Jones, B. S., [ST] **stcox**, [ST] **streg**

K

Kahn, H. A., [ST] **ltable**, [ST] **stcox**
Kalbfleisch, J. D., [ST] **ltable**, [ST] **stcox**, [ST] **stcox diagnostics**, [ST] **streg**, [ST] **sts**, [ST] **sts test**,
    [ST] **stset**
Kaplan, E. L., [ST] **sts**
Kaplan–Meier
    product-limit estimate, [ST] **glossary**, [ST] **sts**,
        [ST] **sts generate**, [ST] **sts graph**, [ST] **sts list**,
        [ST] **sts test**
    survivor function, [ST] **sts**; [ST] **ltable**, [ST] **stcox diagnostics**
Keiding, N., [ST] **stsplit**
Khan, M. R., [ST] **epitab**
Kimber, A. C., [ST] **streg**
Klein, J. P., [ST] **stci**, [ST] **stcox**, [ST] **stcox postestimation**, [ST] **stpower**, [ST] **stpower cox**,
    [ST] **streg**, [ST] **sts**, [ST] **sts test**
Kleinbaum, D. G., [ST] **epitab**
Krakauer, H., [ST] **ltable**
Krall, J. M., [ST] **stpower cox**
Kreidberg, M. B., [ST] **epitab**
Kupper, L. L., [ST] **epitab**

L

Lachin, J. M., [ST] **intro**, [ST] **stpower**, [ST] **stpower cox**, [ST] **stpower exponential**

Lakatos, E., [ST] **stpower**, [ST] **stpower exponential**, [ST] **stpower logrank**

Lan, K. K. G., [ST] **stpower**, [ST] **stpower exponential**, [ST] **stpower logrank**

Langholz, B., [ST] **sttocc**

Lavori P. W., [ST] **stpower**, [ST] **stpower cox**

Lawless, J. F., [ST] **ltable**, [ST] **stpower**

Lee, E. T., [ST] **streg**

Lee, K. L., [ST] **stcox postestimation**

Lee, P., [ST] **streg**

Lemeshow, S., [ST] **stcox**, [ST] **stpower**, [ST] **stpower cox**, [ST] **streg**

Levin, B., [ST] **epitab**

`lexis` command, [ST] **stsplit**

lexis diagram, [ST] **stsplit**

Lexis, W., [ST] **stsplit**

life tables, [ST] **glossary**, [ST] **ltable**

Lilienfeld, D. E., [ST] **epitab**

Lin, D. Y., [ST] **stcox**

Linhart, J. M., [ST] **sts**

`list, sts` subcommand, [ST] **sts list**

Liu, J.-P., [ST] **stpower**

log-log plot, [ST] **stcox diagnostics**

log-logistic survival regression, [ST] **streg**

log-rank,
    power, [ST] **stpower logrank**
    sample size, [ST] **stpower logrank**

log-rank test, [ST] **stpower logrank**, [ST] **sts test**

lognormal survival regression, [ST] **streg**

`logrank, stpower` subcommand, [ST] **stpower logrank**

longitudinal studies, *see* incidence studies

López-Vizcaíno, M. E., [ST] **epitab**

loss to follow-up, [ST] **glossary**

`ltable` command, [ST] **ltable**

Lumley, T., [ST] **epitab**

M

Machin, D., [ST] **stpower**, [ST] **stpower logrank**

MacMahon, B., [ST] **epitab**

Mander, A., [ST] **stsplit**

Mantel–Cox method, [ST] **strate**

Mantel–Haenszel
    method, [ST] **strate**
    test, [ST] **epitab**, [ST] **stir**

Mantel, N., [ST] **epitab**, [ST] **sts test**

Mark, D. B., [ST] **stcox postestimation**

Marr, J. W., [ST] **stsplit**

Martin, W., [ST] **epitab**

martingale residual, [ST] **stcox**, [ST] **streg**

Marubini, E., [ST] **stpower**, [ST] **stpower logrank**, [ST] **sts test**

matched case–control data, [ST] **epitab**, [ST] **glossary**, [ST] **sttocc**

`mcc` command, [ST] **epitab**

`mcci` command, [ST] **epitab**

McCulloch, C. E., [ST] **stcox**

McGilchrist, C. A., [ST] **stcox**, [ST] **streg**

McNemar, Q., [ST] **epitab**

McNemar's chi-squared test, [ST] **epitab**

Meier, P., [ST] **sts**

Meyer, B. D., [ST] **discrete**

`mhodds` command, [ST] **epitab**

Miettinen, O. S., [ST] **epitab**

minimal
    detectable difference, hazard ratio, [ST] **stpower**
    effect size, hazard ratio, [ST] **stpower**

Moeschberger, M. L., [ST] **stci**, [ST] **stcox**, [ST] **stcox postestimation**, [ST] **stpower**, [ST] **stpower cox**, [ST] **streg**, [ST] **sts**, [ST] **sts test**

Monson, R. R., [ST] **epitab**

Morgenstern, H., [ST] **epitab**

Morris, J. N., [ST] **stsplit**

Morrow, A., [ST] **epitab**

mortality table, *see* life table

Müller, H. G., [ST] **sts graph**

multiarm trial, [ST] **glossary**, [ST] **stpower**

multiple-record st data, [ST] **stfill**, [ST] **stvary**

N

Nardi, G., [ST] **epitab**

Neff, R. K., [ST] **epitab**

Nelson–Aalen cumulative hazard, [ST] **sts**, [ST] **sts generate**, [ST] **sts graph**, [ST] **sts list**

Nelson, W., [ST] **sts**

nested case–control data, [ST] **sttocc**

Newman, S. C., [ST] **stcox**, [ST] **sts**

Newson, R., [ST] **stcox postestimation**

nonparametric test, equality of survivor functions, [ST] **sts test**

O

Oakes, D., [ST] **ltable**, [ST] **stcox**, [ST] **stcox diagnostics**, [ST] **stpower**, [ST] **streg**, [ST] **sts**

odds ratio, [ST] **epitab**, [ST] **glossary**

offset variable, [ST] **glossary**

Olshansky, S. J., [ST] **streg**

P

Pagano, M., [ST] **ltable**, [ST] **sts**

Paik, M. C., [ST] **epitab**

parametric survival models, [ST] **streg**

Parmar, M. K. B., [ST] **stpower**, [ST] **stpower cox**

Pasquini, J., [ST] **epitab**

past history, [ST] **glossary**, [ST] **stset**

Pearce, M. S., [ST] **epitab**

penalized log-likelihood function, [ST] **glossary**, [ST] **stcox**

Pérez-Hoyos, S., [ST] **epitab**

person time, [ST] **stptime**

Peto, J., [ST] **sts test**

Peto, R., [ST] **stcox**, [ST] **streg**, [ST] **sts test**

phtest, estat subcommand, [ST] **stcox postestimation**

Pike, M. C., [ST] **ltable**, [ST] **streg**

Pinol, A., [ST] **stpower**, [ST] **stpower logrank**

Pitblado, J. S., [ST] **sts**

Plummer, D., [ST] **epitab**

pooled estimates, [ST] **epitab**

population attributable risk, [ST] **epitab**

postestimation command, [ST] **stcurve**

power, [ST] **glossary**
    Cox proportional hazards regression, [ST] **stpower**, [ST] **stpower cox**
    exponential survival, [ST] **stpower**, [ST] **stpower exponential**
    exponential test, [ST] **stpower**, [ST] **stpower exponential**
    log-rank, [ST] **stpower**, [ST] **stpower logrank**

Prentice, R. L., [ST] **discrete**, [ST] **ltable**, [ST] **stcox**, [ST] **stcox diagnostics**, [ST] **streg**, [ST] **sts**, [ST] **sts test**, [ST] **stset**

prevalence studies, *see* cross-sectional studies

prevented fraction, [ST] **epitab**, [ST] **glossary**

proportional hazards model, [ST] **glossary**, *also see* Cox proportional hazards model

prospective study, [ST] **epitab**, [ST] **glossary**

Pryor, D. B., [ST] **stcox postestimation**

R

Radmacher, R. D., [ST] **stpower**

Ramalheira, C., [ST] **ltable**

rate ratio, [ST] **epitab**, [ST] **stci**, [ST] **stir**, [ST] **stptime**, [ST] **stsum**

recruitment period, *see* accrual period

Reid, N., [ST] **stcox**

Reilly, M., [ST] **epitab**

relative risk, [ST] **epitab**

Richter, J. R., [ST] **stpower**

risk
    difference, [ST] **epitab**
    factor, [ST] **epitab**, [ST] **glossary**
    pool, [ST] **glossary**, [ST] **stcox**, [ST] **stset**
    ratio, [ST] **epitab**, [ST] **glossary**

Robins, J. M., [ST] **epitab**

robust, Huber/White/sandwich estimator of variance,
    Cox proportional hazards model, [ST] **stcox**
    parametric survival models, [ST] **streg**

Rogers, W. H., [ST] **stcox diagnostics**, [ST] **stcox postestimation**

Rosati, R. A., [ST] **stcox postestimation**

Rothman, K. J., [ST] **epitab**

Royston, P., [ST] **epitab**, [ST] **stcox**, [ST] **stcox diagnostics**, [ST] **stpower**, [ST] **stpower cox**, [ST] **streg**

Rubinstein, L. V., [ST] **intro**, [ST] **stpower**, [ST] **stpower exponential**

S

Salim, A., [ST] **epitab**

sample size,
    Cox proportional hazards regression, [ST] **stpower**, [ST] **stpower cox**
    exponential survival, [ST] **stpower**, [ST] **stpower exponential**
    exponential test, [ST] **stpower**, [ST] **stpower exponential**
    log-rank, [ST] **stpower**, [ST] **stpower logrank**

Santner, T. J., [ST] **intro**, [ST] **stpower**, [ST] **stpower exponential**

Sasieni, P., [ST] **stcox**

Savage, I. R., [ST] **sts test**

Schlesselman, J. J., [ST] **epitab**

Schoenfeld, D., [ST] **intro**, [ST] **stcox**, [ST] **stcox postestimation**, [ST] **stpower**, [ST] **stpower cox**, [ST] **stpower exponential**, [ST] **stpower logrank**, [ST] **streg**

Schoenfeld residual, [ST] **stcox**, [ST] **streg**

Scotto, M. G., [ST] **streg**

Sears, R. R., [ST] **epitab**

Selvin, S., [ST] **ltable**, [ST] **stcox**

semiparametric model, [ST] **glossary**, [ST] **stcox**, [ST] **stset**

Sempos, C. T., [ST] **ltable**, [ST] **stcox**

Shao, J., [ST] **stpower**, [ST] **stpower exponential**

Shapiro, S., [ST] **epitab**

Shiboski, S. C., [ST] **stcox**

Simon, R., [ST] **stpower**

singleton-group data, [ST] **glossary**, [ST] **stcox**

Skovlund, E., [ST] **stpower**, [ST] **stpower cox**

Slone, D., [ST] **epitab**

Smith, R. L., [ST] **streg**

SMR, [ST] **epitab**, [ST] **glossary**, [ST] **stptime**

Smythe, B., [ST] **sts**

snapshot data, [ST] **glossary**, [ST] **snapspan**, [ST] **stset**

snapspan command, [ST] **snapspan**

Snell, E. J., [ST] **stcox**, [ST] **stcox diagnostics**, [ST] **streg postestimation**

spell data, [ST] **glossary**

splitting time-span records, [ST] **stsplit**

st data, [ST] **glossary**

standardized
    mortality ratio, *see* SMR
    rates, [ST] **epitab**

stbase command, [ST] **stbase**

stci command, [ST] **stci**

stcox command, [ST] **stcox**

stcoxkm command, [ST] **stcox diagnostics**

st_ct, [ST] **st_is**

stcurve command, [ST] **stcurve**
stdescribe command, [ST] **stdescribe**
Sterne, J. A. C., [ST] **stcox**
Stewart, J., [ST] **ltable**
stfill command, [ST] **stfill**
stgen command, [ST] **stgen**
stir command, [ST] **stir**
st_is 2, [ST] **st_is**
stjoin command, [ST] **stsplit**
stmc command, [ST] **strate**
stmh command, [ST] **strate**
Stoll, B. J., [ST] **epitab**
Stolley, P. D., [ST] **epitab**
stphplot command, [ST] **stcox diagnostics**
stpower cox command, [ST] **stpower cox**
stpower exponential command, [ST] **stpower exponential**
stpower logrank command, [ST] **stpower logrank**
stptime command, [ST] **stptime**
strate command, [ST] **strate**
stratification, [ST] **epitab**, [ST] **stcox**, [ST] **streg**
stratified tables, [ST] **epitab**
streg command, [ST] **streg**
Stryhn, H., [ST] **epitab**
sts command, [ST] **sts**, [ST] **sts generate**, [ST] **sts graph**, [ST] **sts list**, [ST] **sts test**, [ST] **stset**
sts generate command, [ST] **sts**, [ST] **sts generate**
sts graph command, [ST] **sts**, [ST] **sts graph**
sts list command, [ST] **sts**, [ST] **sts list**
sts test command, [ST] **sts**, [ST] **sts test**
stset command, [ST] **stset**
st_show, [ST] **st_is**
stsplit command, [ST] **stsplit**
stsum command, [ST] **stsum**
sttocc command, [ST] **sttocc**
stvary command, [ST] **stvary**
survey sampling, [ST] **stcox**, [ST] **streg**, [ST] **sts**
survival analysis, [ST] **cttost**, [ST] **st**, [ST] **stdescribe**, [ST] **stset**, [ST] **sttoct**
survival clinical trial, [ST] **stpower**
survival-time data, *see* st data
survivor function, [ST] **glossary**, [ST] **sts**, [ST] **sts generate**, [ST] **sts list**, [ST] **sts test**
    graph of, [ST] **stcurve**, [ST] **sts graph**
Svennerholm, A. M., [ST] **epitab**
Sweeting, T. J., [ST] **streg**

T

tables,
    actuarial, *see* life tables
    epidemiological, *see* epidemiological tables
    failure, *see* failure tables
    fourfold, *see* fourfold tables
    hazard, *see* hazard tables
    life, *see* life tables
tabodds command, [ST] **epitab**

Tarone, R. E., [ST] **epitab**, [ST] **intro**, [ST] **sts test**
test, sts subcommand, [ST] **sts test**
test,
    association, *see* association test
    Cox proportional hazards model, assumption, *see* Cox proportional hazards model, test of assumption
    equality of survivor functions, *see* equality test, survivor functions
    Fisher's exact, *see* Fisher's exact test
    heterogeneity, *see* heterogeneity test
    homogeneity, *see* homogeneity test
    independence, *see* independence test
    log-rank, *see* log-rank test
    Mantel–Haenszel, *see* Mantel–Haenszel test
    McNemar's chi-squared test, *see* McNemar's chi-squared test
    trend, *see* trend test
test-based confidence intervals, [ST] **epitab**
Therneau, T. M., [ST] **stcox**, [ST] **stcox postestimation**
Thomas, D. C., [ST] **sttocc**
Tilling, K., [ST] **stcox**
time-span data, [ST] **snapspan**
time-varying covariates, [ST] **glossary**
Tippett, L. H. C., [ST] **streg**
Tobias, A., [ST] **streg**
trend test, [ST] **epitab**, [ST] **sts test**
Trichopoulos, D., [ST] **epitab**
truncation, [ST] **glossary**
type I error, [ST] **glossary**
type II error, [ST] **glossary**

U

under observation, [ST] **glossary**
University Group Diabetes Program, [ST] **epitab**
Uthoff, V. A., [ST] **stpower cox**

V

Væth, M., [ST] **stpower**, [ST] **stpower cox**
Valsecchi, M. G., [ST] **stpower**, [ST] **stpower logrank**
van Belle, G., [ST] **epitab**
variables, generating, [ST] **stgen**
varying variables, [ST] **stvary**
Vidmar, S., [ST] **epitab**
Vittinghoff, E., [ST] **stcox**

W

Walker, A. M., [ST] **epitab**
Walker, S., [ST] **sts test**
Wang, H., [ST] **stpower**, [ST] **stpower exponential**
Wang, J. L., [ST] **sts graph**
Wang, J. W., [ST] **streg**
Wang, Z., [ST] **epitab**
Ware, J. H., [ST] **sts test**